Neuromuscular transmission

Studies in neuroscience *No. 12*

Series editor Dr William Winlow, *Dept. of Physiology, University of Leeds, LS2 9NQ, UK*

Neuroscience is one of the major growth areas in the biological sciences and draws both techniques and ideas from many other scientific disciplines. *Studies in neuroscience* presents both monographs and multi-author volumes drawn from the whole range of the subject and brings together the subdisciplines that have arisen from the recent explosive development of the neurosciences.

Studies in neuroscience includes contributions from molecular and cellular neurobiology, developmental neuroscience (including tissue culture), neural networks and systems research (both clinical and basic) and behavioural neuroscience (including ethology). The series is designed to appeal to research workers in clinical and basic neuroscience, their graduate students and advanced undergraduates with an interest in the subject.

Neuromuscular transmission: basic and applied aspects

edited by Angela Vincent
and Dennis Wray

Manchester University Press

Manchester and New York
Distributed exclusively in the USA and Canada by St. Martin's Press

Published by Manchester University Press
Oxford Road, Manchester M13 9PL, UK
and Room 400, 175 Fifth Avenue,
New York, NY 10010, USA

Distributed exclusively in the USA and Canada
by St. Martin's Press, Inc.,
175 Fifth Avenue, New York, NY 10010, USA

British Library cataloguing in publication data
Neuromuscular transmission.
   1. Man. Muscles. Nerves
   I. Vincent, Angela   II. Wray, Dennis.   III. Series
   612.8

Library of Congress cataloging in publication data
Neuromuscular transmission: basic and applied aspects/edited by
   Angela Vincent and Dennis Wray.
        p.   cm. — (Studies in neuroscience: no. 12)
      Includes index.
      ISBN 0-7190-2598-2 (hardback)
      1. Neuromuscular transmission.   I. Vincent, Angela.   II. Wray.
   Dennis.   III. Series.
      [DNLM: 1. Acetylcholine — physiology.   2. Myasthenia Gravis.
   3. Neural Transmission.   4. Neuromuscular Junction — physiology.
   5. Receptors, Cholinergic. W1 ST927K no. 12/WL 102.9 N4936]
   OP369.5.N483 1990
   616.7'44 — dc20
   DNLM/DLC   90-6121
   ISBN 0 7190 2598 2 *hardback*

Printed in Great Britain by Biddles Ltd., Guildford & King's Lynn

Contents

Contributors

Professor Eric Barnard, Medical Research Council Molecular Neurobiology Unit, University of Cambridge Medical School, Hills Road, Cambridge CB2 2QH

Dr David Beeson, Neurosciences Group, Institute of Molecular Medicine, John Radcliffe Hospital, Headington, Oxford OX3 9DU

Professor David Colquhoun, Dept of Pharmacology, University College, Gower Street, London WC1

Dr Marc de Baets, The University of Limburg, Dept of Immunology, PO Box 616, 6200 MD Maastricht, The Netherlands

Professor J. Oliver Dolly, Dept of Biochemistry, Imperial College, University of London, Prince Consort Road, London SW7

Dr Andrew G. Engel, Mayo Clinic, Dept of Neurology, Rochester, Minnesota 55905, USA

Dr Jon Lindstrom, Institute of Neurological Sciences, University of Pennsylvania School of Medicine, 452 Medical Education Building, 36th & Hamilton Walk, Philadelphia, PA 19104–6074, USA

Dr Peter Molenaar, Sylvius Laboratorium, Faculteit der Geneeskunde, Postbus 9503, 2300 RA, Leiden

Dr Robert Norman, Dept of Medicine, Clinical Sciences Building, Leicester Royal Infirmary, PO Box 65, Leicester LE2 7LX

Dr Clarke Slater, Division of Neurobiology, Newcastle General Hospital, Westgate Road, Newcastle upon Tyne NE4 6BE

Dr Angela Vincent, Neurosciences Group, Institute of Molecular Medicine, John Radcliffe Hospital, Headington, Oxford OX3 9DU

Professor Dennis Wray, Dept of Pharmacology, University of Leeds, Leeds LS2 9JT

Preface

This book arose from our enthusiasm for the multidisciplinary approaches employed in the study of neuromuscular transmission. The neuromuscular junction (NMJ) presents us with a unique situation by virtue of its isolation from the rest of the nervous system and its accessibility to the investigator. Modern techniques of electrophysiology, biochemistry and molecular biology have now been combined in the study of its functional components: for instance, recordings of single channel currents by the patch clamp technique can be made not only in muscle cells, but also in *in vitro* systems after cloning and expression of the relevant genes. The existence of two diseases which fulfil the criteria for autoimmunity has drawn immunology into the arena and extended even further the scope of this book.

We asked active workers to write with enthusiasm and without excessive detail from a wide viewpoint. We tried to restrict references to a few 'classics', several recent reviews and recent important refereed publications. However, the contributors were given a fairly free rein and each chapter reflects the interests of its author, and the way in which they wished to present their material. For this reason each chapter can be read in isolation, but there is perforce some overlap.

The book is roughly divided into three sections. First, three introductory chapters in which we try to draw a molecular picture of the structure and development of the NMJ, and summarise basic electrophysiology and general techniques. Then chapters on the biochemistry of ACh and the biophysics of the ACh/AChR interactions; followed by the molecular biology of the AChR and of the various voltage-dependent ion channels, with particular reference to the use of neurotoxins and antibodies in characterisation and structural analysis. The remaining chapters cover the application of this knowledge to congenital and autoimmune human disorders and an experimental autoimmune model.

We have tried to achieve a readable account of different aspects of neuromuscular transmission, including the diseases that affect it. We hope that this book will be useful to basic science students and serve as an introductory guide for postgraduates and clinical research workers. We are very grateful to the contributors, many of whom were badgered incessantly, and to our colleagues, particularly Dr Bethan Lang, for their help and encouragement.

A.V

D.W.

1 *Clarke Slater and Angela Vincent*

Introduction I: Structure and development of the neuromuscular junction

1.1. Introduction

The transmission of impulses from nerve to muscle depends on the release of acetylcholine (ACh) from the motor nerve ending and its interaction with acetylcholine receptors (AChR) on the muscle fibre. This chemical transmission takes place at the neuromuscular junction (NMJ), a highly structured region of contact between the peripheral nerve terminal of the motor axon and the postsynaptic surface of the muscle fibre.

In this Introductory chapter we will describe briefly the functional organisation of the NMJ and a few of the experimental studies that have helped to shape current views about the development and maintenance of this highly differentiated region of cell–cell contact. Many of the observations referred to have depended on non-mammalian sources, for instance the NMJ of the frog sartorius muscle, and even non-muscle tissue such as the electric organ of the electric ray, *Torpedo*. Fortunately the lessons learnt from examination of diverse species seem to be applicable in principle to mammals, including man. Much of the material summarised here is covered in greater detail by Salpeter (1987a, b).

1.2. Functional Organisation of the neuromuscular junction

The myelinated motor axon originates from the nerve cell body within the ventral horn of the spinal cord and runs to the target muscle in the peripheral nerve. At the nearest point of contact with the muscle fibre it forms an elaborate terminal arborisation enclosed in a region of about 250–1000 μm^2 (Fig. 1.1). The area of true synaptic contact within this zone is less and may represent less than 0.01% of the total muscle fibre surface. The axon terminal is not myelinated but is covered by layered Schwann cell processes where it is not in apposition to the muscle (Fig. 1.2). With the electron microscope it can be seen that the surface of the muscle fibre beneath the nerve terminal is extensively folded (Fig. 1.2) and many studies indicate that the associated plasma membrane is specialised to enable the muscle to respond to the ACh released by the nerve.

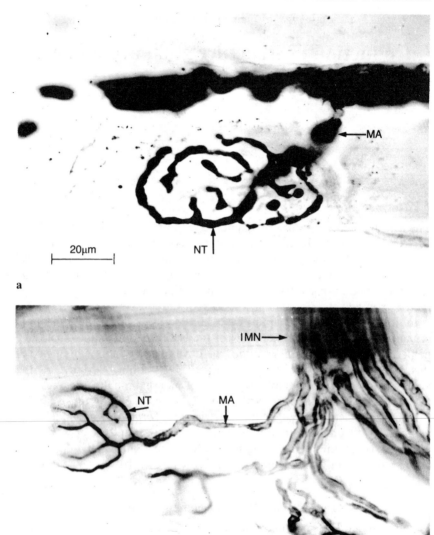

a

b

Fig. 1.1.   The presynaptic nerve terminal at mammalian NMJs. **(a)** Rat soleus muscle, stained with zinc oxide/osmium tetroxide to reveal the full extent of the highly branched terminal arborisation. **(b)** Mouse epitrochleoanconeus muscle, impregnated with silver to reveal the core of neurofilaments within the terminal branches. NT, nerve terminal; MA, myelinated preterminal axon; IMN, intramuscular nerve bundle.

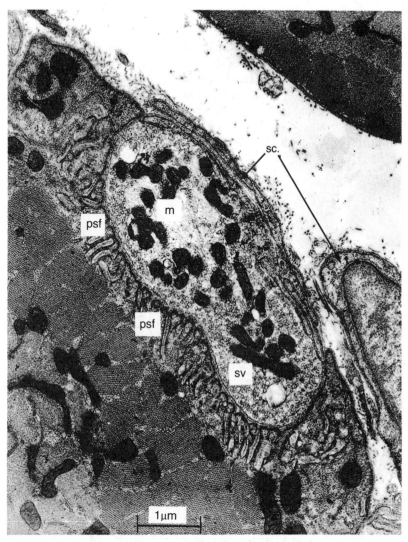

Fig. 1.2.　Electron microscopic section through a mouse neuromuscular junction showing the nerve terminal with mitochondria (m), synaptic vesicles (sv), covered by the Schwann cell (sc). The postsynaptic membrane is thrown into extensive folds (psf). The membrane at the top of the folds is denser due to the presence of acetylcholine receptors. Scale bar 1 μm.

1.2.1.　*The presynaptic nerve terminal*

The most characteristic structural features of the nerve terminal are the synaptic vesicles and the mitochondria, microtubules and actin microfila-ments (Hirokawa *et al.*, 1989). The vesicles are about 50 nm in diameter and are clustered particularly within electron-dense regions of the cytoplasm adjacent to the presynaptic membrane. These 'active zones', opposite the postsynaptic folds, are thought to be the sites of ACh release.

The generally accepted view of the synthesis and release of ACh involves a complex cycle of events (for details see Molenaar, this volume; Jones, 1987) (Fig. 1.3). ACh is first formed in the cytoplasm of the nerve terminal from acetyl CoA and choline in a reaction catalysed by the soluble enzyme choline acetyltransferase (Tucek, 1984). It is then accumulated by an ACh 'transporter' to a high concentration within the vesicles by an energy-

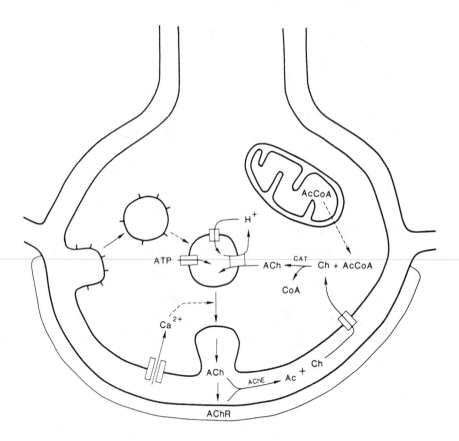

Fig. 1.3. Molecular events involved in transmitter synthesis and release. ACh is formed in the cytoplasm and taken up into synaptic vesicles in exchange for H^+. On depolarisation Ca^{2+} enters through voltage-gated Ca^{2+} channels resulting in the fusion of synaptic vesicles with the plasma membrane, and release of ACh. ACh binds to the postsynaptic AChRs but is soon hydrolysed by acetylcholine esterase to acetate and choline. The choline is recovered by a high-affinity uptake system into the nerve terminal. The synaptic vesicle membrane is also recovered, by coated vesicles. Reproduced with permission from Jones (1987).

dependent uptake system. Release of ACh, a strongly Ca^{2+}-dependent process, involves fusion of the vesicles with the synaptic membrane of the nerve terminal, resulting in the release of a 'quantum' of several thousand ACh molecules into the synaptic cleft. Some of these bind to the AChRs on the postsynaptic membrane while the rest are rapidly hydrolysed by the acetylcholinesterase (AChE) present in the synaptic cleft. The choline thus formed is taken back up into the terminal by a high-affinity uptake system, making it available for resynthesis of ACh.

Following exocytosis, proteins of the vesicle appear in the membrane of the nerve terminal (Valtorta *et al.*, 1988) and may influence its properties. For example, a continuous 'non-quantal' leakage of ACh from the nerve is likely to result from the action of the vesicular ACh transporter during its stay in the nerve terminal membrane (Vyskocil *et al.*, 1988). In order to maintain the constant size of the nerve terminal, membrane is recovered by endocytosis in association with coated pits (Heuser and Reese, 1973; see Fig. 1.3). It is likely that the specialised proteins of the vesicle membrane are also recovered during this process. The key events in ACh release, therefore, involve at least two identifiable structural elements within the nerve terminal, the synaptic vesicles and the active zones.

1.2.1.1. *Synaptic vesicles.* The synaptic vesicles contain a number of specialised proteins. A structural model of the vesicle membrane, based on current information (Smith and Augustine, 1988), is shown in Fig 1.4. The

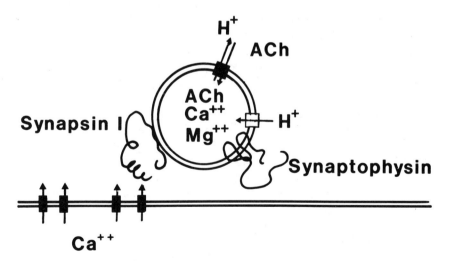

Fig. 1.4 Schematic illustration of a synaptic vesicle and its contents. The membrane must contain both an active H^+ pump and an H^+/ACh exchanger. At least one ion channel exists in the membrane, possibly synaptophysin. Synapsin I is attached to the outer surface of the vesicle. Based on reviews by Marshall and Parsons (1987) and Smith and Augustine (1988).

energy-dependent uptake of ACh appears to involve both an uptake protein and a separate ATPase which may act to pump H^+ ions into the vesicles so that they can be excluded in exchange for ACh (Marshall and Parsons, 1987). Although cytoplasmic ACh is at a high concentration, 30 mM, ACh is packed at super-osmotic concentrations (about 300 mM) within the lumen of the vesicle, together with ATP, proteoglycans and H^+, Ca^{2+} and Mg^{2+} ions.

There is increasing evidence that the membrane of synaptic vesicles contains ion channels. The best documented of these, physiologically, is a Ca^{2+}-dependent K^+ channel (Rahamimoff *et al.*, 1988). What role these channels play in the function of the vesicles is not yet clear, but several have been identified which are likely to be involved in the calcium-dependent process of exocytosis. One of these, synaptophysin, is an integral membrane phosphoprotein, closely associated with synaptic vesicles at many chemical synapses. It forms ion channels when incorporated into phospholipid bilayers and is one of the major calcium-binding proteins in presynaptic nerve terminals (Thomas *et al.*, 1988). It is thought that early during exocytosis synaptophysin binds in a calcium-dependent manner to a complementary 'docking' protein in the presynaptic terminal to form a 'fusion pore'.

Another protein, synapsin I, is also associated with synaptic vesicles but it projects largely towards the cytoplasm (Smith and Augustine, 1988). It can be phosphorylated by cAMP-dependent protein kinase and by calcium-calmodulin activated protein kinases I and II, present within the nerve terminal (McGuinness and Greengard, 1988). Synapsin I is also an actin binding protein (Bahler and Greengard, 1987) and may serve to link vesicles to the presynaptic cytoskeleton (Hirokawa *et al.*, 1989). A recent model of the organisation of the presynaptic cytoskeleton, based on the studies of Hirokawa *et al.* (1989), is illustrated in Fig. 1.5.

1.2.1.2. *Active zones and the presynaptic nerve terminal*. There is convincing evidence that ACh is normally released by exocytosis of synaptic vesicles at the active zones (Jones, 1987; Smith and Augustine, 1988). This evidence includes the appearance near the active zones of 'fusion profiles', corresponding to fused vesicles (Heuser *et al.*, 1979), and the presence of specific vesicle antigens in the presynaptic membrane particularly after nerve stimulation at high rates (Valtorta *et al.*, 1988).

The molecular analysis of the active zones is at an early stage. Most work on the fusion and release of substances from cells has been done on endocrine cells. There, Ca^{2+} entry is thought to activate a calmodulin-dependent kinase which then phosphorylates synapsin I and releases the cytoskeletal restraints that hold the synaptic vesicle away from the membrane, thus allowing fusion to occur (Linstedt and Kelly, 1987). The rapidity with which Ca^{2+} influx results in ACh release at the NMJ (*ca.* 200

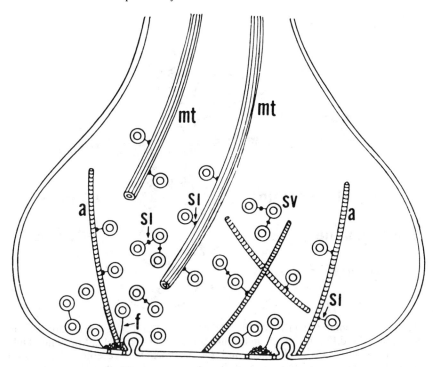

Fig. 1.5. Schematic diagram of the inside of presynaptic nerve terminals. Actin filaments (a) and microtubules (mt) are the main cytoskeletal elements. Synapsin 1 (S1) links synaptic vesicles (sv) with actin and microtubules, and possibly cross-links synaptic vesicles as well. There are also longer strands which might be fodrin. Reproduced with permission from Hirokawa *et al.* (1989).

μs), however, makes it unlikely that protein phosphorylation, which occurs on the time-scale of milliseconds, plays a role in the events immediately associated with synaptic transmitter release. However, it may be important in longer-term regulation of the amount of transmitter available for release.

In spite of the evidence supporting exocytosis as the key event in quantal ACh release, an alternative view has been put forward; that cytoplasmic ACh is released through specialised pores in the presynaptic membrane. A membrane protein, the mediatophore, has been purified from *Torpedo* electric organ and reincorporated into *Torpedo* lipid membranes where it appears to mediate a Ca^{2+}-dependent release of ACh (Israël *et al.*, 1986). Although the Ca^{2+}-dependency is consistent with its involvement in ACh release, it is too early to say what the role of this protein is.

A number of additional membrane proteins must also be present in the nerve terminal membrane. These include Na^+ channels responsible for the

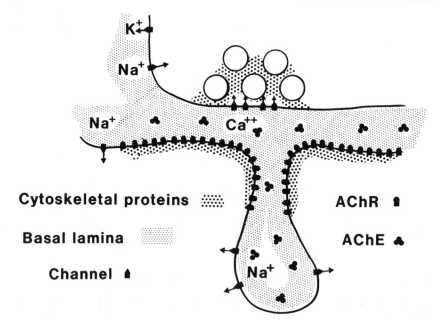

Fig. 1.6. Schematic diagram of the nerve terminal and postsynaptic membrane illustrating the different ion channels and presence of cytoskeletal proteins. Only the voltage-gated Ca^{2+} channels and the acetylcholine receptors have been identified at the ultrastructural level. The presence of the other ion channels is inferred from physiological studies, and of AChE and structural proteins by histochemistry and antibody staining.

propagation of the nerve action potential to the nerve terminal, rectifying K^+ channels that serve to restore the membrane potential after each wave of excitation, and the voltage-dependent Ca^{2+} channels that control release of transmitter (see Norman, this volume). The former two have not been localised but there is strong circumstantial evidence that the active zone particles are the Ca^{2+} channels (see Wray, this volume). There is also pharmacological evidence for the presence of many receptors on the nerve terminal surface to account for the observed modulation of ACh release in response to opiates, ATP, adenosine, ACTH and VIP (see Molenaar, this volume). A schematic illustration of the neuromuscular junction is shown in Fig. 1.6 and some of the specialised proteins are listed in Table 1.1.

1.2.2. *The synaptic cleft*

At the NMJ the nerve and muscle cells are separated by a cleft of about 50 nm. A condensed form of extracellular matrix, the basal lamina, forms a

Table 1.1.   Some specialised proteins at the neuromuscular junction

	Structural	*Functional*
Cytoplasm	Actin Fodrin	ChAT enzyme
Synaptic vesicles		ACh translocator ATPase Synaptophysin Synapsin I
Nerve terminal membrane		Voltage-sensitive Na^+, K^+ and Ca^{2+} channels, receptors for other ligands ? Mediatophore
Synaptic cleft	Agrin NCAM Heparan sulphate proteoglycan S-laminin	AChE
Postsynaptic	43 kDa Actin Spectrin-like NCAM α-actinin	AChR Voltage-sensitive Na^+ and K^+ channels Receptors for trophic factors

sheath some 20–30 nm thick around each muscle and myelinated nerve fibre, and at the NMJ a common basal lamina extends into the synaptic cleft, following the contours of the folds (Fig. 1.7a). In deep-etched, rotary shadowed preparations, projections from the synaptic basal lamina to both nerve and muscle can be clearly seen (Fig. 1.7b; Hirokawa and Heuser 1982), suggesting that it may serve to hold them together. This view is reinforced by the observation that digestion of the basal lamina with collagenase allows the nerve to be detached from the muscle.

Two important structural components of the basal lamina appear to be type IV collagen and laminin (Sanes, 1989). The best-known functional protein is an asymmetric form of acetylcholinesterase (AChE) (Massoulie and Bon, 1982; Rotondo, 1987). This form, consisting of three tetramers, and a collagen-like tail which attaches it to the basal lamina, sediments at 16–18S. Genes coding for several forms of AChE have recently been cloned and sequenced (see Beeson and Barnard, this volume; Rotundo, 1987).

The total number of AChE active sites per NMJ is about the same as that of AChRs (i.e. about 10^7, see below) and more than enough to hydrolyse all the ACh that is released per nerve impulse (see Molenaar, this volume). However, while the AChRs are concentrated at the tops of the folds at a density of some $15–20 \times 10^3/\mu m^2$, the AChE molecules appear to be

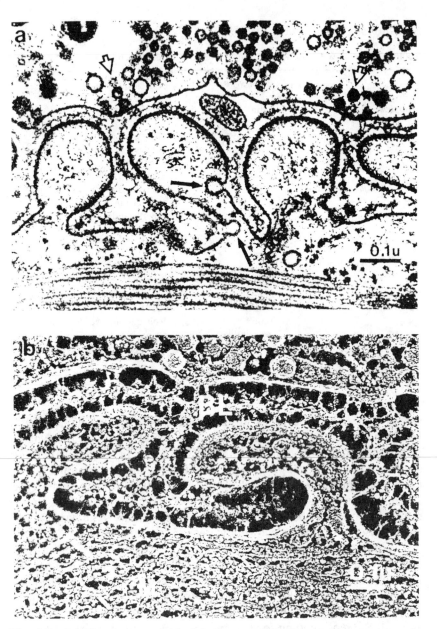

Fig. 1.7. (a) Membrane and basal lamina specialisation at the neuromuscular junction. Synaptic vesicles can be seen clustering near the active zones (open arrows). The dense membrane of the AChR-rich postsynaptic membrane is clearly seen and the double layers of basal lamina in the secondary folds. Endocytotic vesicles (arrows) are present in the postsynaptic cytoplasm, probably recycling acetylcholine receptors. (b) Deep-etched and rotary-shadowed preparation clearly indicates the presence of strands of basal lamina stretching between the nerve terminal membrane and the postsynaptic membrane. Reproduced with permission from Hirokawa and Heuser, 1982.

uniformly distributed throughout the synaptic basal lamina at a density of some $2-3 \times 10^3/\mu m^2$ (Salpeter, 1987a). Thus in the immediate vicinity of the sites of transmitter release, the local density of AChR molecules is 5–10 times greater than that of AChE sites.

Various other molecules have been found to be more or less specifically associated with the synaptic basal lamina. Two of the best characterised are agrin (Nitkin *et al.*, 1987), and S-laminin (Hunter *et al.*, 1989). Agrin is thought to be involved with AChR localisation (see below).

The discovery and characterisation of S-laminin represents an excellent demonstration of the power of modern techniques (for details see Hunter *et al.*, 1989). Its presence at the NMJ was first inferred from the binding of an antiserum raised against an extract of lens capsule basal lamina but also showing specificity for the NMJ. The gene was cloned and its sequence found to show extensive similarity with laminin, which is known to play a role in the control of neural outgrowth. Surfaces coated with purified S-laminin are preferred substrates for neuronal adhesion, suggesting that S-laminin is involved in the formation and maintenance of nerve–muscle contacts.

In addition to these proteins a heparan sulphate proteoglycan of unknown function has also been identified as specific to the extracellular matrix of the NMJ (Anderson and Fambrough, 1983). While the functions of these molecules are not known in detail, it is clear that the junctional basal lamina is highly specialised at the molecular level and is likely to play an important role in maintaining the long-term integrity of the NMJ.

1.2.3. *The postsynaptic membrane*

The most characteristic morphological features of the postsynaptic surface of the muscle cell are the deep infoldings of the plasma membrane, increasing its surface area by up to eight times. At the tops of the folds the membrane is clearly thickened, and many autoradiographic and immuno-histochemical studies have shown that this is where the AChRs are situated (Figs 1.2 and 1.7a; see Salpeter, 1987a). Other molecules, such as the voltage-dependent Na^+ channels, responsible for generation of the muscle fibre action potential, are also concentrated at the NMJ (Angelides, 1986). It seems likely that, in addition to ACh, factors that have a long-term influence on the local properties of muscle fibres are released from the presynaptic terminal. If so, receptors for these factors may also be present in the postsynaptic membrane.

The AChRs, described fully by Beeson and Barnard in a later chapter, are cylindrical, membrane-spanning proteins with a central ion channel. Each functional molecule contains five homologous subunits of four distinct types, with a stoichiometry of 'α_2, β, δ, ε' at adult mammalian NMJs. Each complete molecule has two ACh binding sites, both of which must be occupied for the ion channel to open. The genes for each of the AChR subunits from a wide variety of species have now been cloned and sequenced, and the functional properties of different domains of the subunits are being elucidated.

In addition to proteins involved in the process of neuromuscular transmission itself, the postsynaptic membrane contains specialised proteins, e.g. the nerve cell adhesion molecule, NCAM (Hoffman *et al.*, 1982: Couvalt and Sanes, 1986). NCAM is one of a family of partly related proteins that are involved in cell–cell interactions and show some structural homology with immunoglobulin molecules (see Lander, 1989). It is also found, extracellularly, in association with the presynaptic nerve terminal and may help to mediate nerve–muscle adhesion during early synaptogenesis (Bloch and Pumplin, 1988).

1.2.4. *The postsynaptic cytoplasm*

In most mammalian muscle the NMJ occupies a dome of cytoplasm on the muscle fibre surface. This dome is free of organised contractile proteins but contains many other cytoskeletal proteins (Burden, 1987; Bloch and Pumplin, 1988). While it is likely that these proteins are important in maintaining the general structure of the junctional region, most attention has so far been focused on the possibility that they play a specific role in maintaining the high density and distribution of AChRs.

Most clearly associated with the AChRs is a 43 kDa protein, originally isolated from the electric organ of the electric fish *Torpedo* (Froehner *et al.*, 1981). This '43 kDa protein' binds to the cytoplasmic domain of the β subunit of AChR (Burden *et al.*, 1983). Two cDNAs coding for forms of this protein, also known as 'RAPsyn' (receptor associated protein-synaptic), have recently been cloned (Frail *et al.*, 1987).

A membrane-associated cytoskeleton, based on the heterodimeric protein spectrin, is present in skeletal muscle (Morrow, 1989). A monomeric form of β spectrin, which is preferentially located at the NMJ, has recently been described (Bloch and Morrow, 1989). Actin plays a central role in linking together the dimeric spectrin molecules in many cells. A form of cytoplasmic actin is also present at the NMJ, as are a number of proteins frequently associated with it, including α-actinin, filamin, vinculin, talin (Bloch and Pumplin, 1988) and tropomyosin 2 (Marazzi *et al.*, 1989).

The details of the spatial and functional relationships between the various components of the cytoskeleton at the NMJ are not known. Intracellular injection of antibodies to tropomyosin 2 prevents the formation of new AChR clusters on cultured chick myotubes, suggesting that this protein plays a role in AChR localisation (Marazzi *et al.*, 1989). Dissociation of RAPsyn (using high pH) leaves AChR function intact

(Froehner, 1986). This suggests that the postsynaptic cytoskeleton is more concerned with maintenance of the organisation of the synaptic region in the long term, rather than with any role in the process of neuromuscular transmission itself.

In addition to an accumulation of cytoskeletal proteins, the postsynaptic cytoplasm usually contains a cluster of 5–10 myonuclei. It is an obvious possibility that these nuclei synthesise mRNA coding for the specialised proteins of the NMJ. This view is supported by the finding that mRNA coding for AChRs is concentrated at the NMJ (Merlie and Sanes, 1985; Fontaine and Changeux, 1988). The local factors that cause nuclei to accumulate at the NMJ remain unidentified. Studies of cultured muscle cells show that myonuclei are 'trapped' at sites of AChR clusters, possibly as a result of an interaction with the associated cytoplasm (Englander and Rubin, 1987). This suggests one important structural role for the postsynaptic cytoskeleton.

1.2.5. *Neuromuscular junctions in different muscle types*

The description above applies principally to voluntary striated muscle of the so-called fast and slow *twitch* types. In lower vertebrates, and in a few muscles in mammals, muscle fibres are present that contract directly in response to the nerve-evoked depolarisation (see Salpeter, 1987a). These slow, *tonic* muscle fibres are innervated at multiple sites and their presynaptic terminals have only a single row of active zone particles (Walrond and Reese, 1985). There are fewer junctional folds and less sarcoplasmic reticulum than in twitch fibres. The multi-site endplate potentials (see Chapter 2) activate Ca^{2+} release from the sarcoplasmic reticulum directly and thus initiate contraction in the absence of an action potential. These fibres are not frequent in humans but are found predominantly in the extraocular and some laryngeal muscles. Their importance lies in their distinctive mechanism of neuromuscular transmission, based on a graded response between ACh release and muscle contraction rather than depending on an all-or-none action potential, which may partly account for the frequent involvement of eye muscle in certain neuromuscular diseases (see Vincent, this volume).

1.3. **Development of the neuromuscular junction**

It should be clear from even the brief description given above, that development of the mature NMJ must depend on a complex series of interactions between nerve and muscle. These are not yet fully understood (Salpeter, 1987b), but appear to depend on both muscle activity and on trophic substances released from the nerve and from the muscle.

In humans, the formation of synapses between developing muscle and ingrowing axons starts at about 8 weeks of gestation, and further maturation of the junction continues throughout much of pregnancy (Juntunen and Teravainen, 1972). In rats and mice, on which the following account is primarily based, many features of the mature NMJ are similar to those in humans but their development starts only about a week before birth and is not complete until the fourth postnatal week, making them much more accessible for study.

Motor neurones are amongst the earliest neurones to be 'born' and their axons soon grow out into the regions where muscle will form (Jacobson, 1978; Purves and Lichtman, 1985). The 'growth cones' at the tip of these axons lack many of the characteristic features of synaptic terminals, such as synaptic vesicles and 'active zones', yet they are still capable of releasing ACh (Hume *et al.*, 1983; Young and Poo, 1983) and possibly other factors that may play a role in the formation and maintenance of nerve–muscle contacts.

Skeletal muscle fibres have many nuclei and form by fusion of mononucleated myogenic cells. This process starts just as motor axons arrive, and the immature 'myotubes' soon become innervated, probably within a day of their formation. Each muscle fibre becomes innervated at only a single synaptic site, but initially several axons contact that site ('polyneuronal innervation') and are able to evoke muscle contraction (Redfern, 1970; Brown *et al.*, 1976; Bennett, 1983).

When muscle fibres are first innervated AChRs are present over most of their surface at a density of about $500/\mu^2$ (Diamond and Miledi, 1962; Bevan and Steinbach, 1977). Soon after nerve contact, AChRs accumulate at the immature NMJ (Anderson and Cohen, 1977; Bevan and Steinbach, 1977), and come to occupy the entire zone contacted by nerve terminals at a density of about $2000–3000/\mu m^2$. At the same time the basal lamina begins to form around both the nerve and muscle fibres, with a common layer appearing particularly early in the synaptic cleft. In mammals this is associated with an increase in the activity of the endplate-specific form of AChE (Vigny *et al.*, 1976; see below). By the time of birth the density of AChRs in the synaptic cluster is already close to that at adult junctions $(10,000–20,000/\mu m^2)$ while that in the non-junctional region has begun to decline (Diamond and Miledi, 1962; Bevan and Steinbach, 1977).

During the first postnatal month in rats and mice, the immature junction is transformed into its adult form (Fig. 1.8). This process involves the withdrawal of all but one of the axons innervating each muscle fibre (Betz, 1987), the myelination of the one remaining axon and enlargement of its synaptic terminal, and the elaboration of the synaptic folds (Matthews-Bellinger and Salpeter, 1983). As the folds form, the AChR molecules become highly concentrated at their tops $(20,000/\mu^2)$ close to the axon

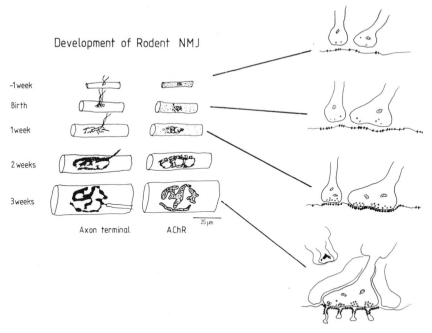

Development of Rodent NMJ

-1week
Birth
1week
2 weeks
3weeks

Axon terminal   AChR

Fig. 1.8. Development of the rodent NMJ. On the left the appearance under the light microscope; on the right schematic illustration of the developing NMJ showing distribution of AChRs.

terminal, and the high density of both AChRs and AChE becomes closely aligned with the maturing presynaptic terminals (Steinbach, 1981; Slater, 1982a).

The AChRs present at the immature NMJs and in the non-junctional region differ in two main ways from those present at the mature NMJ. Firstly, AChRs have a half-life of about 1 day in the immature muscle membrane but, shortly before birth, their metabolic stability increases and the half-life becomes about 10 days (Salpeter, 1987b). Secondly, the ion channels opened by ACh in embryonic muscle differ in having a lower conductance but a longer mean channel open time (see Chapter 2) than in the adult. Channels with the adult properties gradually replace the immature ones during the first 2 weeks after birth (Brenner and Sakmann, 1983; Vicini and Schuetze, 1985). A consequence of the longer open time of the immature channels is that individual miniature endplate currents (see Chapter 2) are able to trigger spontaneous contractile activity in immature muscle fibres (Jaramillo *et al.*, 1988). This activitiy may help to bring about maturation of muscle fibre properties.

The distinctive channel properties of the embryonic AChR molecules

Table 1.2. Changes in AChR properties during development

	Age	Density	Open time	Turnover	Antigenic type	Subunits
Pre-innervation	<14 d i.u.	$500/\mu m^2$	Long	Fast	EJ	$\alpha, \beta, \gamma, \delta$
Neuromuscular junction	16 d i.u.	$2\text{--}4 \times 10^3/\mu m^2$	Long	Fast	EJ	$\alpha, \beta, \gamma, \delta$
	birth	$8\text{--}20 \times 10^3/\mu m^2$	Long	Slow	EJ	$\alpha, \beta, \gamma, \delta$
	2 weeks–adult	$8\text{--}20 \times 10^3/\mu m^2$	Short	Slow	J	$\alpha, \beta, \delta, \varepsilon$
Denervated extrajunctional		$500/\mu m^2$	Long	Fast	EJ	$\alpha, \beta, \gamma, \delta$

result, at least partly, from the presence of a γ subunit in place of the ε subunit of the adult (Mishina *et al.*, 1986). The appearance of mRNA for the 'ε' subunit and a reciprocal loss of that coded for by the 'γ' subunit occur during the first postnatal week (Witzemann *et al.*, 1989), shortly before the changes in channel properties. Both these changes in AChR subunit composition are paralleled by changes in their immunological properties (Hall *et al.*, 1985; Gu and Hall 1988). In the human fetus the immunological change takes palce at around 33 weeks *in utero* (Hessel-mans *et al.*, 1989).

As the junctional AChRs change their properties the non-junctional AChRs disappear completely. These changes are associated with a more general decline in the total amount of AChR mRNA to the steady-state levels found in the adult. There is good reason to think that the increased activity of the maturing muscle is one important factor in mediating the changes in AChR gene expression (see below). However, studies of the expression of the genes for the different subunits during postnatal development show that the synthesis of each is controlled independently (Witzemann *et al.*, 1989). The properties of AChRs in mammalian muscle at various stages of development are summarised in Table 1.2.

The cellular and molecular mechanisms that lead to the local differentia-tion of the NMJ are not well understood. Most work so far has been directed at understanding how AChRs come to be concentrated at the developing NMJ. Two mechanisms have been suggested. One is that substances released from the nerve act directly on the muscle to cause a local increase in the synthesis and insertion of AChRs. Calcitonin gene-related peptide (CGRP) is one candidate (New and Mudge, 1986; Fontaine *et al.*, 1986). ARIA ('AChR-inducing activity'), a glycoprotein from chick brain whose cDNA has recently been cloned (Harris *et al.*, 1989), is another. In very low concentrations ARIA increases AChR synthesis in cultured chick myotubes by increasing the amount of mRNA for the alpha subunit of the AChR (Fischbach *et al.*, 1989).

Other evidence demonstrates that mobile AChRs in the plasma membrane are 'trapped' at sites of nerve contact (Anderson and Cohen, 1977). Factors in the synaptic basal lamina have the ability to localise AChRs and may mediate such trapping. One such factor is agrin (see below), which may be released from the nerve during development and become fixed to the basal lamina identifying it as 'synaptic', and endowing it with the ability to cause the accumulation of a number of key molecular components of the synapse.

Whatever the mechanisms, the effect on the maturation of the junction is to transform it from one which allows the immature muscle to respond with great sensitivity to the small amounts of transmitter released from the immature nerve terminals, to one which is specialised for highly reliable transmission of signals from the nerve, repeated at high frequency.

1.4. **Experimental manipulations of the NMJ**

Mature NMJs in mammals are stable structures, changing little in form over a period of months (Lichtman *et al.*, 1987), Experiments in which one or both of the two principal cellular constituents of the NMJ have been damaged have revealed much about the basis of that stability. These have been comprehensively reviewed elsewhere (e.g. Salpeter, 1987b; Sanes, 1989) and will only be described breifly here.

1.4.1. *Denervation*

When peripheral nerves are transected, the isolated distal portions of the axons degenerate. The first part of the motor axon to degenerate is the presynaptic terminal, which in rodents breaks down completely within less than 24 h (Miledi and Slater, 1970), attesting to its very immediate dependence on factors synthesised in the cell body and transported to the periphery. After denervation, many properties of the muscle fibre change. The membrane potential falls by about 10 mV and becomes unstable, leading to spontaneous fibrillations; and the voltage-dependent Na^+ channels responsible for the action potential (see Norman, this volume) become less sensitive to the blocking action of tetrodotoxin (Redfern and Thesleff, 1971). Within the cytoplasm the pattern of synthesis of the proteins governing contraction is also changed, leading to slowed contractile speed (Pette and Vrbova, 1985).

One of the best-known of the response to denervation is the great increase in sensitivity of the membrane to ACh (Axelsson and Thesleff, 1959; Miledi, 1960). This increased sensitivity is due to the appearance of AChRs all over the muscle fibre surface at a density of about $500/\mu m^2$, and a substantial increase in AChR mRNA (Merlie *et al.*, 1984; Goldman *et al.*, 1985; Tsay and Schmidt, 1989). The AChRs that appear on the non-junctional regions of denervated muscle are similar to those in embryonic muscle in their channel properties, in having a γ subunit in place of the adult ε (Witzemann *et al.*, 1987) and in their short metabolic half-life (Scheutze and Role, 1987).

The initiation of AChR gene expression and the appearance of AChRs in the extrajunctional membrane following denervation is primarily the result of the cessation of muscle activity. The effects of denervation on general muscle fibre properties also seem to be caused largely by the resulting inactivity of the muscle. When denervated muscles are directly stimulated with implanted electrodes the post-denervation increase in ACh sensitivity is lost as are many of the other effects of denervation (Lømo and Rosenthal, 1972; Lømo and Westgaard, 1975). Although other factors can induce an increase in ACh sensitivity, such as an inflammatory reaction at the muscle cell surface (Jones and Vrbova, 1974), it is clear that the normal state is primarily maintained by the continued use of the muscle.

Following partial denervation, the surviving axons put out sprouts which may reinnervate the paralysed muscle fibres (Brown, 1984). A number of factors appear to be involved in the induction and control of that sprouting. Several identified molecules, including NCAM, change in abundance and distribution following denervation (in parallel with AChRs) appearing in the extrajunctional region (Sanes *et al.*, 1986). The appearance of NCAM may directly promote sprouting and may also enhance the association between regenerating or sprouting axons and the denervated muscle fibres. On reinnervation the normal distribution of NCAM is re-established.

In spite of these widespread changes in muscle properties, the NMJ remains as a specialised region of the muscle fibre for weeks after denervation. The junctional folds persist (Miledi and Slater, 1968) and the density of AChRs at the NMJ remains near normal, even though there is a continuous turnover of individual AChR molecules consisting, at least partly, of those with embryonic properties (Loring and Salpeter, 1980; Gu and Hall, 1988). Similarly, while AChE remains concentrated at the synaptic site, the endplate-specific form is selectively lost (Hall, 1973), leaving other forms to predominate. Interestingly, the stability of these postsynaptic features is not present at birth. Neonatal denervation leads to dispersal of the clustered AChR (Slater, 1982b), AChE and other components of the synaptic basal lamina (Slater, unpublished observations); but as the mature form of the junction develops the postsynaptic specialisations become increasingly stable features of the muscle fibre and increasingly independent of interaction with the nerve.

If the nerve is damaged by crushing, so that the basal lamina sheath around each axon remains intact, the axons regenerate and rapidly grow back to the muscle. In most cases the regenerating axons reinnervate the muscle precisely at the sites of the original NMJs (Letinsky *et al.*, 1976; Rich and Lichtman, 1989). The effectiveness and precision of reinnervation appear to result in part from the persistence of adhesive molecules such as NCAM and S-laminin at the synaptic site. These molecules may survive from the original NMJ or be newly synthesised either by the muscle or by nearby fibroblasts (Gatchalian *et al.*, 1989). When reinnervation of original synaptic sites fails to occur, the growing axon may induce the formation of completely new postsynaptic specialisations, essentially identical in function and ultrastructure to normal NMJs (Lømo, 1988). The receptivity of denervated muscles to such 'ectopic' innervation is prevented or abolished if they are made active by direct electrical stimulation. While the molecular basis for this receptivity is not known, its control clearly resembles that of AChRs and NCAM in the extrajunctional region.

1.4.2. *Muscle damage*

Muscle fibres are very sensitive to mechanical, thermal or chemical damage and may degenerate when most of the mononucleated cells around them

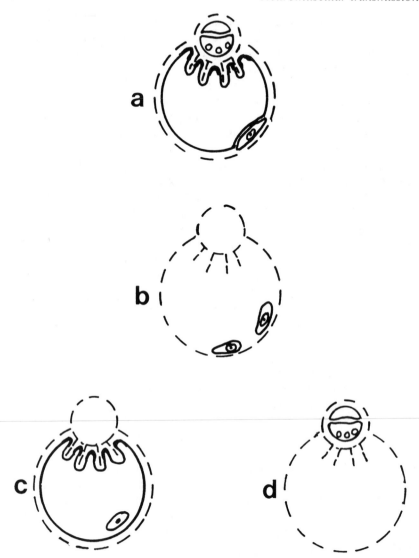

Fig. 1.9.   Destruction of the muscle fibre (**a**) leaves the muscle basal laminal sheath intact (**b**). Proliferation of myosatellite cells reforms the muscle fibre even in the absence of reinnervation (**c**). If the nerve is allowed to regenerate it will grow back to the original endplate due to the persistence of specialised basal lamina proteins. (**d**).

survive. When the basal lamina sheaths of the muscle fibres remain intact, mononucleated myosatellite cells, normally present in small numbers between the muscle fibres and the sheath, rapidly divide several times and then fuse to form a new muscle fibre. Following chemically induced damage of mammalian muscles, the structural properties of the NMJ are rapidly restored on the new muscle fibres (Jirmanova and Thesleff, 1972). A striking series of experiments on the frog has shown that factors stably associated with the synaptic basal lamina can direct the reconstruction of many features of the NMJ (Sanes, 1989) (Fig. 1.9).

On the presynaptic side, the sites of the original NMJ are selectively 'reinnervated' by regenerating axons, even if muscle regeneration is prevented by X-irradiation so that only a basal laminal 'tube' remains (Sanes *et al.*, 1978). Not only is the growth of the axons arrested when they encounter the original synaptic sites, but their terminals develop the structural features of presynaptic terminals, including vesicles and correctly placed active zones. It is likely that, as after denervation, molecules such as NCAM and S-laminin help to mediate this effect.

On the postsynaptic side the folds re-form and AChRs accumulate at their tops even when the muscle is allowed to regenerate in the absence of innervation or Schwann cells (Burden *et al.*, 1979; McMahan and Slater, 1984). Agrins (see above), which are present in motor neurones and may be incorporated into the basal lamina after release from the axon terminal (Magill-Solc and McMahan, 1988), can cause AChR accumulation in experimental systems and may play an important role in directly AChR accumulation on regenerating muscle fibres.

The stability of the normal NMJ is thus best viewed as a result of dynamic interactions between the nerve and the muscle and the fixed clues that come to be associated with the basal lamina during development. The importance of this arrangement is seen following partial denervation, as in local injury or in some diseases of the motor neurone; when the growth of surviving axons is activated, reinnervation of vacated synaptic regions leads to restoration of functional innervation.

Acknowledgements

We thank Carol Young for preparation of the micrographs in Figs 1.1 and 1.2.

References

Anderson, M. J. and Cohen, M. W. (1977) Nerve-induced and spontaneous redistribution of acetylcholine receptors on cultured muscle cells. *J. Physiol. (Lond.)* **268**: 731–756.

Anderson, M. J. and Fambrough, D. M. (1983) Aggregates of acetylcholine receptors are associated with plaques of a basal lamina heparan sulfate proteoglycan on the surface of skeletal muscle fibres. *J. Cell Biol.* **97**: 1396–1411.

Angelides, K. J. (1986) Fluorescently labelled Na$^+$ channels are localized and immboilized to synapses of innervated muscle fibres. *Nature* **321**: 63–66.

Axelsson, J. and Thesleff, S. (1959) A study of supersensitivity in denervated mammalian skeletal muscle. *J. Physiol. (Lond.)* **147**: 178–193.

Bahler, M. and Greengard, P. (1987) Synapsin I binds F-actin in a phosphorylation-dependent manner. *Nature* **326**: 704–707.

Bennett, M. R. (1983) Development of neuromuscular synapses. *Physiol. Rev.* **63**: 915–1048.

Betz, W. J. (1987) Motoneuron death and synapse elimination in vertebrates. In: *The Vertebrate Neuromuscular Junction*, Salpeter, M. M. ed. Alan Liss, New York, pp. 117–162.

Bevan, S. and Steinbach, J. H. (1977) The distribution of α-bungarotoxin binding sites on mammalian skeletal muscle developing *in vitro*. *J. Physiol. (Lond.)* **267**: 195–213.

Bloch, R. J. and Morrow, J. S. (1989) An unusual β-spectrin associated with clustered acetylcholine receptors. *J. Cell Biol.* **108**: 481–493.

Bloch, R. J. and Pumplin, D. W. (1988) Molecular events in synaptogenesis: nerve-muscle adhesion and postynaptic differentiation. *Am. J. Physiol.* **254**: C345–364.

Brenner, H. R. and Sakmann, B. (1983) Neurotrophic control of channel properties at neuromuscular synapses of rat muscle. *J. Physiol. (Lond.)* **337**: 159–171.

Brown, M. C. (1984) Sprouting of motor nerves in adult muscles: a recapitulation of ontogeny. *Trends Neurosci.* **7**: 10–13.

Brown, M. C., Jansen, J. K. S. and Van Essen, D. (1976) Polyneuronal innervation of skeletal muscle in new-born rats and its elimination during maturation. *J. Physiol. (Lond.)* **261**: 387–422.

Burden, S. J. (1987) The extracellular matrix and subsynaptic sarcoplasm at nerve-muscle synapses. In: *The Vertebrate Neuromuscular Junction*, Salpeter, M. M. ed., Alan Liss, New York, pp. 163–186.

Burden, S. J., DaPalma, R. L. and Gottesman, G. S. (1983) Cross-linking of proteins in acetylcholine receptor-rich membranes: association between the β-subunit and the 43Da subsynaptic protein. *Cell* **35**: 687–692.

Burden, S. J. Sargent, P. B. and McMahan, U. J. (1979) Acetylcholine receptors in regenerating muscle accumulate at original synaptic sites in the absence of the nerve. *J. Cell Biol.* **82**: 412–425.

Couvalt, J. and Sanes, J. R. (1986) Distribution of N-CAM in synaptic and extrasynaptic portions of developing and adult skeletal muscle. *J. Cell Biol.* **102**; 716–730.

Diamond, J. and Miledi, R. (1962) A study of foetal and newborn rat muscle fibers. *J. Physiol. (Lond.)* **162**: 393–408.

Englander, L. L. and Rubin, L. (1987) Acetylcholine receptor clustering and nuclear movement in muscle fibres in culture. *J. Cell Biol.* **104**: 87–95.

Fischbach, G. D., Harris, D. S., Falls, D. L., Dubinsky, J. M., Morgan, M., Englisch, K. L. and Johnson, F. A. (1989) The accumulation of acetylcholine receptors at developing chick nerve-muscle synapses. In *Neuromuscular Junction*, Sellin, L. C., Libelius, R. and Thesleff, S. eds., Elsevier, Amsterdam, pp. 515–532.

Fontaine, B. and Changeux, J.-P. (1988) Localization of nicotinic acetylcholine receptor α-subunit transcripts during myogenesis and motor endplate development in the chick. *J. Cell Biol.* **108**: 1025–1037.

Fontaine, E. B., Klarsfeld, A., Hockfelt, T. and Changeux, J.-P. (1986) Calcitonin gene-related peptide, a peptide present in spinal cord motorneurons increases the number of acetylcholine receptors in primary cultures of chick embryo myotubules. *Neurosci. Lett.* **71**: 59–65.

Frial, D. E., Mudd, J., Shah, V., Carr, C., Cohen, J. B. and Merlie, J. P. (1987)

cDNAs for the postsynpatic 43-kDa protein of *Torpedo* electric organ encode two proteins with different carboxyl termini. *Proc. Natl. Acad. Sci.* **84**: 6302–6306.

Froehner, S. C. (1986) The role of the postsynaptic cytoskeleton in acetylcholine receptor organisation. *Trends Neurosci.* **9**: 37–41.

Froehner, S. C., Gulbrandsen, V., Hyman, C., Jeng, A. Y., Neubig, R. R. and Cohen, J. B. (1981) Immunofluorescence localization at the mammalian neuromuscular junction of the Mr 43,000 protein of *Torpedo* postsynaptic membranes. *Proc. Natl. Acad. Sci. USA* **78**: 5230–5234.

Gatchalian, C. L., Schachner, M. and Sanes, J. R. (1989) Fibroblasts that proliferate near denervated synaptic sites in skeletal muscle synthesize the adhesive molecules tenascin (J1), NCAM, fibronectin and heparan sulfate proteoglycan. *J. Cell, Biol.* **108**: 1873–1890.

Goldman, D., Boulter, S., Heinemann, S. and Patrick, J. (1985) Muscle denervation increases the levels of two mRNAs coding for the acetylcholine receptor α-subunit. *J. Neurosci.* **5**: 2553–2558.

Gu, Y, and Hall, Z. W. (1988) Immunological evidence for a change in subunits of the acetylcholine receptor in developing and denervated rat muscle. *Neuron*, **1**: 117–125.

Hall. Z. W. (1973) Multiple forms of acetylcholinesterase and their distribution in endplate and non-endplate regions of rat diaphragm muscle. *J. Neurobiol.* **4**: 343–361.

Hall, Z. W., Gorin, P. D. Silbestein, L. and Bennett, C. (1985) A postnatal change in the immunological properties of the acetylcholine receptor at rat muscle endplates. *J. Neurosci.* **5**: 730–734.

Harris, D. A., Falls, D. L., Walsh, W. and Fischbach, G. D. (1989) Molecular cloning of an acetylcholine receptor-inducing protein. *Soc. Neurosci. Abstr.* **15**: 164.

Hesslemans, L. F. G. M., Jennekens, F. G. I., van den Oord, C. J. M., Veldman, H. and Vincent, A. (1989) Immunoreactivity to acetylcholine receptor in developing human muscle. (Submitted for publication)

Heuser, J. E. and Reese, T. S. (1973). Evidence for recycling of synaptic vesicle membrane during transmitter release at the frog neuromuscular junction. *J. Cell Biol.* **57**: 315–344.

Heuser, J. E., Reese, T. S., Dennis, M. J., Jan, Y., Jan, L. and Evans, L. (1979) Synaptic vesicle exocytosis captured by quick freezing and correlated with quantal transmitter release. *J. Cell Biol.* **81**: 275–300.

Hirokawa, N. and Heuser, J. E. (1982) Internal and external differentiations of the postsynaptic membrane at the neuromuscular junction. *J. Neurocytol.* **11**: 487–510.

Hirokawa, N., Sobue, K., Kanda, K., Harada, A. and Yorifuji, H. (1989) The cytoskeletal architecture of the presynaptic terminal and molecular structure of synapsin 1. *J. Cell Biol.* **108**: 111–126.

Hoffman, S., Sorkin, B. C. White, P. C., Brackenbury, R., Mailhammer, R., Rutishauser, U., Cunningham, B. A. and Edelman, G. M. (1982) Chemical characterization of a neural cell adhesion molecule purified from embryonic brain membranes. *J. Biol. Chem.* **257**: 7720–7729.

Hume R. I., Role, L. W. and Fischbach, G. D. (1983) Acetylcholine release from growth cones detected with patches of acetylcholine receptor-rich membrane. *Nature (Lond.)* **305**: 632–634.

Hunter, D. D., Shah, V., Merlie, J. P. and Sanes, J. R. (1989). A laminin-like adhesive protein concentrated in the synaptic cleft of the neuromuscular junction. *Nature (Lond.)* **338**: 229–234.

Israël, M., Morel, N., Lesbats, B., Birman, S. and Manaranche, R. (1986) Purification of a presynaptic membrane protein that mediates a calcium-dependent translocation of acetylcholine. *Proc. Natl. Acad. Sci. USA* **83**: 9226–9230.

Jacobson, M. A. (1978) *Developmental Neurobiology*. Plenum, New York.

Jaramillo, F., Vicini, S. and Schuetze, S. M. (1988) Embryonic acetylcholine receptors guarantee spontaneous contractions in rat developing muscle. *Nature* **335**: 66–68.

Jirmanova, I. and Thesleff, S. (1972) Ultrastructural study of experimental muscle degeneration and regeneration in the adult rat. *Zeit. Zellforsch. Mik. Anat.* **131**: 77–97.

Jones, S. W. (1987) Presynaptic mechanisms at vertebrate neuromuscular junctions. In: *The vertebrate Neuromuscular Junction*, Salpeter, M. M., ed. Alan Liss, New York, pp. 187–245.

Jones, R. and Vrbova, G. (1974) Two factors responsible for the development of denervation hypersensitivity. *J. Physiol. (Lond.)* **236**: 517–538.

Juntunen, J. and Teravainen, H. (1972) Structural development of myoneruonal junctions in the human embryo. *Histochemie* **32**: 107–112.

Lander, A. D. (1989) Understanding the molecules of neural cell contacts: emerging patterns of structure and function. *Trends Neurosci.* **12**: 189–195.

Letinsky, M. S., Fischbeck, K. H. and McMahan, U. J. (1976) Precision of reinnervation of original postsynpatic sites in frog muscle after a nerve crush. *J. Neurocytol.* **5**: 691–718.

Lichtman, J. W., Magrassi, L. and Purves, D. (1987) Visualisation of neuromuscular junctions over periods of several months in living mice. *J. Neurosci.* **7**: 1215–1222.

Linstedt, A. D. and Kelly, R. B. (1987) Overcoming barriers to exocytosis. *Trends Neurosci.* **10**: 446–448.

Lømo, T. (1988) Role of activity and inactivity in synapse formation. In: *Neuromuscular Junction*, Sellin, L. C., Libelius, R. and Thesleff, S., eds, Elsevier, Amsterdam, pp. 533–540.

Lømo, T. and Rosenthal, J. (1972) Control of ACh sensitivity by muscle activity in the rat. *J. Physiol. (Lond.)* **221**: 493–513.

Lømo, T. and Slater, C. R. (1978) Control of acetylcholine sensitivity and synapse formation by muscle activity. *J. Physiol. (Lond.)* **275**: 391–402.

Lømo, T. and Westgaard, R. H. (1975) Further studies on the control of ACh sensitivity by muscle activity in the rat. *J. Physiol. (Lond.)* **252**: 603–626.

Loring, R. and Salpeter, M. M. (1980) Denervation increases turnover rate of junctional acetylcholine receptors. *Proc. Natl. Acad. Sci. USA*, **44**: 2293–2298.

Magill-Solc, C. and McMahan, U. J. (1988). Motor neurons contain agrin-like molecules. *J. Cell Biol.* **107**: 1825–1833.

Marazzi, G., Bard, F., Klymkowsky, M. W. and Rubin, L. L. (1989) Microinjection of a monoclonal antibody against a 37-kDa protein (tropomyosin 2) prevents the formation of new acetylcholine receptor clusters. *J. Cell Biol.* **109**: 2337–2344.

Marshall, L. G. and Parsons, S. M. (1987) The vesicular acetylcholine transport system. *Trends Neurosci.* **10**: 174–177.

Massoulie, J. and Bon, S. (1982). The molecular forms of cholinesterase and acetylcholinesterase in vertebrates. *Annu. Rev. Neurosci.* **5**: 57–106.

Matthews-Bellinger, J. A. and Salpeter, M. M. (1983) Fine structural distribution of acetylcholine receptors at developing mouse neuromuscular junctions. *J. Neurosci.* **3**: 644–657.

McGuinness, T. L. and Greengard, P. (1988) Protein phosphorylation and synaptic transmission. In: *Neuromuscular Junction*, Sellin, L. C., Libelius, R. and Thesleff, S., eds, Elsevier, Amsterdam, pp. 111–124.

McMahan, U. J. and Slater, C. R. (1984) The influence of basal lamina on the accumulation of acetylcholine receptors at synaptic sites in regenerating muscle. *J. Cell Biol.* **98**: 1453–1473.

Merlie, J. P. and Sanes, J. R. (1985) Concentration of acetylcholine recptor mRNA in synaptic regions of adult muscle fibres. *Nature (Lond.)* **317**: 66–68.

Merlie, J. P., Isenberg, K. E. Russell S. D. and Sanes, J. R. (1984) Denervation suspersensitivity in skeletal muscle: analysis with a cloned cDNA probe. *J. Cell Biol.* **99**: 332–335.

Miledi, R. (1960) The acetylcholine sensitivity of frog muscle fibres after complete or partial denervation. *J. Physiol. (Lond.)* **151**: 1–23.

Miledi, R. and Slater, C. R. (1968) Electrophysiology and electron-microscopy of rat neuromuscular junctions after nerve degeneration. *Proc. Roy. Soc. B* **169**: 289–306.

Miledi, R. and Slater, C. R. (1970) On the degeneration of rat neuromuscular junctions after nerve section. *J. Physiol. (Lond.)* **207**: 507–528.

Mishina, M., Takai, T, Imoto, K. Noda, M., Takahashi, T., Numa, S., Methfessel, C. and Sakmann, B. (1986) Molecular distinction between foetal and adult forms of muscle acetylcholine receptor. *Nature (Lond.)* **321**: 406–411.

Morrow, J. S. (1989) The spectrin membrane cytoskeleton. *Curr. Opin. Cell Biol.* **1**: 23–29.

New, H. V. and Mudge, A. W. (1986). Calcitonin gene-related peptide regulates muscle acetylcholine receptor synthesis. *Nature (Lond)* **323**: 809–811.

Nitkin, R. M., Smith, M. A., Magill, C., Fallon, J. R. Yao, R.-M. M., Wallace, B. G. and McMahan, U. J. (1987) Identification of agrin, a synaptic organizing protein from *Torpedo* electric organ. *J. Cell Biol.* **195**: 2471–2478.

Pette, D. and Vrbova, G. (1985) Neural control of phenotypic expression in mammalian muscle fibres. *Muscle Nerve* **8**: 676–689.

Purves, D. and Lichtman, J. W. (1985). *Principles of Neural Development.* Sinauer Associates Inc., Sunderland, MA.

Rahamimoff, R., Abdul-Ghani, M., deRiemer, S. A., Ginsburg, S., Sakmann, B., Shapira, R., Silberberg, S. D., Stadler, H. and Yakir, N. (1988) Regulation of acetylcholine release: calcium, peptide channels and vesicle. In: *Neuromuscular Junction*, Sellin, L. C., Libelius, R. and Thesleff, S., eds, Elsevier, Amsterdam, pp. 125–136.

Redfern, P. A. (1970) Neuromuscular transmission in new-born rats. *J. Physiol. (Lond).* **209**: 701–709.

Redfern, P. A. and Thesleff, S. (1972) Action potential generation in denervated rat skeletal muscle. *Acta Physiol. Scand.* **81**: 557–564.

Rich, M. and Lichtman, J. W. (1989) *In vivo* visulaization of pre- and postsynaptic changes during synapse elimination in reinnervated mouse muscle. *J. Neurosci.* **9**: 1781–1805.

Rotondo, R. (1987) Biogenesis and regulation of acetylcholinesterase. In: *The Vertebrate neuromuscular Junction*, Salpeter, M. M. ed., Alan Liss, New York, pp. 247–284.

Salpeter, M. M. (1987a) Vertebrate Neuromuscular junctions: general morphology, molecular organization, and functional consequences. In: *The Vertebrate Neuromuscular Junction*, Salpeter, M. M. ed., Alan Liss, New York, pp. 1–54.

Salpeter, M. M. (1987b) Development and neural control of the neuromuscular junction and of the junctional acetylcholine receptor. In: *The Vertebrate Neuromuscular Junction*, Salpeter, M. M., ed., Alan Liss, New York, pp. 55–115.

Sanes, J. R. (1989). Extracellular matrix molecules that influence neural development. *Ann. Rev. Neurosci.* **12**: 521–546.

Sanes, J. R., Marshall, L. M. and McMahan, U. J. (1978). Reinnervation of muscle fibre basal lamina after removal of myofibres. *J. Cell Biol.* **78**: 176–198.

Sanes, J. R., Schachner, M. and Couvalt, J. (1986) Expression of several adhesive molecules (N-CAM, L1, J1, NILE, uvomorulin, laminin, fibronectin and a heparan sulfate proteoglycan) in embryonic, adult and denervated adult skeletal muscle. *J. Cell Biol.* **102**: 420–431.

Schuetze, S. M. and Role, L. W. (1987) Developmental regulation of nicotinic acetylcholine receptors. *Ann. Rev. Neurosci.* **10**: 403–457.

Slater, C. R. (1982a) Neuronal influence on postnatal changes in acetylcholine receptor distribution at nerve–muscle junctions in the mouse. *Dev. Biol.* **94**: 23–30.

Slater, C. R. (1982b) Postnatal maturation of nerve–muscle junctions in hindlimb muscles of the mouse. *Dev. Biol.* **94**: 11–22.

Smith, S. J. and Augustine, G. J. (1988) Calcium ions, active zones and synaptic transmitter release. *Trends Neurosci.* **11**: 458–464.

Steinbach, J. H. (1981) Developmental changes in acetylcholine receptor aggregates at rat skeletal neuromuscular junctions. *Dev. Biol.* **841**. 267–276.

Thomas, L., Hartung, K. Langosch, D., Rehm, H., Bamberg, E., Franke, W. W. and Betz, H. (1988). Identification of synaptophysin as a hexameric channel protein of the synaptic vesicle membrane. *Science* **242**: 1050–1053.

Tsay, H.-J. and Schmidt, J. (1989) Skeletal muscle denervation activates acetylcholine receptor genes. *J. Cell Biol.* **108**: 1523–1526.

Tucek, S. (1984) Problems in the organization and control of acetylcholine synthesis in brain neurons. *Prog. Biophys. Mol. Biol.* **44**: 1–46.

Valtorta, F., Jahn, R., Fesce, R., Greengard, P. and Ceccarelli, B. (1988) Synaptophysin (p38) at the frog neuromuscular junction: its incorporation into the axolemma and recycling after intense quantal secretion. *J. Cell Biol.* **107**: 2717–2727.

Vicini, S. and Scheutze, S. M. (1985) Gating properties of acetylcholine receptors at developing rat endplates. *J. Neurosci.* **5**: 2212–2224.

Vigny, M. Koenig, J. and Rieger, F. (1976) The motor endplate specific form of acetylcholinesterase: appearance during embryogenesis and reinnervation of rat muscle. *J. Neurochem.* **27**: 1347–1353.

Vyskocil, F., Zemkova, H. and Edwards, C. (1988) Non-quantal acetylcholine release. In: *Neuromuscular Junction.* Sellin, L. C., Libelius, R. and Thesleff, S., eds, Elsevier, Amsterdam, pp. 197–205.

Walrond, J. P. and Reese, T. S. (1985) Structure of axon terminals and active zones at synapses on lizard twitch and tonic muscle fibers. *J. Neurosci.* **5**: 1118–1131.

Witzemann, V., Barg, B., Nishikawa, Y., Sakmann, B. and Numa, S. (1987) Differential regulation of muscle acetylcholine receptor α- and ε-subunit mRNAs. *FEBS Lett.* **223**: 104–112.

Witzemann, V., Barg, B., Criado, M., Stein, E. and Sakmann, B. (1989) Developmental regulation of five subunit specific mRNAs encoding acetylcholine receptor subtypes in rat muscle. *FEBS Lett.* **242**: 419–424.

Young, S. H. and Poo, M.-M. (1983) Spontaneous release of transmitter from growth cones of embryonic neurons. *Nature (Lond.)* **305**: 634–635.

Introduction II: Electrophysiology of neuromuscular transmission

2.1. Introduction

One of the reasons why the neuromuscular junction (NMJ) has been the subject of so many diverse studies on synaptic transmission is its accessibility to the electrophysiologist. This chapter outlines the main events which take place during neuromuscular transmission, and the observations which can be made, even from a resting muscle cell, when the endplate region is impaled with a microelectrode (for review see Katz, 1966; Hille, 1984; W.-Wray, 1988). A more detailed account of the postsynaptic events is given in the chapter by Colquhoun in this volume.

2.1.1. *The resting membrane potential*

In nerve, as in other tissues, the intracellular K^+ concentration is high relative to Na^+, whereas the reverse is true for the extracellular fluid. These differences are maintained by active pumping through an energy-dependent K^+/Na^+ exchange. Since the resting plasma membrane has some permeability to K^+, but little to Na^+, there is a tendency for K^+ ions to leak out of the cell down their concentration gradient, thus making the interior of the cell more negative, and the membrane polarised. The efflux of K^+ will be restricted, however, by the increasing negativity of the cell interior until an equilibrium is achieved (the 'equilibrium potential' for potassium). This results in a membrane potential of around -70 mV. If Na^+ ion channels in the membrane are opened, as happens when an action potential travels down the nerve, the influx of Na^+ will tend to bring the membrane potential closer to the 'equilibrium potential' for Na^+ ions. This potential is positive (around 50 mV), in contrast to that for potassium, because of the low concentration of soldium intracellularly. Thus the membrane depolarises to more positive values. When the Na^+ channels close the membrane potential is rapidly restored to negative values due to the recruitment of voltage-activated K^+ channels which increase the rate of K^+ efflux.

2.1.2. *Outline of neuromuscular transmission*

When an impulse is initiated in the motor neurone cell body an action potential, i.e. wave of depolarisation, travels down the nerve axon due to the opening of voltage-activated Na^+ channels. When it reaches the peripheral nerve terminal acetylcholine (ACh) is released in multimolecular packets, or 'quanta' (del Castillo and Katz, 1954). ACh diffuses across the narrow synaptic cleft, and binds to acetylcholine receptors (AChRs) on the surface of the postsynaptic membrane of the muscle fibre. Binding of ACh opens the AChR-associated ion channels, allowing Na^+ ions to enter and depolarise the muscle fibre. This depolarisation, the endplate potential (EPP), opens voltage-dependent Na^+ channels through which further Na^+ ions flow, forming an action potential which is propagated along the length of the muscle fibre surface and leads to contraction. Thus the NMJ forms a chemical relay between electrically conducting tissues.

Meanwhile, ACh dissociates from its binding sites on the AChR, the ion channels close and repolarisation of the endplate takes place. Hydrolysis of unbound ACh by the enzyme acetylcholinesterase (AChE), present in the synaptic cleft, prevents rebinding of ACh and rapidly prepares the junction for transmission of another nerve impulse.

2.1.3. *Endplate potentials and miniature endplate potentials*

Useful information on neuromuscular transmission has been obtained by recording voltages intracellularly with fine-tipped glass microelectrodes inserted into single muscle cells (see Chapter 3 in this volume). The resting potential recorded by a microelectrode in the muscle cell is usually around -70 mV (see above). If the microelectrode is placed near an endplate region of an unstimulated muscle fibre, small spontaneous potential changes are observed: miniature endplate potentials (MEPPs) (Fatt and Katz, 1952), see Fig. 2.1. These MEPPs occur at random (approx. one per second in many animals, but less in humans) and have small amplitudes (0.5–1 mV), which are insufficient to trigger action potentials. Each MEPP arises by the release from the nerve terminal of a single packet of ACh (containing around 10,000 ACh molecules), which then acts on the postsynaptic membrane to produce the depolarisation seen as a MEPP.

When the nerve is stimulated, many such packets of ACh are released almost simultaneously from the nerve terminal, producing a much larger depolarisation (of similar time-course to the MEPP) in the muscle fibre at the endplate: the EPP (Fig. 2.1). The number of packets released by each single nerve stimulus varies somewhat; the *mean* number of packets released is perhaps confusingly referred to as the quantal content, m. As each *single* packet of ACh produces a response of magnitude corresponding to the MEPP amplitude, the EPP amplitude is therefore the quantal content times the MEPP amplitude. Thus, if the MEPP and EPP amplitudes are measured, the quantal content can be found but, in

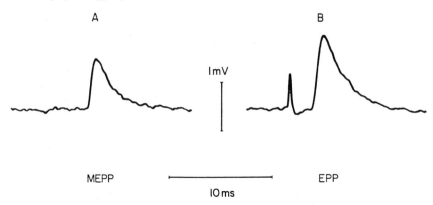

Fig. 2.1. Miniature endplate potential (left) and endplate potential (right) in mouse diaphragm muscle. The EPP was recorded in the presence of d-tubocurarine to reduce the amplitude to sub-threshold values in order to prevent contraction of the muscle fibre and displacement of the recording electrode. Reproduced with permission from W.-Wray, 1988.

practice, corrections to this calculation need to be applied. The practical methods ('direct', 'failures' or 'variance' methods) of calculating quantal content from the EPP data can be found in Katz (1966). Typical values of quantal content are about 60–130 in animals and in humans (see e.g. Lambert and Elmqvist, 1971; Lang *et al.*, 1983).

2.2. Presynaptic events

2.2.1. *Calcium ion influx*

Ca^{2+} ions play a key role in transmitter release. In solutions containing low Ca^{2+} concentrations the number of packets of ACh released per nerve stimulus (i.e. the quantal content) is reduced, leading to reduced EPP amplitude. High Mg^{2+} concentrations have a similar effect because Mg^{2+} ions compete with Ca^{2+}.

Provided that Ca^{2+} ions are present in the bathing solution, any factor causing depolarisation of nerve terminals induces Ca^{2+} entry and subsequent release of ACh. For instance, nerve terminals can be depolarised by increasing the K^+ ion concentration of the bathing solution, leading to an increase in MEPP frequency (Liley, 1956a). Terminals can also be depolarised by passing current pulses from a nearby extracellular electrode, again leading to ACh release. Finally, and most importantly, the action potential itself consists of a brief but large depolarisation, and the associated influx of Ca^{2+} ions is responsible for the nearly simultaneous release of many packets of ACh, forming the EPP. The Na^+ ions themselves (mediators of the nerve action potential; see chapters by

Norman and by Colquhoun in this volume) are not responsible for release (Katz and Miledi, 1969); it is the electrical depolarisation itself which is important.

During the period of depolarisation the Ca^{2+} entry into the nerve terminal occurs because the membrane becomes transiently more permeable to Ca^{2+} ions due to the opening of voltage-dependent Ca^{2+} channels. Intracellular free Ca^{2+} concentration is normally very low (about 0.1 μM) (Baker, 1977), while the physiological concentration of extracellular free Ca^{2+} is about 2 mM. Thus, when the membrane becomes more permeable to Ca^{2+}, these ions flow down their concentration gradient into the nerve terminal.

The presynaptic terminals of the skeletal neuromuscular junction are too small to insert a microelectrode, and most of what we know about Ca^{2+} currents at presynaptic terminals has been obtained by studying those of the squid giant synapse (e.g. Llinas *et al.*, 1976, 1981, Augustine *et al.*, 1985a). The Ca^{2+} permeability of the membrane rises at the beginning of a depolarising pulse, and falls back to normal after the pulse, over a period of milliseconds. The transient increase in Ca^{2+} concentration inside presynaptic terminals during nerve depolarisation has also been detected in the squid giant synapse using Ca^{2+}-sensitive compounds (e.g. Augustine *et al.*, 1985b).

Furthermore, currents produced by single voltage-dependent Ca^{2+} channels have been observed in other (larger) neurones and in heart muscle membranes (Wray *et al.*, 1989; Norman this volume) using the patch clamp technique (see Chapter 3 in this volume). The frequency of the opening of individual Ca^{2+} channels increases when the membrane is suddenly depolarised, leading to an increase in overall Ca^{2+} current.

In general, there appear to be several types of voltage-dependent Ca^{2+} channels (termed T, N and L; see Norman, this volume). The L-type Ca^{2+} channels from skeletal muscle transverse tubulues and from heart, for example, have been purified and their subunit structure is now becoming clear. However, the Ca^{2+} channel present in the nerve terminal membrane at the neuromuscular junction does not appear to fit into the classification of calcium channel types and may be partially different from the above subtypes (see Norman and see Wray, this volume).

2.2.2. *Acetylcholine release*

Following the brief depolarisation of motor nerve terminals there is a time interval ('synaptic delay') of around 0.5 ms (20°C) before the EPP appears (Katz and Miledi, 1965). This occurs mainly because of a *presynaptic* delay in release of ACh following nerve terminal depolarisation. In turn this is due partly to a delay before Ca^{2+} channels open and partly to a further delay once Ca^{2+} current has started to flow before transmitter is released

(Llinas *et al.*, 1981). During the latter very short delay Ca^{2+} ions, which enter the nerve terminal via the Ca^{2+} channels, appear to travel to an intracellular binding site and then cause release. For this to occur, the voltage-dependent Ca^{2+} channels (thought to be the particles found at active zones in freeze-fracture electron micrographs — see morphology discussed in the previous chapter) must be situated very near to the intracellular Ca^{2+} binding sites and to ACh release sites.

As previously mentioned, ACh release depends on the Ca^{2+} concentra-

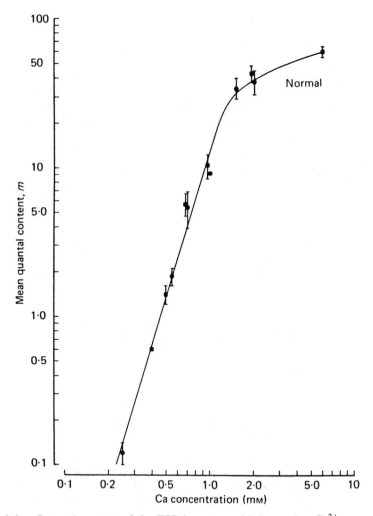

Fig. 2.2.   Quantal content of the EPP increases with increasing Ca^{2+} concentration, measured in human intercostal muscle. Reproduced with permission from Cull-Candy *et al.*, 1980.

tion of the bathing solution; increasing the Ca^{2+} concentration from low levels causes an increase in the number of packets of ACh released by nerve stimulation (Fig. 2.2). However, although Ca^{2+} entry increases linearly with the extracellular Ca^{2+} concentration (Silinsky, 1985), the release of ACh increases more steeply, proportional to $[Ca]^n$, where $n = 3$ to 4. This has been interpreted (Dodge and Rahamimoff, 1967) as the need for cooperation between three or four Ca^{2+} ions at each intracellular binding site to cause the release of ACh.

2.2.3. *Facilitation and depression*

Acetylcholine release depends on the frequency of nerve stimulation (e.g. Ginsborg and Jenkinson, 1976). More specifically, changes in the number of packets of ACh released per nerve impulse can occur. Under normal conditions, if the nerve is stimulated at high frequency, successive EPPs generally decrease in amplitude (Fig. 2.3, top trace, 'depression'). On the other hand, under conditions where only a small number of packets of ACh are released (for instance in low Ca^{2+} or high Mg^{2+} solutions, or in the Lambert–Eaton myasthenic syndrome, see Wray, this volume), successive EPPs generally increase in size during repetitive nerve stimulation (Fig. 2.3, lower trace, 'facilitation').

It is likely that for normal Ca^{2+} concentrations where quantal release is

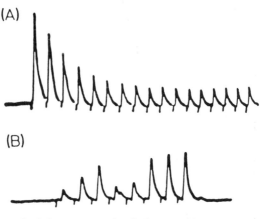

(A)

(B)

Fig. 2.3. EPPs evoked by nerve stimulation at high frequency in the rat diaphragm muscle. Upper: in normal Ca^{2+} concentration there is a steady decrease in the number of packets released per nerve impulse and hence in the EPP amplitude (depression). Recorded in d-tubocurarine. Lower: in 10 mM Mg^{2+} the quantal content is low, but there is an increase in the number of packets released and in the EPP amplitude (facilitation). The variation in EPP amplitudes comes about because of the variation in the number of packets released, particularly evident at these low quantal contents. No d-tubocurarine was needed. Reproduced with permission from Liley, 1956b.

already high, depletion of ACh occurs during high-frequency nerve stimulation (e.g. Martin, 1966; Ginsborg and Jenkinson, 1976). Therefore ACh release and the EPP decrease during repetitive stimulation even though there is an underlying increase in intracellular Ca^{2+}. On the other hand when quantal content is low, for whatever reason, ACh depletion does not occur and then facilitation can be observed due to the progressive summation of intracellular Ca^{2+} levels in the nerve terminal that occurs during repetitive nerve stimulation (Katz and Miledi, 1968; Rahaminoff, 1968).

2.3. Postsynaptic events

2.3.1. *Endplate response*

Following its release from the nerve, ACh reaches the postsynaptic membrane where it binds to acetylcholine receptors (AChR) and causes the AChR channels to open briefly. The 'endplate current' (EPC) flowing into the muscle cell at the endplate via these channels, in turn causes the depolarisation associated with the EPP (Fig. 2.4). When the endplate current has subsided, this depolarisation then decays by a purely passive process determined by the passive electrical properties of the membrane; thus the EPP outlasts the EPC.

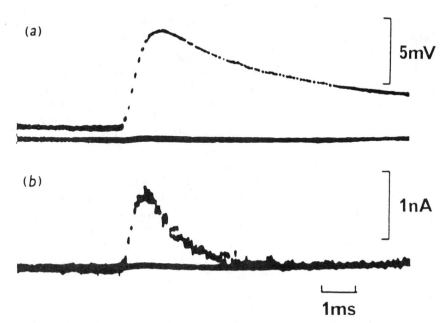

Fig. 2.4. Intracellular recordings of the endplate potential (a) and endplate current (b) in frog muscle. The EPC is shorter in duration (b) than the EPP (a). Reproduced with permission from Takeuchi and Takeuchi, 1959.

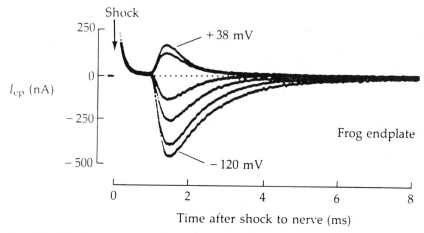

Fig. 2.5.   Endplate currents observed following nerve stimulation while maintaining the endplate at different membrane potentials with the voltage clamp technique. The endplate current is reduced to zero (i.e. the reversal potential) at around 0 mV. Reproduced with permission from Magleby and Stevens, 1972.

The spontaneous release of a *single* packet of ACh leads to a small current, the 'miniature endplate current' (MEPC) with a similar time-course to that of the EPC. This current is in turn responsible for generating the observed potential change, i.e. the MEPP. The currents which flow during the action of ACh (i.e. the EPC or MEPC) can be measured experimentally by the voltage-clamp technique.

During the time that endplate channels are open, ions flow down their concentration and electrical gradients. If the muscle membrane is partially depolarised by holding the membrane potential (using a voltage clamp, see Chapter 3) at less negative voltages, the electrical gradient is decreased so that the EPC amplitude is also decreased. Further depolarisation eventually reverses the EPC from inward to outward currents (Fig. 2.5), and the potential where this (i.e. zero current) occurs is called the reversal potential. The value of the reversal potential is determined by the concentrations and permeabilities of the ions which flow through the channels; ions which do not flow through the channel cannot affect the reversal potential. Varying the concentrations of Na^+ and K^+ ions affects the reversal potential, whereas varying the concentration of Cl^- ions does not (Takeuchi and Takeuchi, 1960). This indicates that the Cl^- ions do not flow through the endplate channels which, however, are permeable to Na^+ ions (usually flowing inwards) and K^+ ions (usually flowing outwards).

The effect of ACh released by nerve stimulation can be mimicked by applying a short pulse of ACh locally by the iontophoretic technique (see Chapter 3 and Fig. 2.6). Unlike nerve-stimulated release, there is almost

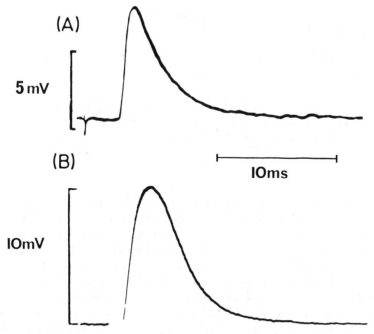

Fig. 2.6. Similarity between the endplate potential following nerve stimulation (**A**) and the potential change evoked by iontophoretic application of ACh (**B**) at the rat diaphragm endplate. Reproduced with permission from Krnjevic and Miledi, 1958.

no delay in the onset of the response after iontophoretic application (Katz and Miledi, 1965), because ACh reacts rapidly with the postsynaptic receptors.

2.3.2. Desensitisation

When ACh or any other agonist is applied continuously to a muscle fibre, after an initial depolarisation the activity of the endplate channels wanes. This effect, desensitisation, is more prevalent at high agonist concentrations and is thought to occur when the AChRs enter a refractory or desensitised state. It is probably not relevant during normal physiological behaviour but can be an important factor during experiments designed to study the action of agonists.

2.3.3. Single channels

Information about single channels was first obtained by 'noise analysis' (Katz and Miledi, 1970; see Chapter 3) and more recently by the patch

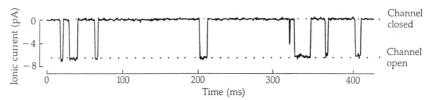

Fig. 2.7. Single-channel currents observed by the patch clamp technique in an excised patch of membrane from a cultured rat myotube exposed to ACh. Note the variable open time and constant amplitude of each current pulse. Reproduced with permission from Hille, 1984.

clamp technique (Neher and Sakmann, 1976; see Colquhoun, this volume). It was found that ACh and other depolarising drugs produce tiny pulses of current corresponding to the opening and closing of single channels (Fig. 2.7). The amplitude, i, of each pulse is fairly constant and equal to a few pA. The conductance of the channel can be found by applying Ohm's law, knowing the voltage, V_m across the membrane; conductance $\gamma = i/V_m$. With i in amps and V_m in volts, the units of conductance are Siemens (S); normal endplate channels usually have a conductance of roughly 50 pS (1 pS $= 10^{-12}$ Siemens). The duration of the open state is not constant; a distribution of open times is seen (see chapter by Colquhoun, this volume). The *average* open time at room temperature and for normal resting potentials is found to be about 1 ms for muscle endplate channels when ACh is the agonist.

From these values of channel conductance and open time, one finds that each channel, while open, passes a quantity of charge equal to about 4×10^{-15} coulombs, equivalent to the passage of roughly 10^4 univalent ions.

The open time of endplate channels depends strongly on temperature, being increased around threefold when the temperature is lowered by 10°C. Open time also depends on membrane potential; as membrane potential is hyperpolarised by 50 mV, channel open time increases by around 50%. On the other hand, the conductance of the channel varies little with temperature or membrane potential.

The rate of decay of both MEPCs and EPCs is determined by the rate of closing of the channel. Thus, the mean channel open time is normally similar to the decay time constant of MEPCs or EPCs (Anderson and Stevens, 1973). This is because, after each nerve stimulation, any ACh which has not bound to receptors is rapidly hydrolysed by acetylcholinesterase and disappears from the synaptic cleft in a time much less than the channel open time. The effect of the acetylcholinesterase is made clear after it has been inhibited with a drug such as neostigmine. In this case ACh molecules persist in the cleft and can act repeatedly to cause channels to open. As a result the endplate currents and potentials are prolonged several-fold, while the open time of the individual channels remains unchanged (Katz and Miledi, 1973).

2.4. Factors affecting MEPPs and EPPs

From the brief description given above we can establish some guidelines which are of considerable use when investigating neuromuscular transmission in preparations treated with novel pharmacological ligands or toxins, in animal models of disease or in human muscle biopsies (see also Chapter 3). The mean number of ACh molecules released in each packet is remarkably constant and not usually affected by drugs or by changes in the ionic environment. Thus the amplitude of the MEPP depends mostly on the sensitivity of the postsynaptic membrane which can be readily varied by postsynaptically acting drugs such as competitive antagonists of ACh (e.g. tubocurarine, see Colquhoun, this volume) or by high-affinity neurotoxins such as α-bungarotoxin. On the other hand, the frequency of spontaneous release of packets of ACh is affected readily by changes in presynaptic conditions. So, for instance, MEPP frequency is increased by a rise in osmolarity or K^+ concentration of the bathing solution (see Ginsborg and Jenkinson, 1976).

The amplitude of the EPP depends both on the postsynaptic sensitivity (which can be varied, as for MEPPs, by postsynaptically acting drugs) and on the number of packets released per nerve impulse (i.e. the quantal content) which depends on presynaptic conditions such as the external Ca^{2+} concentration.

2.5. The safety factor in neuromuscular transmission

The effectiveness of each nerve impulse in eliciting a contraction in the fibre that it innervates depends on the EPP exceeding the threshold for generation of a muscle action potential. Under normal conditions this 'safety factor' (which can be defined as the ratio of EPP amplitude to the depolarisation required to reach the threshold in that particular fibre) is well above one, and even during successive impulses at high frequency, when the number of packets released declines (see above), the EPP remains above threshold.

However, the safety factor varies between species and between muscles in the same species. It seems to be lower for certain human muscles than in, for instance, the mouse diaphragm. Therefore, even a moderate reduction in the efficiency of neuromuscular transmission, such as a reduction in the number of functional AChRs in myasthenia gravis (see Vincent, this volume) or in the quantal content in the Lambert–Eaton Syndrome (see Wray, this volume), may bring about block of muscle contraction at least in some fibres and lead to muscle weakness.

References

Anderson, C. R. and Stevens, C. F. (1973) Voltage clamp analysis of acetylcholine produced end-plate current fluctuations at frog neuromuscular junction. *J. Physiol.* **235**: 655–691.

Augustine, G. J., Charlton, M. P. and Smith, S. J. (1985a) Calcium entry and transmitter release at voltage-clamped nerve terminals of squid. *J. Physiol.* **369**: 163–181.

Augustine, G. J., Charlton, M. P. and Smith, S. J. (1985b) Calcium entry into voltage-clamped presynaptic terminals of squid. *J. Physiol.* **367**: 143–182.

Baker, P. F. 1977 Calcium and the control of neurosecretion. *Sci. Prog., Oxf.*, **64**: 95–115.

Cull-Candy, S. G., Miledi, R., Trautmann, A. and Uchitel, O. D. (1980) On the release of transmitter at normal, myasthenia gravis and myasthenic syndrome affected human end-plates. *J. Physiol.* **299**: 621–638.

del Castillo, J. and Katz, B. (1954) Quantal components of the end-plate potential. *J. Physiol.* **124**: 560–573.

Dodge, Jr, F. A. and Rahamimoff, R. (1967) Co-operative action of Ca ions in the transmitter release at the neuromuscular junction. *J. Physiol.* **193**: 419–432.

Fatt, P. and Katz, B. (1952) Spontaneous subthreshold activitiy at motor nerve endings. *J. Physiol.* **117**: 109–128.

Ginsborg, B. L. and Jenkinson, D. H. (1976) Transmission of impulse from nerve to muscle. In: *Handbook of Experimental Pharmacology*, XLII: *Neuromuscular Junction*, Zaimis, E. ed., Springer-Verlag, Berlin, pp. 229–364.

Hille, B. (1984) *Ionic Channels of Excitable Membranes*, Sinnauer, Sunderland, MA.

Katz, B. 1966 Nerve, muscle and synapse. McGraw-Hill, USA.

Katz, B. and Miledi, R. (1965) The measurement of synaptic delay, and the time course of acetylcholine release at the neuromuscular junction. *Proc. Roy. Soc. B* **161**: 483–495.

Katz, B. and Miledi, R. (1968) The role of calcium in neuromuscular facilitation. *J. Physiol.* **195**: 481–492.

Katz, B. and Miledi, R. (1969) Spontaneous and evoked activity of motor nerve endings in calcium ringer. *J. Physiol.* **203**: 689–706.

Katz, B. and Miledi, R. (1970) Membrane noise produced by acetylcholine. *Nature* **226**: 962–963.

Katz, B. and Miledi, R. (1973) The binding of acetylcholine to receptors and its removal from the synaptic cleft. *J. Physiol.* **231**: 549–574.

Krnjevic, K. and Miledi, R. (1958) Acetylcholine in mammalian neuromuscular transmission. *Nature* **182**: 805–806.

Lambert, E. H. and Elmqvist, D. (1971) Quantal components of end-plate potentials in the myasthenic syndrome. *Ann. N. Y. Acad. Sci.* **183**: 183–199.

Lang, B., Newsom-Davis, J., Prior, C. and Wray, D. (1983) Antibodies to motor nerve terminals: and electrophysiological study of a human myasthenic syndrome transferred to mouse. *J. Physiol.* **344**: 335–345.

Liley, A. W. (1956a) The effects of presynaptic polarization on the spontaneous activity at the mammalian neuromuscular junction. *J. Physiol.* **134**: 427–443.

Liley, A. W. (1956b) The quantal components of the mammalian end-plate potential. *J. Physiol.* **133**: 571–587.

Llinas, R., Steinberg, I. Z. and Walton, K. (1976) Presynaptic calcium currents and their relation to synaptic transmission: voltage clamp study in squid giant synapse and theoretical model for the calcium gate. *Proc. Natl. Acad. Sci., USA*, **73**: 2918–2922.

Llinas, R., Steinberg, I. Z. and Walton, K. (1981) Relationship between presynaptic calcium current and postsynaptic potential in squid giant synapse. *Biophys. J.* **33**: 323–351.

Magleby, K. L. and Stevens, C. F. (1972) The effect of voltage on the time course of end-plate currents. *J. Physiol.* **223**: 151–171.

Martin, A. R. (1966) Quantal nature of synaptic transmission. *Physiol. Rev.* **46**: 51–66.

Neher, E. and Sakmann, B. (1976) Single channel currents recorded from membrane of denervated frog muscle fibres. *Nature* **260**: 799–802.

Rahamimoff, R. (1968) A dual effect of calcium ions on neuromuscular facilitation. *J. Physiol.* **195**: 471–480.

Silinsky, E. M. (1985) The biophysical pharmacology of calcium-dependent acetylcholine secretion. *Pharmacol. Rev.* **37**: 81–131.

Takeuchi, A. and Takeuchi, N. (1959) Active phase of frog's end-plate potential. *J. Neurophysiol.* **22**: 395–411.

Takeuchi, A. and Takeuchi, N. (1960) On the permeability of end-plate membrane during the action of transmitter. *J. Physiol.* **154**: 52–67.

W.-Wray, D. (1988) Neuromuscular transmission. In: (ed) *Disorders of Voluntary Muscle*, 5th edn, Walton, J., ed., Churchill Livingstone, Edinburgh, pp. 74–108.

W.-Wray, D., Norman, R. I. and Hess, P., eds. (1989) Calcium channels: structure and function. *Ann. NY Acad. Sci.* **560**: 1–479.

3 *Dennis Wray, Angela Vincent and David Beeson*

Introduction III: Techniques used in the study of neuromuscular transmission

The advances in understanding neuromuscular function at the molecular level depend entirely on the techniques available in the many different fields of biochemistry, pharmacology, physiology and molecular biology. Since many readers may not be entirely conversant with them all, the following notes are intended as a brief guide.

3.1. **Electrophysiological techniques**

This section summarises some of the more important electrophysiological techniques used in the study of neuromuscular transmission. These techniques are discussed in detail in the books by Katz (1966), Purves (1981), Sakmann and Neher (1983) and Hille (1984). Examples of the use of these techniques can be found in the chapters by Wray and by Colquhoun.

3.1.1. *Intracellular microelectrodes*

The technique of recording intracellular potentials with glass microelectrodes has been successfully used for many years. The principle is shown in Fig. 3.1. Glass microelectrodes are filled with conducting solution (usually 3 M KCl) and connected to a potential measuring device via a chlorided silver wire immersed in the KCl. The resistance of the microelectrodes used to record from muscle fibres is usually of the order of megohms, and so the potential measuring device must also have a high-input resistance in order to record faithfully. The overall result is to measure the potential at the tip of the electrode. Thus, potential differences between the inside and outside of the muscle fibre can be recorded ('membrane potential') by inserting the mircoelectrode into the fibre, and any potential changes occurring in the muscle fibre (such as endplate potentials) can be followed.

3.1.2. *The voltage-clamp technique*

For this technique, two microelectrodes are inserted into the muscle fibre next to each other, usually at the endplate region (Fig. 3.2). One

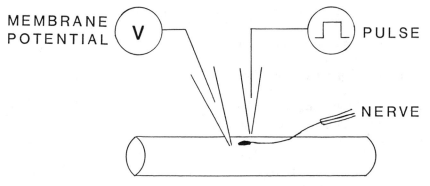

Fig. 3.1. Intracellular recording using a microelectrode to record the membrane potential, and an iontophoretic pipette to apply pulses of drugs to the postsynaptic membrane.

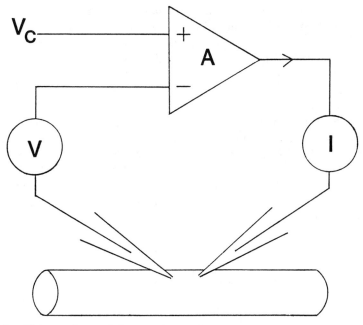

Fig. 3.2. Voltage clamp of the muscle membrane.

microelectrode records the intracellular potential (V) as described above. The other microelectrode is similar, except that it is used to pass current (I) into or out of the muscle fibre. Electronic circuitry (amplifier A, Fig. 3.2) controls the current passed by the latter electrode in order to maintain the intracellular voltage at a constant value (i.e. 'clamped'). The intracellular voltage is set by the command voltage, V_c, applied to the other input of amplifier, A. Currents across the membrane induced by agonists such as ACh can be measured under these conditions; such currents are equal to the current passed in or out of the fibre by the microelectrode. The voltage clamp technique has been routinely used to record endplate currents and miniature endplate currents (see e.g. chapters by Wray and by Colquhoun) following nerve stimulation, as well as currents resulting from experimental application of agonists. This technique is useful not only because the voltage of the membrane can be controlled, but also because passive changes involving charging the capacitance of the membrane cannot occur, thus enabling clear studies of endplate currents uncontaminated by passive currents.

3.1.3. *Patch-clamp recording*

This more recent technique (Neher and Sakmann, 1976) is used to record the current flowing through single channels. A blunt glass microelectrode or 'pipette' (tip diameter anout 1 μm), filled with electrolyte and an agonist such as ACh, is placed in contact with a small patch of membrane (Fig. 3.3). The pipette tip is tightly sealed against the outer face of the membrane. The current flowing across this small patch of membrane can be recorded. This technique can be applied not only to agonist-operated channels (such as endplate channels), but also to other channels such as voltage-operated channels (e.g. Na^+, K^+ and Ca^{2+} channels).

Besides recording single-channel currents with the pipette attached to the whole cell, withdrawal of the pipette from the cell can result in a patch of membrane continuing to be attached to the pipette. Currents can also be recorded across this excised patch of membrane ('inside-out') while investigating the effects of agents applied to it in the bath at known concentrations.

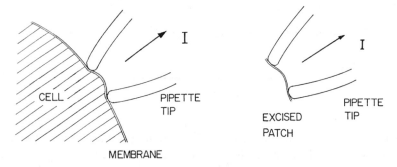

Fig. 3.3. Patch clamp technique for recording single-channel currents with the electrode attached to a cell or attached to a small fragment of membrane excised from the cell.

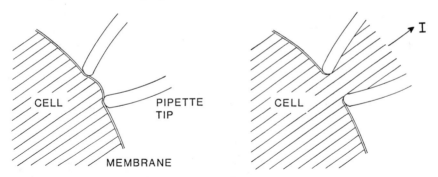

Fig. 3.4. The whole cell patch clamp technique.

The patch-clamp technique can also be used to voltage-clamp the cell, rather than to record single-channel currents. For this, the pipette is first sealed against the membrane, which is then broken by suction (Fig. 3.4). The inside of the pipette is then in electrical contact with the intracellular solution. By electronically controlling the voltage of the pipette, whilst measuring the current flowing via the pipette, the cell can be held at any desired potential (i.e. clamped). This method of voltage-clamping cells has the advantage that cells can be clamped without requiring penetration of two microelectrodes, and is particularly useful for small cells (e.g. cultured cells). Also by changing the composition of the solution in the pipette, the composition of the intracellular solution can be varied, since the intracellular medium is in continuity with the pipette solution.

3.1.4. *Noise analysis*

Before direct recording of single-channel currents by the patch-clamp technique, considerable information about single channels had previously been obtained indirectly by the technique of noise (or fluctuation) analysis (Katz and Miledi, 1972; Anderson and Stevens, 1973; for review see, e.g. Wray, 1980). For this, agonist is applied continuously at an endplate, either in the bath or 'iontophoretically'. The iontophoretic technique consists in electrically ejecting agonist such as ACh, from a micropipette filled with the agonist and placed near the postsynaptic membrane, by applying an appropriate voltage pulse to the micropipette (Fig. 3.1). The current flowing across the endplate membrane induced by the constant application of agonist is measured by the voltage-clamp technique using intracellular microelectrodes. Acetylcholine molecules collide with receptors to open channels randomly; the number of channels open at any one time is not a constant. This creates fluctuations (noise) in the current flowing across the endplate membrane (Fig. 3.5). These current fluctuations

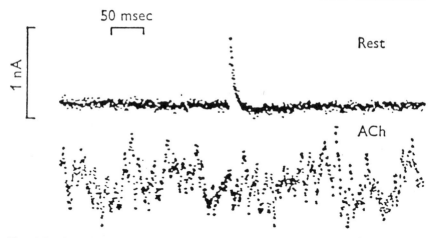

Fig. 3.5. Noise observed in the current during the application of ACh. From Anderson and Stevens (1973) with permission.

can then be analysed to give indirect information about underlying single-channel currents. The mean current passed by a single channel (the mean channel open time), and the mean number of channels open per second (frequency of channel opening) can be obtained by detailed analysis of the current fluctuations.

Useful information can also be obtained using a single intracellular microelectrode to record membrane potentials in unclamped fibres. Continuous application of ACh produces an overall depolarisation while random opening of channels again produces fluctuations which can be seen in the observed potential. Analysis of these voltage fluctuations leads to information on the size of the depolarisation produced by the opening of a single channel as well as the frequency of channel openings.

3.2. General Biochemical techniques

Biochemical techniques have developed particularly fast during the past 20 years and this section, and the following on molecular biology, is only intended as a very simplified description of some of those that have been of value in the study of the molecules concerned in neuromuscular transmission (see Table 3.1). They are illustrated with particular reference to acetylcholine receptors (AChR) largely because the AChR was one of the first membrane ion channel proteins to be purified and cloned. Some general information concerning the AChR and some of the other ion channels is given in Table 3.2. The techniques and approaches touched on here are covered in many textbooks; Stryer (1989) provides a brief and graphical overview.

Table 3.1. Purification and characterisation of membrane proteins

Purify
Identify (physiology)
Characterise (pharmacology)
Find rich source ───────────────────────→ *Apply molecular biology*
Identify high-affinity ligands/toxins   Extract mRNA to make cDNA library
Purify by extraction and affinity chromatograhy

Characterise
SDS polyacrylamide electrophoresis ──────→ Sequence part of each subunit to make oligonucleotide probes to identify
Size, density, glycosylation   the cDNA. Obtain whole cDNA sequence

Confirm identity
Pharmacology   Express in oocytes, *E. coli* or eukaryotic systems. Make synthetic
Reconstitute   peptides
Make antisera and monoclonal antibodies

Table 3.2. Characterisation of some membrane proteins

	Acetylcholine receptor	Na+ channel	Ca2+ channel
Type of channel	Na+, cations	Na+	Ca2+, divalent cations
Source of material	Electric organs, muscle	Electric organs, muscle, brain	Skeletal muscle, brain
Affinity probes	Cholinergic ligands, α-bungarotoxin	Tetrodotoxin, Saxitoxin	Dihydropyridines, ω-conotoxin
Affinity chromatography	α-Cobratoxins	Lectins	Lectins
Number of subunits on PAGE	Four	One or two	Four or five

Further details can be found in the chapters by Beeson and Barnard, and by Norman.

Table 3.3. Toxins and ligands used in the characterisation and purification of functional components involved in neurotransmission

Function	Toxin or Ligand	Action	Target	Chapter
Action potential	STX	Block action potentials	Na+ channel	5
	TTX	Effect activation/inactivation		
	Scorpion toxins			
	μ-Conotoxin			
Ca2+ influx	ω-Conotoxin	Block neurotransmitter release, but not at mammalian NMJ	Ca2+ channels	5
	Dihydropyridines			
Repolarisation	DTX	Blocks K+ currents causing increased transmitter release and repetitive firing	K+ channels	6
Transmitter release	β-Bungarotoxin	Complex action on transmitter release	?	6
Breakdown of ACh	BoTX	Blocks release at NMJ		6
	Fasciculins	Enhance ACh activity	AChE	6
ACh-induced depolarisation	α-Bungarotoxin	Blocks NMJ	AChR	8

NB: Some of these toxins are not effective at the neuromuscular junction, but can be used to characterise and purify related molecules from other tissues.

3.2.1. Radioligand binding

The use of pharmacological compounds and neurotoxins has been of immense help in the purification and characterisation of many functional macromolecules. Table 3.3 summarises the target of some of the toxins that affect neuromuscular transmission.

Radioactively labelled toxins and pharmacological compounds that bind specifically to the protein of interest can be used to characterise, by autoradiography or counting of the radioactivity, the number and distribution of binding sites in whole tissue (see Fig. 3.6). Binding to whole tissue is often complicated by non-specific uptake of the radiolabelled material, but the specificity of binding can be checked by preincubating with non-radioactive ligand or with other ligands that are known to

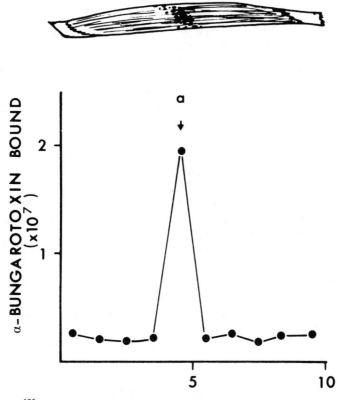

Fig. 3.6. ^{125}I-α-BuTx binding to a small bundle of human muscle. After incubation in the labelled α-BuTx, washing and fixation, the bundle was cut up into 1 mm length segments from tendon to tendon, and each segment counted for radioactivity. The peak of ^{125}I-α-BuTx binding corresponds with the segment which contained the endplates (demonstrated by AChE staining). From Ito *et al.* 1978 with permission.

compete pharmacologically with the radiolabelled form. Radiolabelled ligands can also be used to assay for the protein in solution after extraction, and to label the protein in immunoprecipitation assays as a test for antibodies. Most polypeptide ligands are labelled covalently with ^{125}I, whereas organic compounds are usually labelled by the synthetic incorporation of ^{3}H into the molecule.

Use of radiolabelled ligands for measuring binding in solution usually depends on separation of bound from unbound radioactivity by (a) size difference, (b) charge difference, or (c) precipitation by antibodies directed at the protein. For instance α-bungarotoxin (α-BuTx), which binds specifically and with high affinity to the nicotinic acetylcholine receptor, is both smaller and of opposite charge to the receptor protein. Therefore unbound ^{125}I-α-BuTx can be separated from the ^{125}I-α-BuTx–AChR complex by gel filtration, which fractionates on the basis of size, or by filtration through positively charged filters that bind the negatively charged complex but repel the positively charged free ^{125}I-α-BuTx.

An alternative way of detecting binding of relatively large protein ligands is to covalently attach them to an enzyme such as peroxidase which has an electron-dense product. For instance this has been successfully used to locate AChR at the neuromuscular junction (Engel *et al.*, 1977) and indirectly, to demonstrate the presence of IgG and complement in myasthenia gravis (see Vincent, this volume) and in experimental autoimmune myasthenia (see De Baets, thus volume).

3.2.2. *Purification of membrane proteins*

The most valuable starting point for purifying a membrane protein is a good source of the material. For instance the *Torpedo* electric organ contains about 100 mg AChR protein/kg of starting material (see Lindstrom, this volume). In contrast, even denervated human muscle contains less than 100 μg/kg. Nevertheless even proteins for which there is no good source can be successfully purified using affinity chromatography (see below).

Most of the proteins of interest in studying the neuromuscular junction are embedded in a membrane bilayer and have to be extracted in some form of detergent which substitutes for the lipid in the membrane and frees the protein. Detergents are amphipathic molecules that have a hydrophilic head and a hydrophobic tail. They can be either ionic (e.g. sodium dodecyl sulphate, SDS, which tends to denature proteins harshly) or non-ionic (e.g. Triton X100, which is relatively gentle). These form small vesicles, called micelles, in solution and after extraction each protein is embedded in one such micelle. Fortunately the part of the protein that was exposed to the extracellular medium *in vivo* tends to remain on the outside of the micelle and available for binding of radioactive ligands. Unfortunately, however, many proteins do lose some or all of their reactivity with ligands after extraction (see for example the voltage-dependent Na^+ channel in Norman, this volume) which makes it more difficult to follow them during purification. The AChR retains essentially full binding characteristics.

3.2.3. *Affinity chromatography*

In order to purify the protein of interest from among all the other extracted proteins a highly specific method is required. Many of the compounds that are used as specific radiolabelled ligands for assaying can also be fixed to insoluble supports, such as agarose or sephadex, in order to selectively absorb the protein molecule. After washing, the absorbed material is 'eluted' with a high concentration of the same or a competing ligand. The protein fractions can then be dialysed to remove the soluble ligand. This technique of 'affinity chromatography' (Cuatrecasas, 1969) revolutionised protein purification but is not applicable if moderate affinity ligands cannot be identified, or if the ligand cannot be attached to the gel in an active form. The very high affinity of α-BuTx is a problem for the purification of AChRs, since it would be difficult to elute the receptor. However, nature has provided a variety of lower affinity toxins (for example some α-neurotoxins from the cobra family) which show similar specificity for the AChR and have been used extensively in affinity chromatography. In the absence of a suitable affinity candidate relatively non-specific ligands such as lectins, that bind to carbohydrate attached to the protein surface, can be used to partially purify the material.

3.2.4. *Characterisation of membrane proteins*

Most of the proteins referred to in this book are large, often oligomeric (i.e. made up of more than one non-identical subunit; see Table 3.2), macromolecules. A rough estimate of their molecular size while still in the membrane can be obtained by the technique of radiaction inactivation (see Norman, this volume).

A particularly important technique by which to test for purity and to identify the number of subunits in the protein is polyacrylamide gel electrophoresis (PAGE). The protein is first boiled in the detergent SDS with β-mercaptoethanol, which reduces any inter-subunit disulphide bonds, and then applied to a column or slab of polyacrylamide gel (Laemmli, 1970). An electric current is applied for several hours, during which the denatured protein subunits, which are negatively charged in the presence of SDS, migrate towards the positive electrode, their speed depending mainly on size. The gel is then stained for protein to identify the different subunits (Fig. 3.7). Many membrane proteins, e.g. AChRs or Ca^{2+} channels, can be shown to consist of more than one subunit using this

MW markers   Denatured proteins in SDS

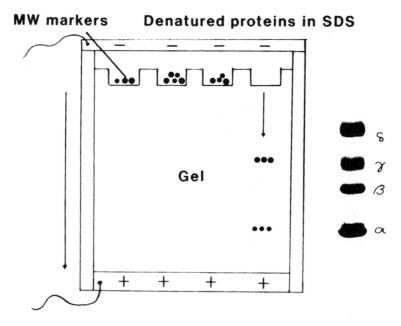

Fig. 3.7. The technique of SDS polyacrylamide gel electrophoresis. The protein subunits separate during application of the current, mainly on the basis of their size. For instance the purified electric organ acetylcholine receptor shows four major bands, denoted α, β, γ, δ. Taken from Tzartos and Lindstrom, 1980, with permission.

technique; but further studies are always needed to confirm that the different subunits do come from the macromolecule rather than being contaminants. In addition the gel can be 'blotted' onto nitrocellulose which can be probed with radioactive ligands or specific antibodies (see below).

Another approach to characterise a newly purified protein is to perform gel filtration and sucrose density gradient centrifugation. These methods give an approximation of the size of the macromolecule in detergent extracts but estimates will depend on the amount of bound detergent or lipid present, which affect both the size and the density, and can be misleading. In addition many membrane proteins are glycosylated with highly branched and complex carbohydrate chains, adding to the bulk of the molecule and tending to make the overall molecule more negatively charged. Their binding to lectins is often used as a secondary purification step.

3.2.5. *Functional studies*

There are several approaches required to identify the extracted and purified membrane protein as the functional molecule. Firstly, ligand binding studies should confirm the pharmacological specificity of the molecule. Secondly, re-incorporation of the protein into artificial membrane lipids often successfully reconstitutes the ligand-activated function of the protein as it was *in vivo*. Thirdly, antibodies raised against the protein may be shown to inhibit its function *in situ*. Fourthly, when the protein has been 'cloned', expression of pure messenger RNA in oocytes will create the appropriate surface membrane protein. Examples of these approaches are given in the chapters by Norman and by Beeson and Barnard.

3.2.6. *Immunological techniques*

Once a protein is purified it can be used to raise specific antibodies which will be of much use in the characterisation of the protein. The protein is injected with an 'adjuvant' into a rabbit or other mammal and antibodies are made against the foreign protein. These are 'polyclonal', being made by many different clones of B lymphocytes and directed at many different 'antigenic determinants' on the surface of the protein. Although useful for some purposes these antibodies are not pure reagents.

Monoclonal antibodies are raised by immunising mice or rats and fusing the antibody-producing cells with a myeloma cell line which is immortal (Kohler and Milstein, 1975). The fused cells are therefore also immortal and can be cultured indefinitely. The cells are 'cloned' in order to obtain highly pure antibody of single specificity. Monoclonal antibodies can be raised against the whole purified (or partially purified) protein, isolated subunits, or peptides synthesised from the known amino acid sequence. Monoclonals against peptides are particularly useful for determining the relative position of the amino acids in the intact, native, protein (see, for example, Lindstrom, this volume).

3.2.7. *Assays for antibody binding*

If a specific high-affinity ligand is available the simplest assay for antibody is probably immunoprecipitation. The protein is preincubated with radioactively labelled ligand followed by the antisera or monoclonal antibody. Addition of an anti-IgG serum precipitates all the antibody(ies) and the radioactivity (Fig. 3.8). However, if no suitable ligand is available the protein, subunits or synthetic peptides, can be attached, by non-covalent interactions, to a microtitre plate or other solid-phase support. The plates are incubated in antibody and, after extensive washing, the presence of bound antibody is detected by addition of radiolabelled (solid-phase radioimmunoassay) or enzyme-linked (ELISA assay) anti-IgG. Binding of monoclonal antibodies raised against the native AChR to short synthetic peptides has been partially successful using these methods (e.g. see Fig. 3.9). Binding to small peptides can also be tested by

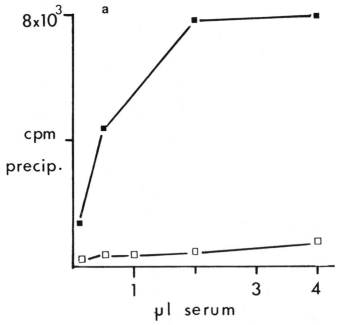

Fig. 3.8. Immunoprecipitation of human AChR prelabelled with ^{125}I-α-Bungarotoxin. Crude detergent extracts of human muscle were incubated with the ^{125}I-α-BuTX before addition of human serum. After overnight incubation the human immunoglobulins were precipitated by anti-human Ig antiserum (made in goats). The precipitate was centrifuged, washed and counted on a gamma counter. ■, Myasthenia gravis serum, □ control serum.

immunoprecipitation if a tyrosine residue (which is the target of iodination techniques) is deliberately added to the NH_2 terminal during synthesis; however, the bulk of an iodinated tyrosine may alter the conformation of the resulting peptide.

Western blotting is a technique to pick up antibodies binding to different proteins or subunits. After PAGE (see above) the polypeptide bands are transferred electrophoretically to a special nitrocellulose paper to which they bind. Strips of the paper are then incubated in a 'blocking' solution of protein, e.g. albumin or gelatine, that blocks the excess charged sites on the nitrocellulose, and then in the relevant antibody. The presence of antibody bound to one or more of the polypeptide bands can be picked up by various methods, e.g. binding of radioactive anti-IgG and autoradiography, or binding of peroxidase-conjugated anti-IgG which, when developed, gives a brown stain. Similarly, the whole protein or synthetic peptides can be 'spotted' onto nitrocellulose and then treated as above to detect antibody binding. Binding of high-affinity radioactive ligands can also be detected by these approaches.

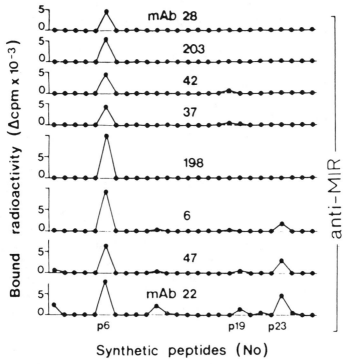

Fig. 3.9. Solid-phase radioimmunoassays used to identify binding of anti-MIR monoclonal antibodies. Synthetic peptides representing the entire AChR α subunit sequence were bound to the wells of a microtitre plate, followed by incubation in each monoclonal antibody. Bound antibody was identified by binding of rat anti-IgG followed by ^{125}I-protein A (which binds to rat immunoglobulins). Antibodies against the main immunogenic region bound to peptide 6 which contained the sequence 67–76. Taken with permission from Tzartos *et al.*, 1988.

3.2.8. *Identifying binding sites for ligands and antibodies*

There are several approaches to the problem of identifying where on a protein ligands (or antibodies) bind. The most logical approach, if binding occurs to denatured protein, is to perform western blotting to identify the subunit involved. The subunit can be purified from the gel and treated with proteolytic enzymes before re-running on western blots to characterise the fragments that bind the ligand or antibody. This approach was used by Lindstrom and his colleagues to map monoclonal antibody binding sites on the AChR subunits (see Fig. 9.6 of Lindstrom, this volume). Alternatively, once cDNAs for the subunits and their amino acid sequence are available, binding to different sized recombinant polypeptides, made in *Escherichia coli* (see below), can be examined, and short synthetic sequences can be tested. In addition antibodies can be raised to short synthetic peptides and tested to see whether they inhibit binding of the ligand or antibody to the native molecule.

Using these approaches it has proved possible to identify sequences involved in ^{125}I-α-BuTx and monoclonal antibody binding to the AChR (see Lindstrom, this volume). However, unfortunately, many areas of functional interest in oligomeric proteins seem to be dependent on three-dimensional structure (conformation), and any antibodies or ligands that bind to denatured material often do so with much lower affinity than to the native molecule.

A powerful technique to identify the position of ligand binding sites is available once the amino acid sequence is known. The radioactive high-affinity label is adapted so that when exposed to light it covalently binds to the nearest suitable amino acid (photoaffinity labelling). Then the protein is purified and cleaved with special peptidases. The resulting peptides are subjected to high-performance liquid chromatography (HPLC), which separates them according to their molecular weight. The radioactive peptide(s) can then be sequenced and their position in the protein deduced by comparison with the known sequence. In this way the channel-forming region of the AChR ion channel has been localised (see Beeson and Barnard, this volume).

3.3. Molecular biology

The use of recombinant techniques has made it possible to obtain the entire sequence of complex proteins, to identify by mutagenesis functional domains, and to investigate the control and expression of the genes that code for them. Stryer (1989) covers many of these approaches in his monograph.

The protein subunits extracted from a PAGE gel should be very pure, and it may be possible to obtain the amino acid sequence of the NH_2 terminus. Alternatively the pure subunits can be cleaved proteolytically (see above) and a single peak from HPLC sequenced. It is not possible to sequence the entire molecule/subunit since this may consist of several hundred amino acids. Once a sequence of 20 or so amino acids is known it is possible to construct oligonucleotide probes complementary to the mRNA sequences coding for the amino acids. These are then used to identify the relevant clones in a 'cDNA library' (Fig. 3.10). A cDNA library is derived by first synthesising complementary strands to mRNA from the relevant source, followed by the removal of the mRNA and synthesis of the second strand of the DNA in order to give double-stranded cDNA. Cloning is achieved by ligating the cDNA into either plasmid or bacteriophage vectors, and the subsequent replication of these vectors after introduction into a bacterial (*E. coli*) host. Only one copy of a vector

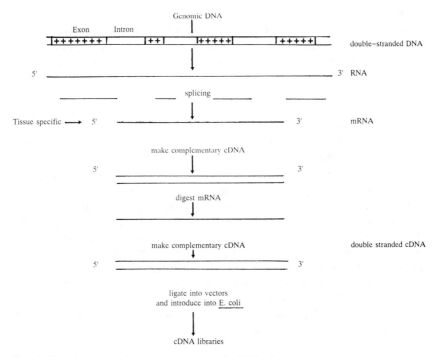

Fig. 3.10.   Diagramatic representation of cDNA cloning.

is introduced into each bacterium, so that when this multiplies to form a colony it contains a single 'cloned' cDNA. A 'cDNA' library usually consists of about 10^4 to 10^6 cloned cDNAs. A bacterial colony or bacteriophage plaque carrying the cDNA coding for the whole or part of the polypeptide can be recognised by hybridisation with the radiolabelled oligonucleotide probe. The cDNA in the relevant clones can be sequenced to derive the amino acid sequence.

Some idea of the secondary and tertiary structure of the polypeptide can be inferred from inspection of the primary amino acid sequence (see for example chapters by Norman, and by Beeson and Barnard, this volume). For instance the presence of a hydrophobic 'leader' sequence at the N terminal of the sequence encoded by the mRNA, but not found in the mature protein, indicates that the N terminus will be translocated across the membrane and will be extracellular. This sequence is cleaved after translocation. Other long stretches of hydrophobic residues are likely to represent transmembrane regions. The presence of cysteine residues may also help to predict tertiary structure, and suitably placed asparagine or serine and tyrosine residues may suggest regions of glycosylation and phosphorylation respectively.

3.3.1. *Gene expression*

Genes in higher animals are frequently discontinuous in that they consist of coding sequences called 'exons', interspersed among non-coding regions called 'introns'. In many cases the exons code for discrete regions of the final gene product.

When a gene is expressed an RNA transcript is formed in the nucleus which contains a sequence complementary to the whole gene, including the introns. Thereafter the primary transcript is spliced in such a way that only the coding regions are retained, producing mRNA. Some genes can be spliced in more than one way, resulting in alternative forms of the mature mRNA and hence of the polypeptide product. This applies in particular to the K^+ channel (see Dolly, this volume), and appears to be the case in the human AChR a subunit (see Beeson and Barnard, this volume).

In order to study the genes it is necessary to break up chromosomal DNA into smaller fragments using sonication or restriction endonucleases. These are highly specific enzymes that recognise unique nucleotide sequences. The fragments that result from restriction enzyme digests can be separated on agarose gels (similar to PAGE), and visualised with ethidium bromide under ultraviolet light. Alternatively they can be denatured with NaOH to separate the double strands, and probed with ^{32}P-cDNA to locate fragments containing a specified coding region(s) (Southern blotting). Using a battery of different enzymes, each producing different fragments, and the relevant probe, one can piece together a map of the genome that contains the gene in question. The AChR genes, for instance, consist of several exons and introns (see Beeson and Barnard). Many complex genes are polymorphic; that is there are minor differences among the normal population. These polymorphisms may be in the exons leading to alternative forms of the protein (for example the HLA molecules), or may be in the introns, in which case the protein that they encode will not differ between individuals.

One way to look for genetic defects is to start by looking for restriction fragment length polymorphisms (RFLPs) in families with the inherited condition. The fragments formed are picked up with radiolabelled probes for different regions on the chromosome. The RFLPs are used as impure markers to an inherited gene defect. If it can be demonstrated that a particular RFLP is inherited in the same way as a gene defect within a family tree, then the probe is likely to be binding close to the defective gene. The degree or tightness of the linkage gives an indication of the distance between the probe and the gene defect. Once a tightly linked probe is established then it is possible to use techniques of 'chromosome walking' to locate the actual gene, and eventually the actual defect responsible for the inherited disorder.

If there is a specific probe for a candidate gene this can be used in the same way. The ability to detect a change in the gene itself depends on the presence of a mutation that coincides with the cutting site for a particular enzyme, or on large deletions or insertions in the DNA which alter the size of the fragments formed. In both cases, however, the change detected may be in an intron and not related to the gene product. This sort of approach is beginning to be applied to the study of congenital myasthenic syndromes (see Beeson and Barnard, this volume).

3.3.2. *Polymerase chain reaction*

One of the major developments in molecular biology of the past few years is a technique to amplify selected DNA or RNA sequences. This technique, called the polymerase chain reaction (PCR), depends largely on the characteristics of a particular enyzme, 'Taq polymerase', which is capable of withstanding relatively high temperatures.

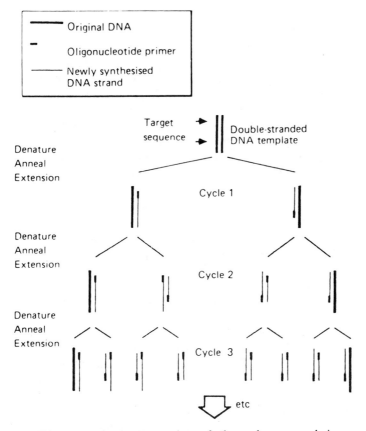

Fig. 3.11. Diagrammatic representation of the polymerase chain reaction. Reproduced with permission from Lynch and Brown (1990).

Two short oligonucleotide 'primers' are synthesised which will hybridise to opposite strands of the DNA, at opposite ends of the sequence that is to be amplified. The DNA is denatured by heating and then the temperature is lowered to allow the primers to anneal to their complementary sequences. In the presence of the polymerase and excess nucleotides, the primers initiate the formation of complementary strands. These are then subjected to another round of heat denaturation, annealing and extension (see Fig. 3.11) resulting in eight strands. Because of the thermostability of the enzyme the cycle can be repeated many times without additional enzyme, and this results in the rapid and exponential amplification of the sequences between the two primers. This technique is being used, for instance, to amplify specified regions of the DNA sequence in individuals with defects in the acetylcholine receptor (see Beeson and Barnard, this volume). There are, however, many other applications, which are discussed in White *et al.* (1989) and Lynch and Brown (1990).

3.3.3. Expression systems

Once a cDNA coding for the entire subunit has been identified, it can be expressed in a number of different systems in order to study the polypeptide produced. There are several different types of expression system. The simplest is probably the *Xenopus* oocyte, which is large enough to be penetrated by a needle. Purified RNA extracted from a rich source of the protein will contain specific messenger RNA for the protein in question. When injected into *Xenopus* oocytes the membrane protein is frequently made by the oocyte and expressed on the surface of the egg where it can be detected by appropriate physiological or pharmacological techniques (see Snutch, 1988, for a review).

Oocyte expression has also been used to investigate the requirement for the different subunits of the proteins. If a single subunit synthetic mRNA, derived from the appropriate cDNA, can direct the synthesis of functional protein then any other subunits which co-purify with the protein may be contaminants or perform some other function. Oocyte expression is also used to investigate the importance of different amino acids in the primary sequence by injecting mRNA which is copied from cDNA after site-directed mutagenesis.

A stable expression system can be obtained by inserting vectors containing the relevant cDNA into *Escherichia coli*. These bacteria can then be induced to make large quantities of the relevant polypeptide, but the protein tends to aggregate into 'inclusion bodies' from which it is very difficult to extract except by drastic means that tend to destroy any of the molecule's native properties. Nevertheless recombinant proteins purified from PAGE gels can be used to study ligand binding by Western blotting, and are proving to be of exceptional use in the study of autoimmune T cell responses (see Vincent, this volume).

Systems are now available for expression in various eukaryotic cell lines, using vectors which incorporate the cDNAs into the genome. These can be stable and make functional protein if all the polypeptide subunits are co-expressed (for example see Claudio *et al.*, 1987). In others the cDNA is not stably integrated into the genome but relatively native polypeptides may be secreted, short-term, into the culture medium in reasonable quantities. One great advantage of eukaryotic systems is that the polypeptide chains are glycosylated as they are transported to the cell surface. Glycosylation is probably essential for the normal conformation and surface expression of a membrane protein.

3.4. Investigation of neuromuscular transmission in human disease

One of the major impacts of the work described in the main part of this book is its application to human disease. It is now clear that there are several different disorders affecting neuromuscular transmission, both inherited and autoimmune (see the chapters by Engel, by Vincent and by W.-Wray). Since the study of the basic abnormalities in these diseases has to be conducted on rather small specimens of human muscle, we conclude with a brief outline of the approaches that have been used successfully to investigate abnormalities in these patients.

Intercostal muscle biopsies are usually preferred in order to obtain intact muscle fibres, suitable for electrophysiological investigation. However, motor-point biopsies from, for instance, the deltoid muscle have also been used. The muscle is maintained in Krebs' solution with oxygenation and dissected into small bundles.

Electrophysiology: the quantal content gives useful information on the release process itself, probably more useful than measurement of acetylcholine release (see below) since there is a continuous background release of ACh (see chapter by Molenaar, this volume). The quantal content can be calculated by a number of methods which give similar, but not identical results (see Chapter 2).

The amplitude of the MEPPs give a good indication of the number of functional AChRs, which can be confirmed by ^{125}I-α-Bungarotoxin binding.

α-Bungarotoxin (α-BuTX) binding: this is performed at about 1 μg/ml of high specific activity ^{125}I-α-BuTX. The muscle is washed thoroughly for several hours and the endplates located by staining for acetylcholinesterase. The amount of radioactivity in the endplate region can then be compared with that in non-endplate areas of the muscle fibres, and the results expressed as the number of ^{125}I-α-BuTX-binding sites/endplate (e.g. Fig. 3.6).

Choline acetylase (ChAT) and acetylcholine esterase (AChE) activity: these enzymes can be measured in homogenates of muscle bundles which have been cut into segments to separate the region containing endplates from non-endplate areas. The endplate-containing segment(s) should contain most of the activity. ChAT is measured by a radiochemical method using ^{14}C-acetyl CoA and unlabelled choline (see Molenaar *et al.*, 1981).

Acetylcholine (ACh) content and synthesis: the ACh content of tissue can be determined by extraction and measurement by gas chromatography/mass spectrometry (Polak and Molenaar, 1979). The synthesis of ACh is derived by measuring the ACh content of the tissue and that of the medium during stimulation of ACh release by incubation in high K^+ solutions.

Morphological techniques: considerable information has been obtained from quantitative morphology, freeze-fracture and immunohistochemistry of the neuromuscular junction. These techniques are referred to in the chapter by Engel.

References

Anderson, C. R. Stevens, C. F. (1973) Voltage clamp analysis of acetylcholine produced end-plate current fluctuations at frog neuromuscular junction. *J. Physiol (Lond)* **235**: 655–691.

Claudio, T., Green, W. N., Hartman, D. S. M., Hayden, D., Paulson, H. L., Sigworth, F. J., Sine, S. M. and Swedlund, A. (1987) Genetic reconstitution of functional acetylcholine receptor channels in mouse fibroblasts. *Science* **238**: 1688–1694.

Cuatrecasas, P., Wilchek, M. and Anfinse, C. (1968) Selective enzyme purification by affinity chromatography *Proc. Natl. Acad. Sci., USA* **61**: 636–643.

Engel, A. G., Lindstrom, J., Lambert, E. H. and Lennon, V. A. (1977) Ultrastructural localization of the acetylcholine receptor in myasthenia gravis and its experimental autoimmune model. *Neurology* **27**: 307–315.

Hille, B. (1984) *Ionic Channels of Excitable Membranes*, Sinauer, Sunderland, MA.

Ito, Y, Miledi, R., Vincent, A. and Newsom-Davis, J. (1978) Acetylcholine receptors and endplate electrophysiology in myasthenia gravis. *Brain* **101**: 345–368.

Katz, B. (1966) *Nerve, Muscle and Synapse*, McGraw-Hill, New York.

Katz, B. and Miledi, R. (1972) The statistical nature of the acetylcholine potential and its molecular components. *J. Physiol.* **224**: 665–699.

Kohler, G. and Milstein, C. (1975) Continuous cultures of fused cells secreting antibody of predefined specificity *Nature* **256**: 495–497.

Laemmli, U. K. (1970) Cleavage of structural proteins during assembly of the head of Bacteriophage T4. *Nature* **227**: 680–685.

Lynch, J. and Brown, J. (1990) The polymerase chain reaction. *J. Med. Gen.* **27**: 2–6.

Molenaar, P. C. M., Newsom-Davis, J., Polak, R. L. and Vincent, A. (1981) Choline acetyltransferase in skeletal muscle from patients with myasthenia gravis. *J. Neurochem.* **37**: 1081–1088.

Neher, E. and Sakmann, B. (1976) Single channel currents recorded from membrane of denervated frog muscle fibres. *Nature* **260**: 799–802.

Polak, R. L. and Molenaar, P. C. (1979) A method for determination of acetylcholine by slow pyrolysis combined with mass fragmentography on a packed capillary column. *J. Neurochem.* **32**: 407–412.

Purves, R. D. (1981) *Microelectrode Methods for Intracellular Recording and Ionophoresis.* Academic Press, New York.

Sakmann, B. and Neher, E. (1983) *Single Channel Recording.* Plenum Press, New York.

Snutch, T. (1988) The use of *Xenopus* oocytes to probe synaptic communication. *Trends Neurosci.* **11**: 250–256.

Stryer, L. (1989) *Molecular Design of Life.* Freeman, New York.

Tzartos, S. and Lindstrom, J. (1980) Monoclonal antibodies used to probe acetylcholine receptor structure; localization of the main immunogenic region and detection of similarities between subunits. *Proc. Natl. Acad. Sci. USA* **77**: 755–759.

Tzartos, S., Kordossi, A., Walgrave, S. L., Kokla, A. and Conti-Tronconi, B. M. (1988) Determination of antibody binding sites on the three-dimensional and primary structure of acetylcholine receptor. In: *Myasthenia Gravis*, M. H. De Baets, H. J. G. H. Oosterhuis and K V Toyka, eds, *Monogr. Allergy*, vol. 25, pp. 20–32.

White, T. J., Arnheim, N. and Erlich, H. A. (1989) The polymerase chain reaction. *Trends Genet.* **5**: 185–188.

Wray, D. (1980) Noise analysis and channels at the postsynaptic membrane of skeletal muscle. *Progr. Drug Res.*, **24**: 9–56.

W.-Wray, D. (1988) Neuromuscular transmission. In: *Disorders of Voluntary Muscle*, 5th edn, Walton, J., ed., Churchill Livingstone, Edinburgh, pp. 74–108.

Synthesis, storage and release of acetylcholine

4.1. **Introduction**

Electrophysiological events recorded from the neuromuscular junction reflect the culmination of many biochemical processes in the nerve terminal. Over the past decade or so many workers have applied biochemical techniques to study the synthesis, storage and release of acetylcholine in electric organ, nerve and muscle. This chapter outlines some of the findings and their relationship to morphological and physiological studies.

As outlined in Chapter 1 the main nerve trunk ramifies within the muscle and splits up into nerve cells which innervate the individual muscle cells of the motor unit. At the endplate the nerve cell loses its myelin sheath, and branches into several 'terminals', which are covered by a Schwann cell for protection and biochemical support. At higher magnification more detail can be seen in the nerve terminals: notably mitochondria and numerous synaptic vesicles. The postsynaptic membrane has large infoldings, called postsynaptic folds or secondary clefts, that are characteristic of the neuromuscular junction. In electron micrographs a hazy band can be seen which runs along the middle of the synaptic cleft and down to the bottom of the postsynaptic folds. This is the basal lamina, a loose matrix of collagen in which the enzyme acetylcholinesterase and several specialised proteins are anchored.

With some skill it is possible to cut endplates into longitudinal sections for electron microscopy, enabling one to inspect junctions over a relatively long distance. In such micrographs specialised regions, consisting of synaptic vesicles at a high density, clustered near thickened areas of the presynaptic membrane can be seen. These regions, the so-called active zones, form a repetitive pattern and it is believed that transmitter release takes place exclusively or principally at these sites.

The nerve terminal seems to have much in common with other cholinergic synapses including those of the muscarinic type. Figure 4.1 illustrates the metabolic processes involving ACh at the motor endplate. These include uptake of choline by the nerve terminals, synthesis of ACh from choline and acetyl CoA, uptake of the newly formed transmitter into and storage in synaptic vesicles, and finally the release of ACh followed by

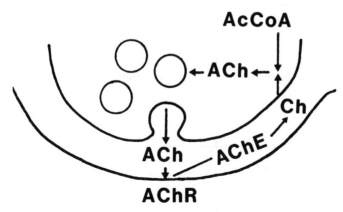

Fig. 4.1.   Rough outline of the biochemistry of the neuromuscular junction. ACh is synthesised in the cytoplasm and taken up into the synaptic vesicles. After its release and binding to the AChRs it is hydrolysed by acetylcholinesterase.

its destruction by the enzyme acetylcholinesterase. The structural basis for these processes is beginning to be resolved (see Chapter 1).

A few words should be said about a technical problem encountered in many biochemical investigations of the neuromuscular junction. The problem has its roots in the fact that the total volume of the nerve terminals is very small compared to the total muscle mass, the ratio being typically of the order of 1:100,000. Consequently, when a muscle is ground up for biochemical studies, the contents of the nerve terminals are heavily contaminated with substances or enzymes derived from the muscle fibres, even if the concentrations of the substances involved are relatively low. For this reason biochemical studies concerning the metabolism of ACh at the neuromuscular junction are often difficult, in contrast to electrophysiological and morphological studies for which skeletal muscle is a model preparation *par excellence*. Therefore, much of the information has been obtained from other cholinergic systems, notably the electric organ of the ray, *Torpedo marmorata*, a purely cholinergic system that is extremely rich in nerve terminals and ACh (cf. Table 4.1).

In 50 years the literature on cholinergic presynaptic function has grown

Table 4.1.   ACh content of endplate-containing segments of muscles from rat and frog and of the electroplaque of *Torpedo*

	ACh (nmol per gram wet weight)	*Reference*
Rat Diaphragm	2.0 ± 0.16	Miledi *et al.* (1982a)
Frog sartorius	0.8 ± 0.06	Miledi *et al.* (1977)
Torpedo electroplaque	500–1000	Dunant *et al.* (1972)

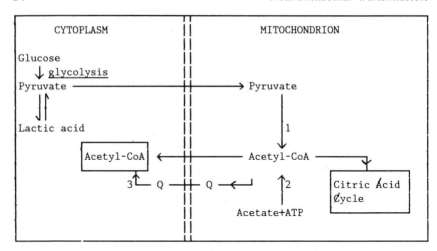

Fig. 4.2. Supply of acetyl groups in the nerve ending. There are different possible routes of transfer of the acetyl moiety through the membrane of the mitochondrion.

to proportions which greatly exceed the space available for this review. Several recent more detailed reviews are available (e.g. Ceccarelli and Hurlbut, 1980; Whittaker 1987).

4.2. Synthesis of ACh

4.2.1. *Supply of choline*

ACh is synthesised from choline and acetyl CoA by the enzyme acetyltransferase (see Fig. 4.2). Choline is an important substance for the metabolism of phospholipids and much more of it is present in the body than is needed for the biosynthesis of ACh. It is mainly chemically bound in lipid form in body fat and cell membranes. The blood contains some choline at a relatively steady concentration (*ca.* 10 µM), so that all tissues, including cholinergic neurones, have a more or less constant supply of free choline.

Substances with a quaternary ammonium group, such as choline, have difficulty crossing the membrane of the living cell, and for uptake to take place a carrier protein is needed. Such a system was demonstrated 20 years ago, with an apparent K_m of 50–200 µM. However, later studies, in which isolated cells or subcellular fractions were used, e.g. synaptosomes from brain, revealed that cholinergic nerve terminals also possess a 'high-affinity' uptake system with K_m usually between 1 and 5 µM (see Jope, 1979), which seems to be an exclusive feature of cholinergic terminals devoted to the synthesis of ACh. High-affinity choline uptake requires the presence of external Na^+ ions; it is not directly dependent on the expenditure of energy since the uptake of positively charged choline ions proceeds down their electrochemical gradient. Unfortunately it is not possible to study the high-affinity uptake of choline at the neuromuscular junction since such uptake tends to be overshadowed by uptake of choline by the bulk of muscle fibres.

4.2.2. *Supply of acetyl CoA*

It is quite clear from enzymological studies that cytoplasmic acetyl CoA is the immediate donor of the acetyl moiety of ACh. On the other hand, most acetyl CoA is formed from pyruvate in the mitochondrion, and considerable uncertainty exists about the identity of the cytoplasmic precursor of acetyl CoA. Several precursors have been proposed, e.g. pyruvate, acetate or citrate (Fig. 4.2, see Tucek, 1978). Another possibility is that enough acetyl CoA gets through the mitochondrial wall to support ACh synthesis directly, although it is known to penetrate poorly.

4.2.3. *Choline acetyltransferase (ChAT)*

The enzyme responsible for ACh synthesis from choline and acetyl CoA, first demonstrated in 1943 by Nachmansohn and Machado, is almost exclusively found in the cytoplasmic compartment of cholinergic nerve terminals where it probably exists in a soluble form (Fonnum, 1967).

The reaction catalysed by ChAT is reversible, i.e. the enzyme can both form and hydrolyse ACh, dependent on the concentrations of the reactants (Fig. 4.3). The affinity of ChAT for acetyl CoA is much greater than for choline (for reviews see Macintosh and Collier, 1976; Tucek, 1978). It is likely that the enzyme binds acetyl CoA before it binds choline, and that the end-products, ACh and CoA, are released in that order.

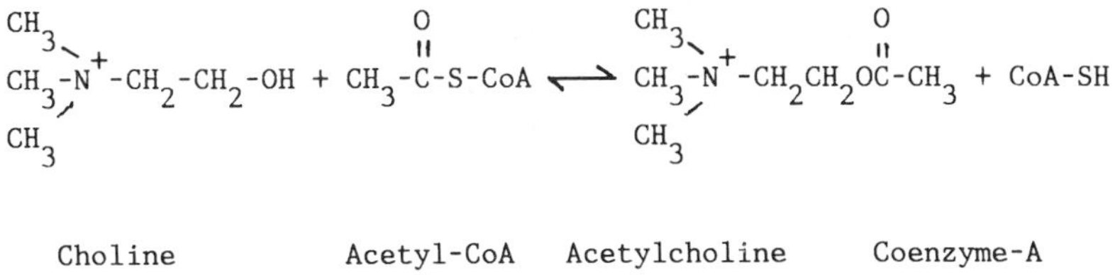

$$CH_3-\underset{\underset{CH_3}{|}}{\overset{\overset{CH_3}{|}}{N^+}}-CH_2-CH_2-OH \; + \; CH_3-\overset{\overset{O}{\parallel}}{C}-S-CoA \; \rightleftharpoons \; CH_3-\underset{\underset{CH_3}{|}}{\overset{\overset{CH_3}{|}}{N^+}}-CH_2CH_2O\overset{\overset{O}{\parallel}}{C}-CH_3 \; + \; CoA-SH$$

| Choline | Acetyl-CoA | Acetylcholine | Coenzyme-A |

$$K_m = [ACh][CoA] \, / \, [choline][acetyl\text{-}CoA] = 40 \; (\text{GLOVER and POTTER, 1971})$$

$$K_m(acetyl\text{-}CoA) = 10\text{-}25 \; \mu M \qquad K_m(choline) = 400\text{-}1000 \; \mu M$$

Fig. 4.3.   Reaction catalysed by choline acetyltransferase.

In nerve muscle preparations, homogenised for determination of ChAT activity, some ACh synthesis is usually found at regions of the muscle that are devoid of nerves and endplates. It appears that this extrajunctional synthesis of ACh is brought about by an enzyme other than ChAT, as has been demonstrated for muscles of amphibia and mammals, including humans (Molenaar and Polak, 1980; Molenaar *et al.*, 1981; Tucek, 1982). Since muscle fibres contain carnitine acetyltransferase, which to some extent accepts choline as a substrate, it is quite possible that this enzyme is responsible for the synthesis of ACh by muscle fibres.

The true enzyme ChAT is predominantly present in the nerve terminals. The remaining part (about 30% of total) is stored in the motor axon branches of the nerve muscle preparation (Miledi *et al.*, 1981, 1982a), in agreement with the general observation that ChAT is synthesised in the cell body and transported to the periphery of the nerve cell (see Tucek, 1978). The actual rates of ChAT activity in homogenates show considerable differences depending on the type of muscle and species. Rates range from a low 2 nmol $\cdot$ g^{-1} h^{-1} in the frog sartorius (Molenaar and Polak, 1980) to around 500 nmol.g^{-1}h^{-1} in the rat diaphragm (Hebb *et al.*, 1964). Small densely innervated muscles may score even higher.

One could question what purpose is served by the measurement of ChAT at the neuromuscular junction since the total activity of this enzyme in homogenates is much greater than the amount of ACh synthesised in intact preparations under conditions of vigorous stimulation; differences as great as 50–100 times between homogenate and intact muscle are not unusual. However, it should be borne in mind that ChAT activity in homogenates is determined under optimal conditions (high substrate and low product concentrations), whereas ACh synthesis in the nerve terminal probably takes place in the presence of substrate at concentrations far below the K_m values of the enzyme, and of end-products at such high concentration that the backward reaction begins to be important. In this connection it is of interest that the concentration of ACh in the cytoplasm of motor nerve terminals has been estimated to be as high as 30 mM (Katz and Miledi, 1977; Miledi *et al.*, 1977). Consequently, it is conceivable that the rate of ACh synthesis, and hence of ACh release, may be limited under certain conditions.

4.2.4. *Regulation of acetylcholine synthesis*

A general feature of cholinergic nerves is that they contain a steady concentration of ACh at rest and that, during a period of stimulation in which the ACh content is decreased, synthesis is turned on until the original ACh level is restored. Apparently, synthesis of ACh is regulated but how this is brought about is still a mystery and the following are some of the possibilities:

1. Inhibition of ChAT by ACh (end-product inhibition) is unlikely since ACh has a relatively weak inhibiting effect on ChAT activity.
2. Regulation by virtue of the equilibrium of the reaction, i.e. any decrease of ACh is replenished by re-equilibration of the reactants (this model implies that ChAT is present in amounts sufficiently high to ensure rapid equilibration times). However, the concentration of ACh is high in motor nerve terminals (about 30 mM, see above), and from the

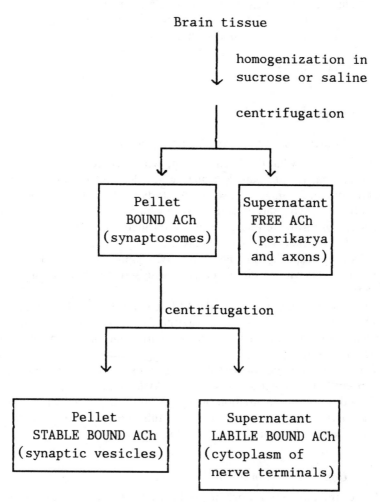

Fig. 4.4. ACh compartment in brain. Free and labile bound ACh can be extracted, provided the homogenisation medium contains an anti-acetylcholinesterase to prevent hydrolysis. The fractionation scheme by centrifugation is oversimplified for reasons of clarity (see Whittaker, 1969, for procedures and interpretation of the meaning of the ACh fractions). The fractions stem to some extent from anatomically defined compartments as indicated in this scheme between brackets.

value of the equilibrium constant ($K_m = 40$, Fig. 4.3) we can calculate that the concentrations of choline and acetyl CoA must be relatively low. Thus a substantial loss of ACh cannot be replaced by synthesis from the precursors unless these are replenished very rapidly. In other words, regulation by 'mass action', does not give a simple answer to the problem.

3. This concerns direct regulation by the availability of the precursors: choline and acetyl CoA may be regulated by ACh or by activation via another substance intimately related to neurotransmitter metabolism, such as internal Ca^{2+}. Indeed there is some evidence that mitochondria release some acetyl CoA under the influence of Ca^{2+} (see Tucek, 1978 and Jope, 1979).

4.3. Storage of acetylcholine

4.3.1. *Vesicular ACh and other ACh compartments*

On the basis of what has been said one would expect to find two principal ACh compartments, namely synaptic vesicles and the cytoplasm of the nerve ending. If things were so simple studying ACh storage would involve mainly a detailed analysis of the way in which ACh is taken up by synaptic vesicles. Unfortunately suspensions of purified synaptic vesicles (e.g. from *Torpedo* electric organ) take up ACh to only a small proportion of their total storage capacity. Furthermore, ACh is present in a number of other compartments which cannot clearly be assessed in relation to physiological function.

ACh compartments can be studied at several levels depending on the technique used. These include: (a) the forceps-and-scissors approach in which compartments have a clear anatomical basis; (b) biochemical fractionation techniques, usually consisting of homogenisation of the tissue followed by a number of centrifugation steps; or (c) following differences in specific radioactivities between the ACh found in the tissue and that released into the incubation medium, after exposure to a 'pulse' of radioactive precursor. The origin of this metabolic compartmentation cannot be clearly related to morphological structures.

4.3.2. *Compartments in the brain*

Most of the pioneering work on ACh was done with brain tissue which for a long time served as a model biochemical preparation for cholinergic neurons in general.

Figure 4.4 illustrates how different ACh compartments can be isolated by homogenisation and centrifugation of brain tissue. After homogenisa-tion, some ACh (about 20% of the total acid-extractable ACh) is lost when saline medium or sucrose medium is used (see Whittaker, 1969; Macintosh and Collier, 1976). The fraction of the lost ACh, designated 'free' ACh, could be preserved in the presence of a cholinesterase inhibitor and separated from the bulk of 'bound' ACh by centrifugation, a procedure in which nerve endings are sedimented together with the mitochondria (De Robertis *et al.*, 1961; Gray and Whittaker, 1962). It thus appears that the nerve endings, after being removed mechanically from the axons, are sealed off, behaving as separate cell-like structures. These 'synaptosomes' can be broken down by the addition of distilled water (osmotic lysis) and the ACh thus liberated can be detected if a cholinesterase inhibitor is present ('labile bound' fraction). Not all the ACh is released in this way; the remaining ACh ('stable bound') can be sedimented by another centrifugation step. It is likely that the fractions free, labile bound and stable bound ACh are derived from perikarya and axons, the cytoplasm of the nerve ending and the synaptic vesicles, respectively (see Whittaker, 1969).

4.3.3. *Compartments of skeletal muscle*

About 30 years ago it was noted that following denervation of skeletal muscle not all ACh was lost from the tissue (Bhatnagar and Macintosh, 1960; Hebb, 1962). This was an unexpected observation because it implied that some ACh may occur in non-cholinergic tissue, in this case the muscle fibres. While these amounts of ACh were low and barely detectable with the bioassay procedures used at that time, the presence of ACh in skeletal muscle fibres was later confirmed by means of highly sensitive mass spectrometric methods (Miledi *et al.*, 1977, 1982a). On the other hand the intramuscular branches of the motor nerve contain negligible amounts of ACh compared to the ACh contained in the nerve terminals (Miledi *et al.*, 1982a).

Another possible compartment for ACh is the Schwann cell, and there is good electrophysiological evidence that Schwann cells under certain conditions synthesise and release ACh (Birks *et al.*, 1960; Dennis and Miledi, 1974), but direct biochemical evidence is lacking, probably because this ACh compartment is too small (Miledi *et al.*, 1982a).

Figure 4.5 gives a schematic representation of the ACh stores in muscles together with the amounts of ACh contained in them, as estimated for the frog sartorius and the rat hemidiaphragm.

4.3.4. *Compartments of the motor nerve terminal*

Unfortunately 'direct' measurements of vesicular and cytoplasmic ACh in the nerve terminal by means of centrifugation methods on homogenised tissue tend to be unreliable, because such procedures take a long time and

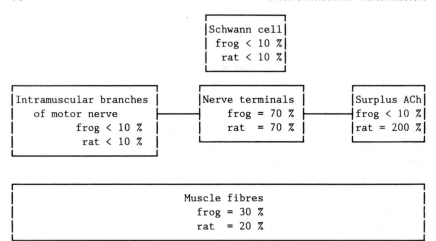

Fig. 4.5.   ACh compartments of skeletal muscle preparations as determined by 'mechanical' procedures (denervation, division of the tissue with scissors). Values indicated are percentage points relative to the total fresh ACh content of the frog sartorius and the rat diaphragm. Taken from Miledi *et al.* (1977, 1982a) and Molenaar *et al.* (1987).

ACh may become redistributed between these two pools, e.g. by leakage of ACh from the vesicles. Israël and co-workers (1979) avoided this problem by using a rapid determination of free and bound ACh, a method which is reminiscent of the procedure for brain tissue mentioned above.

Two 'fractions' from electroplaque tissue were thus obtained almost instantaneously, the one containing *total* ACh (homogenisation in acid) and the other consisting of *bound* ACh (homogenisation in saline, Dunant *et al.*, 1972), which probably derives from synaptic vesicles because their ACh is protected against the action of the acetylcholinesterase by the vesicular membrane (Marchbanks and Israël, 1971). The 'free' ACh (total minus bound ACh) probably corresponds to cytoplasmic ACh. For skeletal muscle a similar fractionation procedure has been described, in which the bound ACh is isolated within minutes (Miledi *et al.*, 1982b). The amounts

Table 4.2.   Free and bound ACh in nerve terminal

	Ach (nmol per gram fresh tissue) *Frog sartorius*	Torpedo *electroplaque*
Total	0.7	470
Bound	0.4	230
Free	0.3	240

Data taken from Miledi *et al.*, 1982b, and from Dunant *et al.*, 1972.

of free and bound ACh in *Torpedo* electroplaque and frog sartorius muscle are compared in Table 4.2. It is clear that the ratio of free to bound ACh is similar in the two preparations, although there is a roughly 1000-fold difference between the absolute levels.

4.3.5. *ACh storage by vesicles*

The number of synaptic vesicles per nerve terminal as estimated by electron microscopic studies (around one million in the frog sartorius) and the amount of bound ACh in the nerve terminals (about 20 femtomoles per endplate) indicate that vesicles in skeletal muscle contain between 11,000 and 15,000 molecules ACh (Miledi *et al.*, 1982b). This is much less than the number estimated for *Torpedo* vesicles, 50,000 or more, as deduced from studies on purified vesicle preparations. However, synaptic vesicles from electroplaque tissue are larger than those found in the cholinergic system from other animals, and therefore the higher content does not imply a higher *concentration* of ACh in the *Torpedo* vesicle.

An amount of 12,000 molecules of ACh chloride would, at isotonic solution, correspond to a sphere with a diameter of 70 nm, i.e. a larger sphere than the vesicles from muscle as observed by electron microscopy (40–60 nm). Consequently, it is possible that synaptic vesicles contain ACh at a *hypertonic* concentration, and the question arises as to how vesicles manage to accumulate ACh and to withstand the osmotic pressure.

Much has been learned from other systems, and secretory vesicles such as (nor)adrenaline-containing granules have been found to hold an ATPase system embedded in the membrane which pumps H^+ ions into the vesicle. As a result the inside of the vesicle becomes acidic, pH 5 or so, and a positive potential difference is established across the membrane with regard to the cytoplasm (see for instance Johnson, 1987). Vesicles formed by receptor-mediated endocytosis similarly possess such a proton pump (e.g. the endocytosis of insulin and ferritin, reviewed by Wileman *et al.*, 1985), so it may be a common feature of all types of vesicles, including those in cholinergic neurones. Consequently, the minimal equipment for a cholinergic vesicle would be that its membrane contains a proton pumping ATPase and a carrier protein which exchanges vesicular protons against cytoplasmic ACh^+ ions.

In fact the situation is more complex (see Whittaker, 1987; Parsons *et al.*, 1987; Michaelson and Wien-Naor, 1987). *Torpedo* vesicles also contain a proteoglycan, synapsin I and II, synaptophysin and a number of small molecules, ATP, Ca^{2+}, Mg^{2+} (and of course ACh itself). The function of ATP is unclear. It is unlikely to be a substrate for the ATPase because the active site of proton pumps in secretory organelles has been established to be at the cytoplasmic face of the membrane. Instead, the polyvalent negative ATP ion may be just a suitable counterion for the ACh packed in a vesicle. The possible function of vesicular Ca^{2+} is also intriguing. The vesicular Ca^{2+} is present at a ratio of about 1:5 with regard to ACh, and this implies that a lot of Ca^{2+} (a 'rare metal' for the cytosol of the nerve terminal!), is bound in vesicles. It can be calculated that if this were to be released into the cytoplasm the free cytosolic Ca^{2+} would rise at least 1000 times. It is quite possible that exocytosis gets rid of the Ca^{2+} which has entered the nerve terminal during previous stimuli. This would be an elegant solution for Ca^{2+} elimination from the cell in view of the fact (see below) that ACh release and Ca^{2+} entry appear to occur in a more or less constant ratio. However, one would then have to add a Ca^{2+} pump or exchanger to the scheme of the vesicle membrane. Current ideas about the specialisation of the synaptic vesicle membrane are discussed briefly in Chapter 1.

4.3.6. *Surplus ACh*

This is a somewhat mysterious compartment, first described for an autonomic ganglion. It becomes manifest when tissue is incubated in the presence of a cholinesterase inhibitor, a treatment which causes typically a doubling of the ACh content (Birks and Macintosh, 1961; Collier and Katz, 1971). The 'surplus' ACh is thought to reside in a cytoplasmic compartment, where in the absence of inhibitor it is continuously destroyed by a cholinesterase with an *intracellular* localisation. In some other cholinergic preparations, including mammalian skeletal muscle, surplus ACh is also formed under the influence of a cholinesterase inhibitor (frog muscles, however, do not form surplus ACh, Molenaar *et al.*, 1987). Surplus ACh is localised in an extravesicular compartment, probably in, or very near, the motor nerve terminals (Molenaar *et al.*, 1987).

4.3.7. *Effects of nerve stimulation on ACh compartments*

Stimulation of ACh release, by electric impulses or by direct depolarisation of nerve terminals in high potassium, causes a depletion of ACh in the nerve terminals mostly of bound ACh (Miledi *et al.*, 1982b; Molenaar and Polak, 1983). On the other hand, the ACh contained in muscle fibres remains unaffected by several forms of chemical stimulation (Miledi *et al.*, 1980, 1981, 1982a) although some reduction occurs during prolonged incubation in the presence of high K^+ (Molenaar *et al.*, 1987). While these data underline the importance of nerve terminal ACh in neuromuscular transmission, especially the compartment of bound ACh, the meaning of the other compartments remains unclear, but has to be taken into account, since their sizes can be considerable.

Table 4.3. Stimulation of acetylcholine release as seen by chemical and electrophysiological methods

	Chemical assay moles/sec/endplate	Electrophysiological MEPPs/sec
Normal Ringer (2 mM − K$^+$) (a)	2.5×10^{-19}	0.1
High K-Ringer (17 mM − K$^+$) (b)	12.2×10^{-19}	59
Stimulation factor (b/a)	4.9	590

Non-quantal release of ACh is revealed by chemical methods but not by electrophysiological techniques which specifically show only quantal release. Frog sartorius muscle 4°C: results taken from Miledi *et al.*, 1983.

4.4. **Release of ACh**

When a glass microelectrode is inserted into a muscle cell at the endplate region, small discharges can be seen of a more or less uniform amplitude. These MEPPs are due to the spontaneous release of packets or quanta of ACh (see Chapter 2). For some time it was thought that this was the only type of transmitter release. However, when investigators began measuring the ACh release into the bathing fluid with bioassay or chemical methods, in the presence of the AChE inhibitors, it became clear that quanta did not account for all ACh that was found in the bath (see for an example the results in Table 4.3) In fact the ACh released in many muscles at rest is often 100 times higher than can be accounted for by the release associated with ACh quanta. We now know that as well as quantal ACh release, ACh molecules can also be released on an individual basis (non-quantal release).

4.4.1. *Quantal transmitter release*

It is not clear whether the spontaneous MEPPs have a physiological role at the muscle membrane, or whether they merely represent a random spill-over. At any rate they convey information that is very helpful to the electrophysiologist. Among other things the amplitude of the MEPP is dependent on the number of ACh molecules in a quantum (this may change in the course of an experiment) and also on the density of the ACh receptors. The frequency of the MEPPs can be increased by various methods that lead to depolarisation of the nerve terminals, e.g. by incubating muscles with potassium at elevated concentrations. Alternatively, procedures that directly or indirectly cause an increase of the intraterminal concentration of free Ca^{2+} also lead to increased frequency of MEPPs. The relation between depolarisation, Ca^{2+} and transmitter release will be discussed below (see also Chapter 2).

In addition to 'normal' MEPPs of about 0.5–1.0 mV amplitude, other spontaneous potentials may be encountered that are either very small (sub-or dwarf MEPPs; Ceccarelli and Hurlbut, 1975; Kriebel and Florey, 1983) or large (giant MEPPs up to 10 mV; Pécot-Dechavassine and Couteaux, 1972). They are usually seen after a period of nerve stimulation, albeit their frequency is much less than that of the normal MEPPs. Normal MEPP amplitudes have an approximately normal (Gaussian) distribution but dwarf and giant MEPPs do not, and their origins are uncertain. One possibility is that dwarf MEPPs are caused by the release of immature quanta, in other words quanta that have not had enough time to gather up sufficient ACh molecules. Giants may originate from large vesicles which are occasionally observed in electron micrographs, but their frequency, in contrast to that of the MEPPs does not increase in the presence of high potassium.

Upon the arrival of an action potential the nerve terminal becomes depolarised for a very short time, less than one millisecond, and voltage-dependent Ca^{2+} channels open transiently, allowing Ca^{2+} ions to flow inwards. The amount of Ca^{2+} internalised determines how many transmitter quanta will be released. The internal Ca^{2+} is then rapidly taken up by a process in which several organelles are involved, e.g. the vesicles as suggested above, and the mitochondrion. The number of packets released per nerve stimulation varies. For instance whereas in normal Ca^{2+} solutions the quantal content (mean number of packets released) is around 100, when repolarisation of the nerve terminals is retarded (e.g. by drugs that block K^+ channels) the quantal content may increase dramatically (up to 80,000, Katz and Miledi, 1979). On the other hand at low external Ca^{2+} or in the presence of Mg^{2+} which blocks Ca^{2+} entry, there may be no release at all ('failure') or the release of one, two or three packets.

Under normal conditions when the nerve is stimulated the muscle contraction that follows dislodges the microelectrode from the impaled cell and prevents further recordings. Only when the postsynaptic depolarisa-tion is reduced below the firing threshold of the muscle fibre is it possible to monitor the so-called 'endplate potential' (EPP) that derives from the released ACh. To achieve this end, muscle spikes can be prevented by reduction in postsynaptic sensitivity by application of curare (e.g. see Chapter 2, Fig. 2.1); by reduction of the quantal content in low Ca^{2+} or high Mg^{2+}; or by cutting the muscle fibres away from the endplates. The resulting steady depolarisation of the muscle fibres causes inactivation of the voltage-dependent Na^+ channels of the muscle fibre so that an action potential does not occur.

There is good evidence (see Katz, 1966; Gage, 1976) that the EPP is caused by electrical summation of many MEPPs synchronously discharged from the active zones. Under normal circumstances more ACh is released than actually needed to bring about neuromuscular transmission, and the EPP is larger than the firing threshold. The extra depolarisation caused by

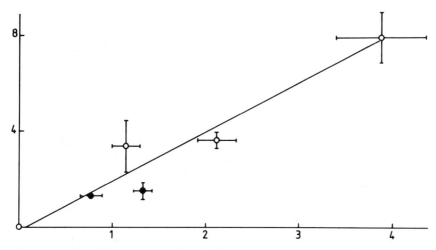

Fig. 4.6. Correlation between chemically detectable ACh release (ordinate) and MEPCs (MEP currents) in frog sartorius muscle treated with the cholinesterase inhibitor DEPP. Temperature 5°C. The frequency of the MEPCs was increased by KCl (15, 17 and 18.5 nM; open symbols) or by hypertonic NaCl (216 and 241mM; filled symbols). Means$^{\pm}$ SE From Miledi *et al.*, 1983, with permission of the *Journal of Physiology*.

the surplus of quanta is called the safety factor of neuromuscular transmission (see Chapter 2 and the chapter by Engel).

It has been possible to estimate the number of ACh molecules in a quantum in a series of experiments in which electrophysiological and chemical assays of ACh were combined. In these experiments the quantal release was stimulated by K^+ ions. The results, summarized in Fig. 4.6, indicate that about 12,000 molecules are contained in a quantum. This agrees with a similar figure for the content of a vesicle (see above) and strongly supports the vesicular theory of quantal release.

Stimulated ACh release can, to a moderate extent, be 'modulated' by substances that affect ACh receptors and cholinesterase activity. The physiological significance of these phenomena is unclear, but it is possible that some regulation is effected through ACh receptors located on the presynaptic membrane (see Molenaar and Polak, 1980) although the evidence for presynaptic AChRs at the neuromuscular junction is not strong.

4.4.2. *Non-quantal transmitter release*

It is now well established that only a small percentage of the ACh released under resting conditions, 'resting release', can be accounted for by ACh quanta (see Vizi and Vyskocil, 1979; Miledi *et al.*, 1983). Apparently, the

ACh from resting muscle is released mainly in a non-quantal form (see above).

Non-quantal ACh release has a small, steady depolarising effect on the muscle membrane of 1 mV or less (Katz and Miledi, 1977) which reveals itself as a *hyperpolarisation* when curare, which blocks ACh action, is applied to the endplate. Clearly, measurements of non-quantal ACh release based on such hyperpolarisation tend to be inaccurate.

As mentioned above, skeletal muscle fibres contain some ACh and therefore it is not surprising that part of the resting release originates from muscle fibres. The remainder (50–80%, depending on the type of muscle) originates from the nerve terminals themselves, whereas the main nerve trunk does not seem to be involved (Molenaar and Polak, 1986).

It has been suggested that a *carrier* is involved in non-quantal ACh release because it is not increased when the membrane potential of the nerve terminal is depolarised, as would be expected if the non-quantal release were the result of ACh leaking down an electrochemical gradient through pores in the membrane (Katz and Miledi, 1981; Miledi *et al.*, 1983). Furthermore the non-quantal release is partly dependent on Ca^{2+} (Molenaar and Polak, 1986) and in some way dependent on the activity of membrane Na/K ATPase (Vizi and Vyskocil, 1979). These features could be partly explained by the presence of vesicular proteins in the nerve terminal membrane following vesicle fusion (see Chapter 1).

The physiological significance of non-quantal release is unclear. It may be thought that it serves a trophic role at the muscle membrane, especially since the bulk of the ACh in resting muscle is released in that way, and because muscle fibres in the living animal may be under 'resting' conditions during much of the time. However, the postsynaptic effect of non-quantal release more or less vanishes if the cholinesterase inhibition is omitted. So it is quite possible that under normal conditions very little non-quantal ACh reaches the AChRs. At any rate the non-quantal release cannot be ignored, because its share in total turnover of ACh is so large, especially in mammals.

4.4.3. *Hydrolysis of released transmitter*

Acetylcholinesterase (AChE) in the synaptic cleft is anchored in the basal lamina which runs between the nerve terminal and the muscle membrane. Consequently, a quantum of ACh released at an active zone has to cross this barrier and thereby a considerable part of it is lost. The rest of the quantum reaches the receptors and is hydrolysed a few milliseconds later when the ACh becomes unbound. The hydrolysis of ACh therefore occurs in two phases. When the activity of the AChE is decreased by inhibitors such as neostigmine, inhibition of the first phase leads to an increase of the MEPP amplitude whereas inhibition of the second phase leads to a

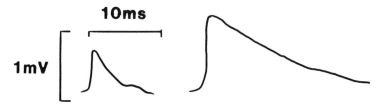

Fig. 4.7. Electrophysiology at the motor endplate. MEPPs before (left) and after (right) potentiation by cholinesterase inhibition.

considerable prolongation of the decay time of the MEPP (Fig. 4.7); many repetitive interactions occur between ACh and AChRs until ACh is finally lost by diffusion out of the synaptic cleft.

AChE is extremely rapid in its action and enough active sites are present to destroy all of the released ACh in a fraction of a millisecond. However, only about 20% of the AChE actually lies between the presynaptic active zones and the postsynaptic AChRs. The rest is present in the secondary folds where it is unlikely to affect the initial binding of ACh.

It is often thought that the function of the AChE is to enable the junction to transmit impulses at a high frequency without interference by ACh left over from previous events. However, clearance of ACh by diffusion alone is rather rapid, 5 ms or so, and it may be that the main function of AChE is to protect the endplate against the repeated binding of ACh and the damage caused by excessive Ca^{2+} entry into the muscle at the endplate.

4.4.4. *Mechanisms of transmitter release*

While there seems to be general agreement that the nerve action potential releases the transmitter in the form of quanta it has been difficult so far to obtain direct unequivocal evidence that the quanta are derived from synaptic vesicles and that vesicles, through the action of internal calcium, fuse with the presynaptic membrane. However, as far as the neuromuscular junction is concerned, many observations are in accordance with the vesicular hypothesis. In particular the reduction of bound ACh upon stimulation (Molenaar and Polak, 1983), the formation of omega-shaped profiles in the synaptic membrane coinciding with the stimulus-induced release process (Torri-Tarelli *et al.*, 1985) and the disappearance of evoked quantal transmitter release under conditions which lead to disappearance of synaptic vesicles (Miledi *et al.*, 1983).

However, other results, mainly obtained in experiments on the electric organ of *Torpedo*, indicate involvement of the free, cytosolic ACh, instead of vesicular ACh, and an alternative theory has been proposed (see reviews by Israël *et al.*, 1979). In this theory 'operator' or 'mediatophore'

Table 4.4.   Effect of drugs and toxins

	Mode of action
Synthesis	
Hemicholinium-3	Blockage of high-affinity uptake
Bromoacetylcholine	Inhibitor of ChAT
Storage	
Vesamicol (AH5183)	Blockage of ACh uptake in vesicles
La^{3+}; propionate; black widow spider venom	Inhibition of endocytotic formation of vesicles
Release	
Mg^{2+} and other divalent ions	Block of Ca^{2+} uptake
Botulinum toxins	Inhibition of quantal release
b-Bungarotoxin	Mixed action; interfers with ACh release
Black widow spider venom; La^{3+} ions	Promote ACh release
Diaminopyridines; Tetraethylammonium	Potentiate stimulus-evoked ACh release by inhibition of K^+ channels
Hydrolysis	
Carbamate-compounds, e.g. Neostigmine	Slowly reversible inhibition of AChE
Organophosphorus, e.g. DFP	Irreversible inhibition of AChE

For reviews see Gage, 1976; Katz & Miledi, 1979; Ceccarelli & Hurlbut, 1980; Tucek, 1982.

molecules in or near the presynaptic membrane bind sub-quantal amounts of ACh which are released in concert as a quantum. Up to this stage the idea has features which are rather similar to the vesicular theory. The main difference, however, is that in the operator theory the vesicles merely have the function of an ACh store, to be used only in times of need, whereas the operator, which has no storage capacity of its own, recruits its ACh directly from the cytosol, and continuously repeats this action. Further studies are required to clarify the role of this molecule.

4.4.5. *Drugs and toxins on ACh metabolism*

Table 4.4 summarises the wide range of drugs and toxins that have been found to affect ACh synthesis, storage, release and hydrolysis. Some are used in research (see for instance Dolly, this volume) and others, e.g. acetylcholine esterase inhibitors and aminopyridines, have proved invaluable in the treatment of human neuromuscular disorders.

Acknowledgements

The generous support by the foundations MEDIGON/ZWO and the Prinses Beatrix Fonds is gratefully acknowledged.

References

Bhatnager, S. P. and MacIntosh, F. C. (1960) Acetylcholine content of striated muscle. *Proc. Canad. Fed. Biol. Soc.* **3**: 12–13.

Birks, R. and MacIntosh, F. C. (1961) Acetylcholine metabolism of a sympathetic ganglion. *Canad. J. Biochem. Physiol.* **39**: 787–827.

Birks, R., Katz, B. and Miledi, R. (1960) Physiological and structural changes at the amphibian myoneural junction, in the course of nerve degeneration. *J. Physiol. Lond.* **150**: 145–168.

Ceccarelli, B., Grohovaz, F. and Hurlbut, W. P. (1979) Freeze-fracture studies of frog neuromuscular junctions during intense release of neurotransmitter. I. Effects of black widow spider venom and Ca^{2+}-free solutions on the structrure of the active zone. *J. Physiol. Lond.* **81**: 163–177.

Ceccarelli, B. and Hurlbut, W. P. (1980) Vesicle hypothesis of the release of quanta of acetylcholine. *Physiol. Rev.* **60**: 396–441.

Collier, B. and Katz, H. S. (1971) The synthesis, turnover and release of surplus acetylcholine in a sympathetic ganglion. *J. Physiol. Lond.* **214**: 537–552.

Dennis, M. J. and Miledi, R. (1974) Electrically induced release of acetylcholine from denervated Schwann cells. *J. Physiol. Lond.* **237**: 431–452.

De Roberts, E., Pellegrino de Iraldi, A., Rodriguez de Lores Arnaiz, G. and Gomez, C. J. (1961) On the isolation of nerve endings and synaptic vesicles. *J. Biophys. Biochem. Cytol.* **9**: 229–235.

Dunant, Y., Gautron, J., Israël, M., Lesbats, B. and Manaranche, R. (1972). Les compartiments d'acetylcholine de l'organe electrique de la Torpille et leurs modifications par la stimulation. *J. Neurochem.* **19**: 1987–2002.

Fonnum, F. (1967) The compartmentation of choline acetyltransferase within the synaptosome. *Biochem. J.* **103**: 262–270.

Gage, P. G. (1976). Generation of end-plate potentials. *Physiol. Rev.* **56**: 177–247.

Gray, E. G. and Whittaker, V. P. (1962) The isolation of nerve endings from brain: an electron-microscopic study of cell fragments derived by homogenization and centrifugation. *J. Anat. Lond.* **96**: 79–87.

Hebb, C. O. (1962) Acetylcholine content of the rabbit planatris muscle after denervation. *J. Physiol. Lond.* **163**: 294–306.

Hebb, C. O., Krnjevic, K. and Silver, A. (1964) Acetylcholine and choline acetyltransferase in the diaphragm of the rat. *J. Physiol. Lond.* **171**: 504–513.

Israël, M., Dunant, Y. and Manaranche, R., (1979) The present status of the vesicular hypothesis. *Progr. Neurobiol.* **13**: 237–275.

Johnson, R. G. (1987) Proton pumps and chemiosmotic coupling as a generalized mechanism for neurotransmitter and hormone transport. *Ann. N. Y. Acad. Sci.* **493**: 162–177.

Jope, R. S. (1979) High affinity choline transport and acetyl-CoA production in brain and their roles in the regulation of acetylcholine synthesis. *Brain Res. Rev.* **1**: 313–344.

Katz, B. (1966) *Nerve, Muscle and Synapse.* McGrow-Hill, New York.

Katz, B. and Miledi, R. (1977) Transmitter leakage from motor nerve endings. *Proc. R. Soc. Lond. B* **196**: 59–72.

Katz, B. and Miledi, R. (1979) Estimates of quantal content during 'chemical potentiation' of transmitter release. *Proc. R. Soc. Lond. B* **205**: 369–378.

Katz, B. and Miledi, R. (1981) Does the motor nerve evoke 'non-quantal' transmitter release? *Proc. R. Soc. Lond. B.* **212**: 131–137.

Kriebel, M. E. and Florey, E. (1983) Effect of lanthanum ions on the amplitude distributions of miniature endplate potentials and on synaptic vesicles in frog neuromuscular junction. *Neuroscience* **9**: 535–547.

MacIntosh, F. C. and Collier, B. (1976) Neuroschemistry of cholinergic terminals. In: *Neuromuscular Junction*, E. Zaimis, ed. Springes, Berlin/Heidelberg/New York, pp. 99–228.

Marchbanks, R. M. and Israël, M. (1971) Aspects of acetylcholine metabolism in the electric organ of *Torpedo marmorata*. *J. Neurochem.* **118**: 439–448.

Michaelson, D. M. and Wien-Naor, J. (1987) Enkephalin uptake into cholinergic synaptic vesicles and nerve terminals. *Ann. N. Y. Acad. Sci.* **493**: 234–251.

Miledi, R., Molenaar, P. C. and Polak, R. L. (1977) An analysis of acetylcholine in frog muscle by mass fragmentography. *Proc. R. Soc. Lond. B* **197**: 285–297.

Miledi, R., Molenaar, P. C. and Polak, R. L. (1980) The effect of lanthanum ions on acetylcholine in frog muscle. *J. Physiol. Lond.* **309**: 199–214.

Mildei, R., Molenaar, P. C. and Polak, R. L. (1981) Early effects of denervation on acetylcholine and choline acetyltransferase. In: *Cholinergic Mechanism*, G. Pepeu and H. Ladinsky, eds, Plenum, New York, pp. 205–214.

Miledi, R., Molenaar, P. C., Polak, R. L., Tas, J. W. M. and van der Laaken, T. (1982a) Neural and non-neural acetylcholine in the rat diaphragm. *Proc. R. Soc. Lond. B* **214**: 153–168.

Miledi, R., Molenaar, P. C. and Polak, R. L. (1982b) Free and bound acetylcholine in frog muscle. *J. Physiol.* **333**: 189–199.

Miledi, R., Molenaar, P. C. and Polak, R. L. (1983) Electrophysiological and chemical determination of acetylcholine release at the frog neuromuscular junction. *J. Physiol. Lond.* **334**: 245–254.

Molenaar, P. C. and Polak, R. L. (1980) Acetylcholine synthesizing enzymes in frog skeletal muscle. *J. Neurochem.* **35**: 1021–1025.

Molenaar, P. C., Newsom-Davis, J., Polak, R. L. and Vincent, A. (1981) Choline acetyltransferase in skeletal muscle from patients with myasthenia gravis. *J. Neurochem.* **37**: 1081–1088.

Molenaar, P. C. and Polak, R. L. (1983) Potassium propionate causes preferential loss of 'bound' acetylcholine in frog muscle. *Neurosci. Lett.*, **43**: 209–213.

Molenaar, P. C. and Polak, R. L. (1986) Resting release of acetylcholine at the motor endplate. In: *Dynamics of Cholinergic Function*, I. Hanin, ed. Plenum, New York, pp. 481–487.

Molenaar, P. C., Oen, B. X. and Polak, R. L. (1987) Surplus acetylcholine and acetylcholine release in the rat diaphragm. *J. Physiol. Lond.* **385**: 147–167.

Nachmanson, D., and Machado, A. L. (1943) The formation of acetylchoine, a new enzyme, choline acetylase'. *J. Neuro physiol.* **6**: 397–403.

Parsons, S. M., Bahr, B. A., Gracz, L. M., Kaugman, R., Kornreich, W. D., Nilsson L. and Rogers, G. A. (1987) Acetycholine transport: fundamental properties and effects pharmacologic agents. *Ann N. Y. Acad. Sci.* **493**: 220–233.

Pécot-Dechavassine, M. and Couteaux, R. (1972) Potentials miniatures d'amplitude anormale obtenues dan des conditions experimentales et changement concomitants des structures presynaptiques. In: *International Symposium on Cholinergic Transmission of the Nerve Impulse*, INSERM, Paris, pp. 177–185.

Torri-Tarelli, F., Grohovaz, F., Fesce, R. and Ceccarelli, B. (1985) Temporal coincidence between synaptic vesicle fusion and quantal secretion of acetylcholine. *J. Cell Biol.* **101**: 1386–1399.

Tucek, S. (1978) *Acetylcholine Synthesis in Neurons*, Champan & Hall, London.

Tucek, S. (1982) The synthesis of acetylcholine in skeletal muscles of the rat. *J. Physiol. Lond.* **322**: 53–69.

Vizi, E. S. and Vyskocil, F. (1979) Changes in total and quantal release of acetylcholine during activation and inhibition of membrane ATPase. *J. Physiol. Lond.* **286**: 1–14.

Whittaker, V. P. (1969) The nature of acetylcholine pools in tissue. *Progr. Brain*

Res. **31**: 211–222.

Whittaker, V. P. (1987) Cholinergic synaptic vesicles from the electromotor nerve terminals of *Torpedo*. Composition and life cycle. *Ann. N. Y. Acad. Sci.* **493**: 77–91.

Wileman, T., Harding, C. and Stahl, P. (1985) Receptor-mediated endocytosis. *Biochem. J.* **232**: 1–14.

5 *Robert Norman*

Properties of ion channels involved in neuromuscular transmission

5.1. Introduction

The transmission of impulses from nerve to muscle is achieved via a chemical messenger, acetylcholine, but the process is critically dependent on the presence of highly selective ion channels in the nerve terminal and postsynaptic membrane. These channels are complex proteins that respond to changes in the membrane potential. Their biochemical characterisation has been made possible largely through the existence of neurotoxins from a wide variety of species. These toxins bind with high affinity to particular ion channels and have enabled scientists to purify, characterise and eventually obtain the primary sequence of several voltage-dependent ion channels. For a more detailed review see Catterall (1988).

5.1.1. Propagation of the action potential

Action potentials in nerve and muscle are due to a wave of depolarisation carried along the plasma membrane. At rest a potential difference is maintained across the membrane with the inside of the cell negative with respect to the outside. This potential difference (the membrane potential) is achieved by the concentration gradient (primarily K^+ ions, resulting from an adenosine triphosphate dependent pump) between inside and outside (see Chapter 2). Depolarisation of the membrane (i.e. a reduction in membrane potential) stimulates the opening of voltage-sensitive Na^+ channels which carry Na^+ ions, down their electrochemical gradient, into the cell. The passage of these positively charged ions depolarises the membrane further, but the Na^+ channels inactivate rapidly so that the inward Na^+ current is only short-lived. Furthermore, in response to the depolarisation, K^+ channels with a slightly delayed activation open and carry K^+ ions out of the cell, down the K^+ concentration gradient. This delayed outward current restores the membrane to its resting potential ready to carry further action potentials. In this way a wave of depolarisation spreads along the fibre.

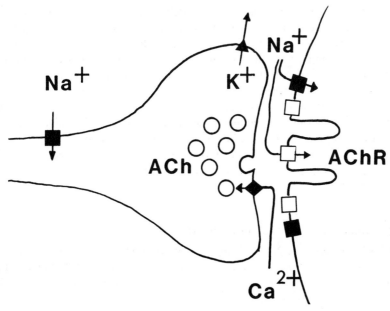

Fig. 5.1. Schematic representation of electrical events at the nerve terminal. Na^+ entering through Na^+ channels during an action potential induces depolarisation of the nerve terminal membrane. Ca^{2+} channels open in response to the depolarisation, resulting in an influx of Ca^{2+} which triggers acetylcholine (ACh) release. The membrane potential of the nerve terminal is rapidly restored by delayed rectifying K^+ channels. ACh binding to specific receptors on the postsynaptic membrane results in depolarisation of the endplate, opening of Na^+ channels and generation of an action potential in the muscle.

5.1.2. Ca^{2+}-dependent release of ACh

When the action potential in the motor nerve arrives at the nerve terminal, voltage-sensitive Ca^{2+} channels located on the presynaptic membrane open and Ca^{2+} ions flow into the cell down the large electrochemical gradient that is maintained for this ion (Fig. 5.1). Ca^{2+} ions entering in this way then trigger the exocytotic mechanism to release acetylcholine into the synaptic cleft (for discussion, see Molenaar, this volume). The acetylcholine diffuses across the synaptic cleft and binds to specific acetylcholine receptors on the postsynaptic membrane. Binding causes a conformational change in the receptor protein which opens an ion channel within its structure and allows ions (mostly Na^+) to enter. This in turn results in the generation of an endplate potential (EPP) in the postsynaptic membrane with triggers an action potential. The muscle surface has deep tubular invaginations known as the transverse tubular system, and passage of action potentials down these stimulates release of Ca^{2+} from the sarcoplasmic reticulum leading to the contraction process.

At least three voltage-sensitive cation channels are therefore involved in the excitation–secretion process that results in neuromuscular transmission, namely Na^+, K^+ and Ca^{2+} channels. However, because the nerve terminal is so small very little is known at the biochemical level about the molecular structure of these channels at the neuromuscular junction. Nevertheless, the Na^+ channel present in the preterminal region is likely to be similar to that in other nervous tissues. This chapter describes the methods and overall conclusions drawn from the study of voltage-sensitive cation channel structures, mainly from electric organ, brain and muscle. Lessons learnt from the study of these channels in other tissues should ultimately facilitate the stuctural characterisation of the channels present at the neuromuscular junction.

5.2. Voltage-sensitive sodium channels

The voltage-sensitive Na^+ channel can be thought of as a gated pore that allows the passage of Na^+ ions in preference to other ionic species. The 'gate', which is normally closed, is caused to open transiently when the

Table 5.1. Neurotoxin binding sites associated with voltage-sensitive sodium channels. Receptor sites are numbered according to the scheme of Catterall (1980).

Toxin receptor site	Toxin	Physiological effect
I	Tetrodotoxin Saxitoxin μ-Conotoxin	Block sodium channels
II	Alkaloids, e.g. veratridine, batracotoxin, aconitine, grayanotoxin	Alter activation and inactivation; cause persistent activation
III	Sea anemone toxins, e.g. *Anemonia sulcata* toxins North American and North African scorpion α-toxins, e.g. *Leirus quinquestralis* toxin	Slow down inactivation Enhance persistent activation by alkaloid toxins
IV	Central and South American scorpion toxins, e.g. *Centruroides suffusus suffusus* β-toxin, *Tityus serrulatus* γ-toxin	Shift activation of sodium channels to lower potentials
?	Pyrethroids Brevetoxins Palytoxin Ciguarotoxin Local anaesthetics	Alter activation and inactivation; cause persistent activation

membrane is depolarised. Several openings and closings may occur before a slightly slower gating mechanism causes the channel to inactivate. The channel then remains closed until reprimed by re-establishment of the potential difference across the membrane.

5.2.1. *Action of specific neurotoxins*

A large number of naturally occurring, highly specific neurotoxins, from a wide range of animal species, have provided essential tools for the characterisation of the electrophysiological and molecular properties of the Na^+ channel. These toxins have been classified according to their sites of interaction and physiological effects into several different categories (Table 5.1, Fig. 5.2) Catterall, 1980, Strichartz *et al.* 1987), and

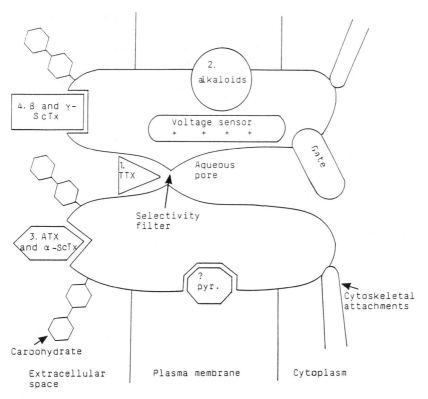

Fig. 5.2. Neurotoxin binding sites on the Na^+ channel. Hypothetical view of a Na^+ channel macromolecule in the plasma membrane. Positioning of the ion coordination site or selectivity filter, the channel gating mechanism and the neurotoxin binding sites are deduced from electrophysiological measurements. Taken from Hille (1984) with permission.

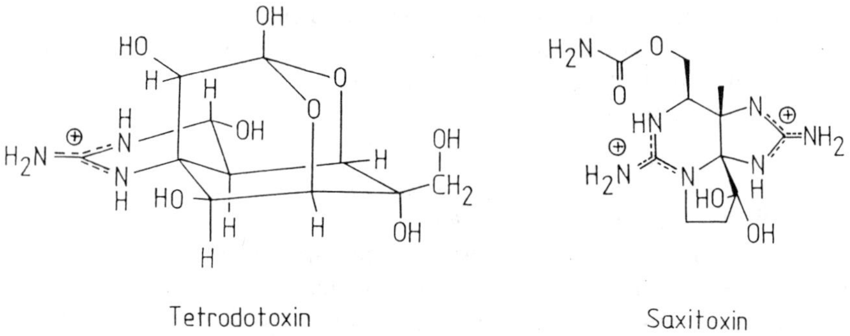

Tetrodotoxin   Saxitoxin

Fig. 5.3.   Structures of the guanidinium blockers of voltage-sensitive Na^+ channels. Tetrodotoxin and saxitoxin bind at neurotoxin site I associated with the selectivity filter of the Na^+ channel.

measurement of their binding to the Na^+ channel during its purification has been an invaluable tool.

The traditional blockers of Na^+ channel permeability are the water-soluble, heterocyclic guanidines, tetrodotoxin and saxitoxin (Fig. 5.3). Blockade by these toxins has been attributed to the binding of the guanidinium moieties at a specific coordination site (site 1; Fig. 5.2) involved in ion selectivity, located near the extracellular opening of the Na^+ channel. μ-Conotoxin, a polypeptide isolated from a fish-hunting snail, also produces block of Na^+ channel permeability by interaction at site I, and competes with saxitoxin for high-affinity receptors. Interestingly, this toxin is selective for skeletal muscle and electric organ Na^+ channels, and has a much weaker potency on neuronal and cardiac channels.

The major group of lipid-soluble Na^+ channel toxins are the alkaloid toxins (Fig. 5.4). These are a group of small, chemically unrelated compounds derived from various species of plants and the skin of a tropical frog. In general their effect is to cause persistent channel opening due to a shift in the voltage-dependence of channel activation, so that channels open in response to smaller depolarisations. There is also a slowing or inhibition of channel inactivation. Competition binding studies indicate that all four commonly studied alkaloids bind at a common site, designated site II (Fig. 5.2).

There are two classes of Na^+ channel-specific polypeptide toxins. One group acts by slowing or inhibiting the inactivation of the Na^+ channel resulting in prolonged openings. Members of this group are the positively charged α-toxins from the venom of North African and North American scorpions, and sea anemone toxins isolated from nematocysts. Even though no amino acid sequence similarity exists between them they bind to a common site on the Na^+ channel (site III) which is accessible only from

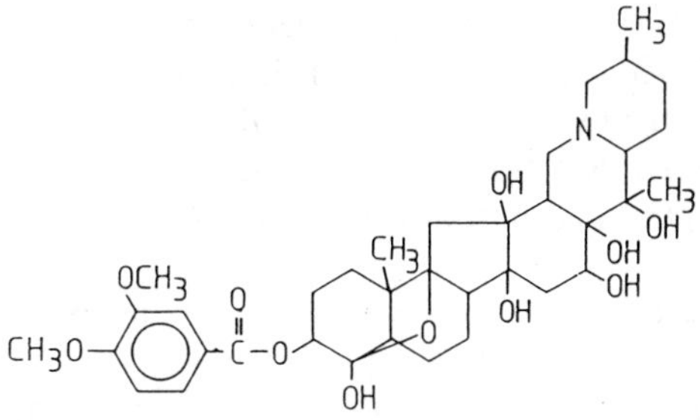

Veratridine

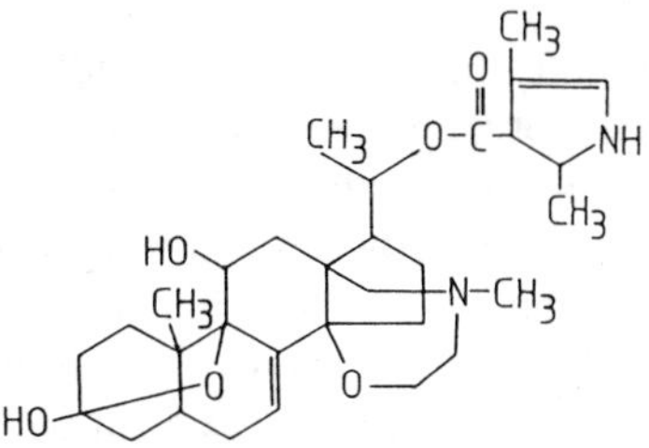

Batrachotoxin

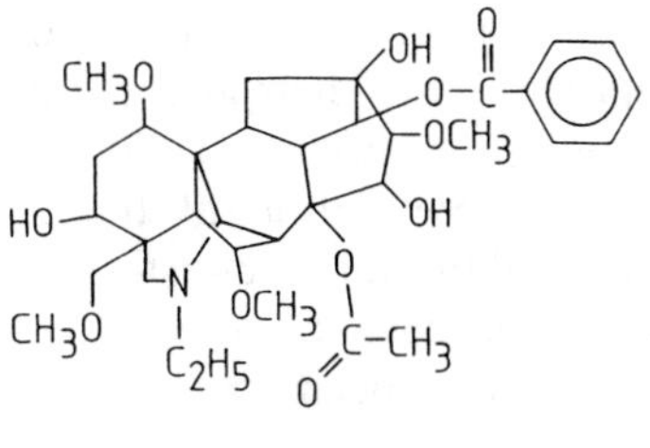

Aconitine

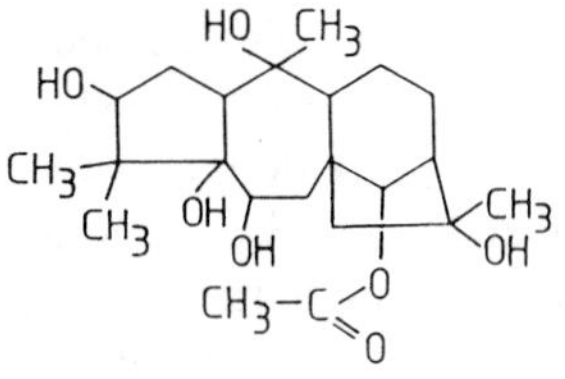

Grayanotoxin I

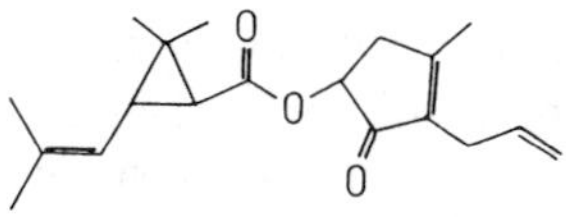

Allethrin

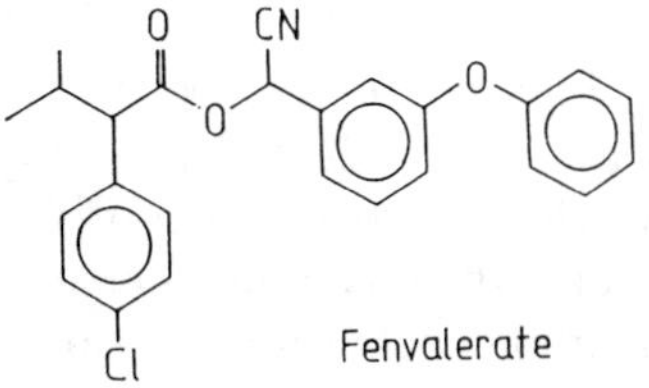

Fenvalerate

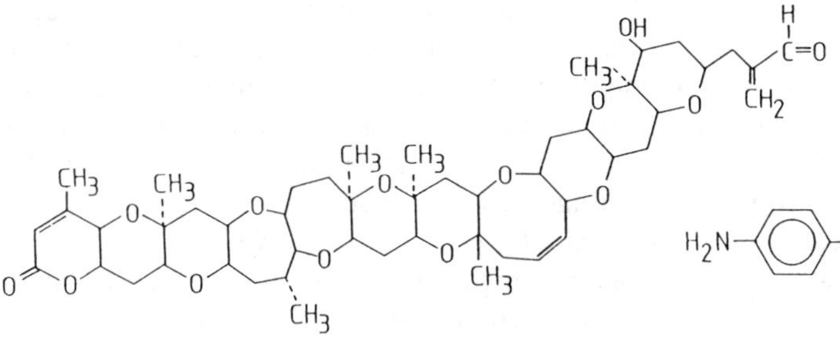

Brevetoxin B

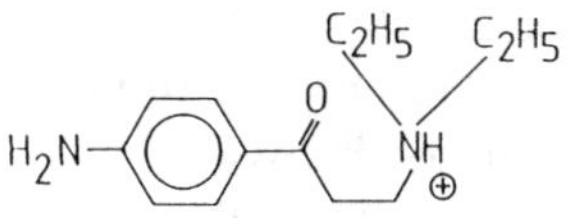

Procaine

Fig. 5.4. Structures of the lipid-soluble Na^+ channel toxins. Veratridine, batrachotoxin, aconitine and grayanotoxin I are the most widely used alkaloid toxins. Allethrin and fenvalerate are examples of pyrethroids. Procaine is a local anaesthetic. The lipid-soluble toxins produce similar alterations on Na^+ channel activation and inactivation but may bind to several distinct binding sites on the Na^+ channel structure.

the extracellular side. Binding to this site is voltage-dependent since the affinity for toxins is markedly reduced on depolarisation. In addition, site III polypeptide toxins act synergistically with the site II alkaloid toxins, resulting in enhanced persistent activation of the Na^+ channel. This group of toxins is therefore thought to act at a region of the channel involved in the inactivation mechanism.

The second class of polypeptide toxins include β-and γ-scorpion toxins from the venom of Central and South American scorpions and bind to site IV. The predominant effect of these toxins is on Na^+ channel activation, although inactivation is also slowed.

In addition to the alkaloid toxins, a number of other classes of lipid-soluble Na^+ channel toxins have been characterised (see Table 5.1). The similarities with respect to lipid solubility, and their effects on Na^+ channel properties, suggest that all the lipophilic toxins interact in a similar way to the alkaloid toxins. However, the potentiation of the effects produced by one class of toxins on another, and the varied allosteric effects that individual classes of lipophilic toxins produce on the other Na^+ channel toxin binding sites, suggest that other sites specific for lipid-soluble toxins may remain to be characterised.

5.2.2. *Neurotoxins as biochemical probes of Na^+ channel structure*

The high degree of specificity in channel function, as evidenced by ion selectivity, conductivity, gating and toxin sensitivity, all suggest that the Na^+ channel structure consists of a channel-forming, intrinsic, membrane protein which is able to respond to changes in membrane potential. The goal of biochemical studies on any ion channel is to determine the detailed molecular structure of the channel in the membrane and then to understand how aspects of the structure contribute to the voltage-dependent gating properties. A necessary part of this analysis is the isolation of channel components from the membrane environment. Since channels are functionally identified by virtue of the ionic currents associated with channel activation or inactivation, removal from the membrane environment no longer allows these parameters to be measured. However, the specific interaction of the various groups of neurotoxins with their respective high-affinity binding sites, described above, provide a wide range of potential tools for the characterisation of the molecular properties of distinct regions of the Na^+ channel.

For a toxin to be of use in biochemical studies, stable, radioactively labelled derivatives of the toxin that retain biological activity must be available. The most widely used toxins in radioactive form have been the group I and group IV neurotoxins. These toxins retain biological activity and bind to the Na^+ channel protein with high affinity even when the channel is solubilised from its membrane environment with detergents.

5.2.3. *Structural studies using neurotoxins*

Using the techniques of radiation inactivation the size of the so-called 'target' protein in a membrane is reflected in the rate of loss of biological activity caused by the irradiation of samples with high-energy electrons. Larger proteins present larger targets in the field of electrons and therefore require lower doses to inactivate them. Using this technique the molecular size of the Na^+ channel has been investigated by observing the radiation-induced loss of the specific binding activity of radiolabelled toxins. Interestingly, use of both the site I and site IV toxins, has indicated a very large binding protein of between 230 and 270 kDa (Barharin *et al.*, 1983). Whether this protein represents the entire Na^+ channel or a subunit of the channel which binds both classes of toxins cannot be resolved by this technique.

Covalent attachment of radiolabelled toxin that is bound specifically to the channel in the membrane, and analysis of the membrane sample by solubilisation and polyacrylamide gel electrophoresis (see Chapter 3), provides a second way to determine the size of a channel protein. Representative toxins for sites I, III and IV have each been shown to label specifically a protein of 270 kDa, suggesting that these three toxin sites all reside on, or very near to, the same large polypeptide molecule (Catterall, 1986). In brain membranes *Leiurus* scorpion toxin, a site III toxin, also labelled a second smaller polypeptide of 39 kDa.

The Na^+ channel can be readily solubilised by treatment of the membrane with non-ionic detergents. Tetrodotoxin binding activity in the detergent extract can be stabilised by maintaining the temperature at 4°C and addition of glycerol and/or phospholipids to the detergent extracts. Interestingly, while these conditions permit the solubilisation and stabilisation of receptor sites I and IV, both sites II and III lose the ability to bind their respective toxins. (This apparent loss of binding sites can be attributed to temporary inactivation in detergent solution, rather than a loss of part of the Na^+ channel complex, since reincorporation of Na^+ channels from detergent extracts into artificial membranes results in their reappearance.) The size of the detergent-solubilised saxitoxin receptor, after correction for bound detergent and phospholipid, has been estimated by centrifugation and gel filtration analyses to be approximately 315 kDa in both brain and skeletal muscle.

Many laboratories have endeavoured to purify the Na^+ channel from a variety of tissues including eel electric organ, brain and skeletal muscle, using classical purification procedures such as ion-exchange chromatogra-

phy, adsorption chromatography, lectin affinity chromatography, gel
filtration and sucrose density gradient centrifugation, in various combinations (Catterall, 1986) (see Chapter 3 of this volume); radiolabelled toxin
being used to label or assay for the Na^+ channel.

From subunit analyses, by SDS polyacrylamide gel electrophoresis of
purified fractions from various tissues, there is now general agreement that
a large glycoprotein of 270 kDa is common to all sodium channel
preparations. In addition to containing the binding sites for site I and site
IV toxins this subunit is heavily glycosylated and contains approximately
30% of its weight in sugar residues. While this is the only polypeptide
identified in preparations from eel electric organ, additional smaller
polypeptides co-purify with the 270 kDa polypeptide in preparations from
mammalian brain and skeletal muscle. It is not yet clear whether these
represent distinct subunits or arise as a result of proteolytic nicking of a
single large' sodium channel polypeptide.

5.2.4. *Functional reconstitution*

To confirm that all Na^+ channel components have been identified it is
necessary to demonstrate that the purified toxin-binding proteins can
reconstitute selective ion fluxes with the appropriate voltage and toxin
sensitivities. These properties have been investigated by reincorporation of
purified Na^+ channel proteins into lipid vesicles or planar bilayers and
measurement of $^{22}Na^+$ fluxes or electrophysiological recordings, respectively (Catterall, 1986).

The 270 kDa protein purified from eel electroplax has been shown to be
sufficient to reconstitute a Na^+ channel with essentially all the biophysical
properties of the physiologically defined channel. Furthermore, reincorporation of the 270kDa electroplax protein alone into artificial lipid
bilayers is sufficient to reconstitute toxin binding sites I, II, III and IV,
even though functional binding sites for site II and III toxins were not
detectable during purification (see above). Since full channel function
appears to be reconstituted by the 270 kDa protein alone (and see also
below) questions are raised regarding the relevance of the additional small
putative subunits, identified in affinity labelling and purification studies.
These proteins could have roles in channel regulation or anchoring of the
channel protein in the membrane (cf. 43 kDa protein, see Chapter 1).
Recently the cytoskeletal proteins ankyrin (220 kDa) and spectrin (260
kDa) have been shown to associate with Na^+ channels in the brain.

5.2.5. *Primary sequence determination*

Before the molecular mechanisms of ion selectivity and voltage-dependent
gating can be fully understood, knowledge of the amino acid sequence of

Na^+ channel components is essential. The very large size of the main Na^+ channel subunit, together with the low yields from protein purification studies, precludes analysis of the primary structure using classical protein sequencing techniques. Recombinant DNA techniques have therefore been employed and the amino acid sequence derived from the nucleotide sequence of cloned cDNA encoding the channel protein (Noda *et al.*, 1984, 1986a). The 270 kDa protein consists of a sequence of 1820–2009 amino acid residues (depending on the tissue source) which contains four repeated units of similar but not identical sequence (Fig. 5.5). Within each repeating structure are found five hydrophobic segments (S1, S2, S3, S5 and S6) and a highly positive charged segment (S4). The four repeats have been assumed to represent four repeated structural units which are oriented in a pseudosymmetric fashion across the membrane. Assuming that the N-terminal is cytoplasmic (because there is no 'leader' sequence,

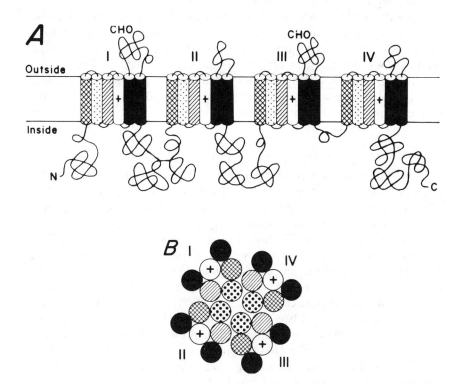

Fig. 5.5. Proposed transmembrane topology of the α-subunit of the voltage-sensitive Na^+ channel. The transmembrane segments are viewed in a direction perpendicular to the membrane. In **A** the four internal repeats (I to IV) are displayed linearly. They probably surround the ionic channel as shown in **B**. Segments S1 to S6 in each repeat are shown by cross-hatched, stippled, hatched, plus-signed or filled-in cylinders, respectively. From Noda *et al.*, 1986a with permission.

see Chapter 3), either four or six transmembrane segments (S1–S6) in each repeat must be postulated to maintain a pseudosymmetric orientation. Thus, models for the transmembrane topology of the large Na^+ channel protein have been proposed (Fig. 5.5).

On the basis of the high conservation of charged residues which align one face of an α-helix of segment S2, it has been postulated that the S2 helical segments of each repeat participate to form the inner wall of the channel at the narrowest point. The highly positive charge of the S4 segment suggests a role as the voltage-sensor of the channel. Electrophysiological recording of gating currents suggests that four to six charges must move fully across the membrane for one channel to open. This consideration would favour a topology in which all six segments of each repeat had intramembranous locations. In this model positive charges in S4 should be stabilised by the formation of ion pairs with negative charges in other segments such as S1 and S3.

Support for this model has been provided by the assignment in the primary structure of extracellular glycosylation sites, a scorpion toxin binding site, a number of intracellular phosphorylation sites and antibody binding sites (Catterall *et al.*, 1988), as well as from studies to map structure to function (see below). Knowledge of the primary structure has, therefore, led to detailed postulates regarding the topology of the various segments and their role in Na^+ channel function.

5.2.6. *Expression of Na^+ channel cDNA*

Perhaps the most exciting development in recent channel research has been the expression of functional channels derived from cloned cDNA. Messenger RNAs generated by *in vitro* transcription of cloned cDNAs encoding the rat brain Na^+ channel large polypeptide were injected into *Xenopus* oocytes. After 3 days tetrodotoxin-sensitive transient Na^+ currents could be measured following depolarisation of the oocyte membrane. Many of the properties of the cDNA encoded channel were comparable with Na^+ channels encoded by rat brain messenger RNA expressed under the same conditions, and also those of the native channels *in vivo* (Noda *et al.*, 1986b). Only the kinetics of inactivation were modified, being slightly slower for the expressed channels. These data argue very strongly that the 270 kDa polypeptide alone is sufficient to form functional sodium channels, raising again the question concerning the function of the putative small channel subunits.

5.2.7. *Structure/function relationships*

The accumulation of structural information available for the Na^+ channel has allowed the design of studies to map functional properties of the channel to discrete regions of the channel structure. One approach has been the use of anti-Na^+ channel antibodies. Some monoclonal antibodies raised against the Na^+ channel protein have been shown to alter the functional properties of Na^+ channels *in vivo* (Barhanin *et al.*, 1985; Meiri *et al.*, 1986). However, mapping of these antibody binding sites to distinct regions of primary sequence is not a straightforward task due to the small amounts of Na^+ channel protein available and the conformational dependence for binding of some of the antibodies (as for the acetylcholine receptor, Lindstrom, this volume).

The production of antibodies with functional effects on the Na^+ channel has, however, stimulated an alternative strategy. In this case antibodies have been generated against short synthetic peptides corresponding to regions of the sodium channel protein and the effect on physiological function assessed. Antibodies directed against the putative transmembrane segment S4 have been shown to alter the inactivation properties of the Na^+ channel when applied to the extracellular medium, suggesting that at least part of the S4 segment is accessible from the outside of the cell (Meiri *et al.*, 1987). In a second study, antibodies directed against a region of the conserved intracellular sequence which links internal repeat structures III and IV have also been shown to produce effects on channel inactivation (Vassilev *et al.*, 1988). Such evidence argues for a conformational change during inactivation which involves both extra- and intracellular regions of the channel structure.

A further approach has been to reconstitute synthetic peptides containing putative channel-forming sequences into artificial bilayers (Oiki *et al.*, 1988; Tosteson *et al.*, 1989). A synthetic peptide corresponding to the S3 transmembrane domain of the Na^+ channel has been shown to reconstitute monovalent ion selective channels with ion conductances similar to those of the native Na^+ channel. However, unlike the native Na^+ channel, opening and closing of the channels formed by the synthetic peptide are voltage-independent. These results argue in favour of a role for segment S3 in the formation of the ion conducting pore of the Na^+ channel and indicate the requirement for additional sequence(s) to confer voltage sensitivity. Interestingly, reconstitution of a monovalent cation-sensitive channel has also been shown with a synthetic peptide corresponding to the S4 segment. In this case the conductance *was* voltage-sensitive.

The availability of cDNA encoding functional channel protein together with the oocyte expression system has opened the way for studies using site-directed mutagenesis. By changing individual amino acids or short regions of sequence in the Na^+ channel structure and characterising the functional properties of the expressed mutant channels, it has been possible to provide further evidence regarding structure/function relationships (Stühmer *et al.*, 1989). Using deletion mutants, all four repeats of the Na^+ channel structure have been shown to be necessary for the expression of functional channels. However, the introduction of cuts between the repeats did not prevent channel formation. Interestingly, when a cut was introduced between repeats III and IV, channels were expressed but with a dramatically decreased rate of inactivation. This result suggests that the cytoplasmic linking region between these repeats is involved in channel inactivation, and is consistent with previous observations on the effects of endopeptidases applied to the cytoplasmic side of wild-type Na^+ channels, and the effects of antibodies directed against this region.

Attention has also been directed towards the transmembrane segment S4 which is postulated to be involved in the voltage-sensing properties. In a number of experiments the net positive charge in the S4 segment of repeat I was reduced by replacement of basic residues with neutral or acidic residues. The resulting mutant channels showed alterations in their voltage dependence of activation, consistent with the involvement of the S4 segment in voltage sensitivity (Stühmer *et al.*, 1989).

Preliminary assignments of channel function to discrete structures have been made using a variety of approaches. These studies have also validated, to some extent, the two-dimensional models predicted from the amino acid sequence. Much further study is required to establish the full structure/function relationships.

5.3. **Voltage-sensitive calcium channels**

5.3.1. Ca^{2+} channel types

Voltage-sensitive Ca^{2+} channels are responsible for the influx of Ca^{2+} at the nerve terminal that results in ACh release, and similar channels are found elsewhere in a variety of different tissues including adrenal medulla, smooth and striated muscle, as well as central, autonomic and peripheral nervous tissue. However, unlike the relative uniformity of Na^+ channel subtypes the situation with Ca^{2+} selective channels is much more complicated. Subdivision has been suggested on the basis of differences in electrophysiological properties and sensitivity to pharmacological agents such as organic Ca^{2+} channel antagonists and Ca^{2+} channel-specific neurotoxins. On the basis of these properties there is now much evidence for at least three distinct Ca^{2+} channel subtypes (Table 5.2) (McClesky *et al.*, 1986).

While three calcium channel subtypes can be distinguished on the basis of electrophysiological measurement it is not clear whether or not they represent different molecular structures. Indirect evidence in favour of, at least, partly discrete molecular entities is provided by their pharmacological properties. While T-type channels appear to be relatively insensitive to

Table 5.2. Distinguishing properties of T, N and L currents in dorsal root ganglion neurones. See McClesky *et al.*, 1986.

Property	T	N	L
Single-channel conductance	8–10 pS	13 pS	25 pS
Selectivity	Ca > Ba		Ba > Ca
Activation range	−70 mV	−10 mV	−10 mV
Peak current	−30 mV	+20 mV	+20 mV
Inactivation rate	Fast (20–50 ms)	Fast (20–50 ms)	Slow (>700 ms)
Sensitivity to 1,4-dihydropyridines	No	No	Yes
Sensitivity to ω-conotoxin	No	Yes	Yes*

*Not in skeletal muscle.

most of the pharmacological agents tested so far, both L and N types display characteristic pharmacological profiles; in particular the L-type channels are sensitive to a whole range of organic Ca^{2+} channel antagonists. Further pharmacological subdivision has been suggested on the basis of the differential effects of a neurotoxin, Omega-conotoxin (ω-CgTx), of the marine snail *Conus geographus*. In the presence of this toxin neuronal L and N currents are blocked, whereas the T current remains unaffected. Thus the fast and slow inactivating channels can be distinguished using this toxin. Interestingly, the action of this toxin also demonstrates possible structural differences between L-type channels from neuronal and skeletal muscle tissues; it only produces block of Ca^{2+} current carried by neuronal L-type channels.

5.3.2. *Pharmacology: agonists, antagonists and toxins*

The vital role played by Ca^{2+} in the contractility of the heart and vascular tissue has attracted the pharmaceutical industry to direct much attention to the identification of compounds able to alter Ca^{2+} currents in these tissues. From this endeavour a large number of structurally diverse compounds have been discovered which modify the properties of L-type voltage-sensitive Ca^{2+} channels (Fig. 5.6) (Glossmann *et al.*, 1985). On the whole Ca^{2+} channel-specific drugs are antagonists although some agonists have been identified, e.g. BAY K 8644 and CGP 28392.

Block of L-type Ca^{2+} channel activity by these antagonists is use-dependent and indicates that these drugs do not act simply to plug the pore from the outside (cf. for instance the action of tetrodotoxin on voltage-sensitive Na^+ channels). Ion channels undergo transitions between different states: resting (closed but available for opening), open (conducting ions) and inactivated (closed and unavailable for opening). Ca^{2+}

1,4-DIHYDROPYRIDINES   (Site I)

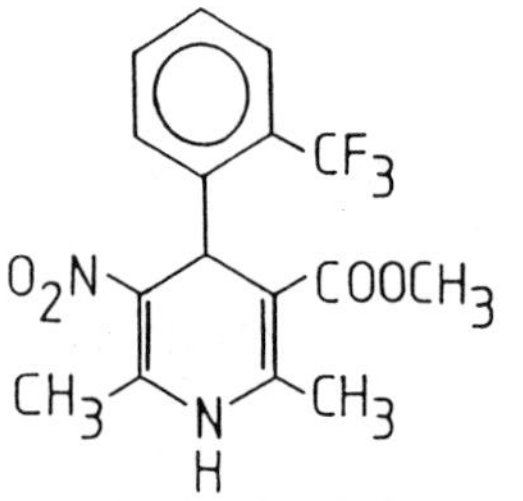

BAY K 8644 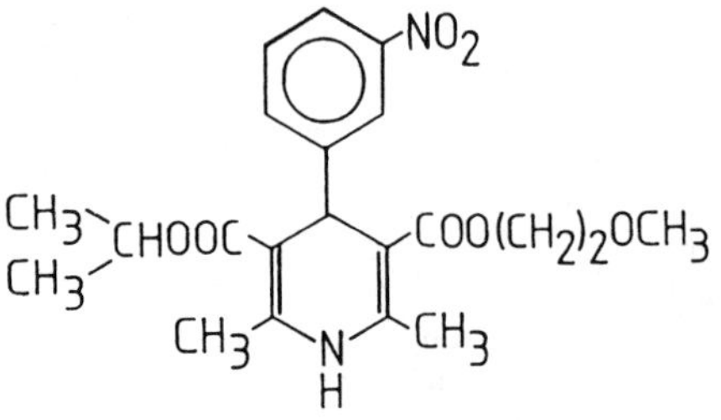   Nimodipine

PHENYLALKYLAMINES   (Site II)

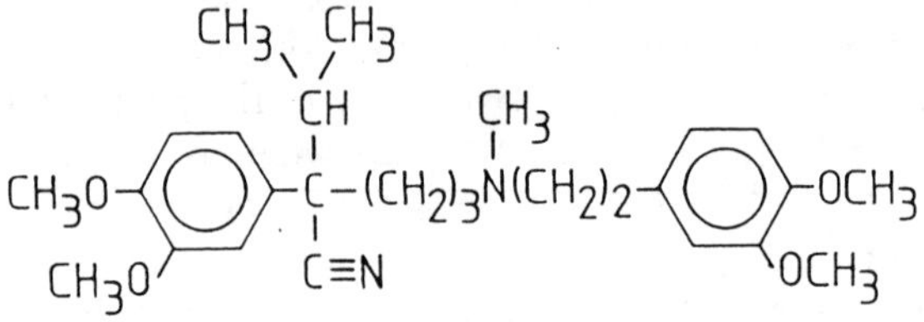

Verapamil

BENZOTHIAZEPINES   (Site III)

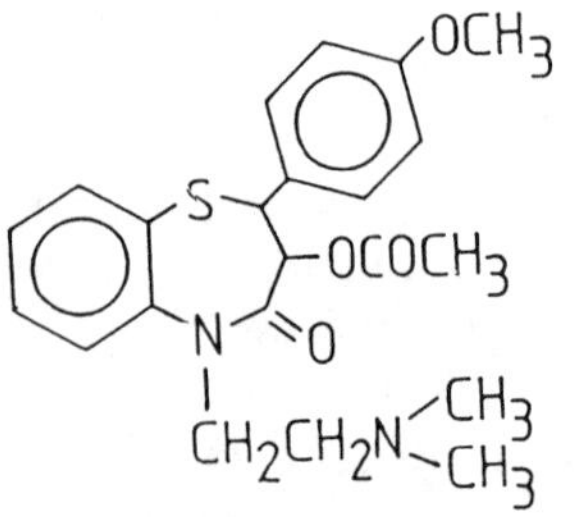

Diltiazem

Fig. 5.6.   Drugs active on L-type, voltage-sensitive Ca^{2+} channels. Representative drugs which bind to sites I, II and III are shown. Bay K 8644 is a Ca^{2+} channel agonist. Nimodipine, verapamil and diltiazem are antagonists.

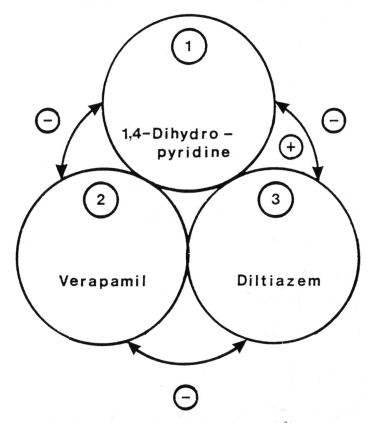

Fig. 5.7.   Allosteric interactions between three distinct Ca^{2+} antagonist receptor sites. ($+$) Stimulation of binding; ($-$) inhibition of binding. Binding of ω-conotoxin from the fish-hunting snail, *Conus geographus*, occurs at a separate site. Taken from Glossmann *et al.* (1985) with permission.

channel antagonists must therefore act by binding to open (or perhaps inactivated) states of the channel. Detailed binding studies of many different ligands have demonstrated the presence of two or three independent, allosterically coupled drug receptor sites on the Ca^{2+} channel structure. A three-site model proposed by Glossmann and colleagues (1985) is shown in Fig. 5.7.

All studies agree that site I is highly specific for both agonist and antagonist 1, 4-dihydropyridines. This has been shown by competitive binding and by the ability of agonists to overcome antagonist blockade of channel opening. The phenylalkylamines, verapamil and desmethoxyverapamil, are Ca^{2+} channel antagonists that bind to site II. These compounds produce non-competitive inhibition of binding of 1, 4-dihydropyridines to site I and vice-versa. Evidence for a third site (III) comes from the interaction of the benzothiazepine, diltiazem. At 37°C the presence of the enantiomer, D-*cis*-diltiazem, stimulates an increase in the apparent number of 1, 4-dihydropyridine binding sites.

Although no endogenous modulators of Ca^{2+} channel function have been identified, one naturally occurring neurotoxic molecule, ω-CgTx (as mentioned above), with antagonistic effects on Ca^{2+} channels, is now well characterised. Like the synthetic Ca^{2+} channel antagonists, ω-conotoxin is an antagonist of L-type channels, at least in neuronal tissue, but in contrast also produces blockade of N-type channels. Binding of ω-conotoxin to neuronal membranes occurs with very high affinity. Furthermore this interaction is not affected by the presence of Ca^{2+} channel antagonists for the L-type receptor sites I, II or III. ω-Conotoxin should, therefore, prove to be an invaluable tool for the identification and purification of Ca^{2+} channel subtypes, and has been used recently as an affinity label for Ca^{2+} channels in an immunoprecipitation assay for autoantibodies (see chapter by Wray).

5.3.3. *Structural studies of L type channels*

Investigators interested in the structure and function of L-type Ca^{2+} channels have been presented with a wide range of potential probes with specificities for three or four discrete regions of the Ca^{2+} channel structure. Compounds specific to each of these sites have been used in structural studies, but by far the most popular probes of L-type Ca^{2+} channels have been the 1,4-dihydropyridines (Glossman *et al.*, 1985). This group of compounds has been selected not only due to their high specificity but also for the relatively high-affinity binding of these drugs compared to those for sites II and III. The availability of suitable probes has meant that the characterisation of L-type channels at the molecular level has far outstripped that of the N- or T-type channels.

Attempts to estimate the molecular size of the L-type Ca^{2+} channel using radiation inactivation analysis have suggested a complicated oligomeric structure for this channel (Glossman *et al.*, 1987). Not only have different molecular sizes been determined for the three drug binding sites but the size determined for the 1,4-dihydropyridine receptor alone ranges from 136 to 278 kDa, depending on the tissue, the particular 1,4-dihydropyridine derivative used, and the conditions of irradiation. While furnishing much data, interpretation has required information from other approaches.

Photoaffinity labelling of the L-type Ca^{2+} channel with 1,4-dihydro-pyridines, phenylalklamines and D-*cis*-diltiazem has identified a large polypeptide of 155 – 170 kDa (Glossman *et al.*, 1987). These results strongly suggest that this large polypeptide, which has been denoted α_1, is involved in the binding of drugs to all three sites in the Ca^{2+} channel structure.

Choice of detergent has proved most important in determining conditions for the solubilisation of the L-type Ca^{2+} channel and it has only been possible to detect 1,4-dihydropyridine-binding after solubilisation in CHAPS or digitonin. The transverse tubule system of skeletal muscle has provided the best starting material for channel isolation since it contains approximately 100-fold more 1,4-dihydropyridine-binding sites than any other membrane preparation (Glossmann *et al.*, 1987). [³H]-1,4-dihydropyridine derivatives have been used extensively to prelabel the channels and to allow them to be followed during purification; classical protein purification techniques, in particular lectin affinity chromatography in the presence of detergent (Catterall *et al.*, 1988), were employed.

The purified 1,4-dihydropyridine receptor contains several polypeptides. Gel electrophoresis under non-reducing conditions reveals three non-covalently associated classes of subunit: α (170 kDa), β (52 kDa), and γ (30 kDa). Under these conditions the α subunit sometimes appears as two bands of very similar molecular weight. Similiar gel analysis under reducing conditions, which cleaves disulphide bonds, confirms the presence of distinct polypeptides. The 170 kDa subunit, designated α_1, is a non-glycosylated polypeptide that does not change its apparent molecular weight in gels under reducing conditions. However, under these conditions the apparent molecular weight of the α_2 subunit decreases from 175 kDa to 140 kDa due to the release of a small disulphide-linked polypeptide, designated δ. In contrast to the α_1 subunit, the α_2 polypeptide is heavily glycosylated and contains about 25% sugar residues. The 1,4-dihydropyridine receptor complex therefore contains five distinct polypeptide components: α_1 (170 kDa), α_2 (140 kDa), β (52 kDa), γ (30 kDa) and δ (27 kDa) (Table 5.3, Fig. 5.8). Tight association of these components under non-denaturing conditions is illustrated both by the co-purification of the various components on lectin affinity columns, by virtue of the carbohydrate on the α_2, δ and γ subunits, and by co-immunoprecipitation of the five putative subunit proteins using anti α_1 and anti-β subunit antibodies.

Table 5.3. Biochemical properties of the L-type calcium channel subunits (see Takahashi *et al.*, 1987).

Property	Subunit				
	a_1	a_2	β	γ	δ
MW × 10^{-3}	170	140	54	30	27
Drug binding	+	−	−	−	−
Channel forming	+	−	−	−	−
Glycoprotein	?	+	−	+	+
Phosphoprotein	+	−	+	−·	−
Hydrophobicity	+++	+	−	+++	+

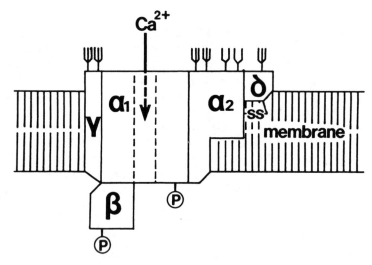

Fig. 5.8. Subunit structure of the L-type Ca^{2+} channel. Proposed model for Ca^{2+} channel structure showing sites of cAMP-dependent phophorylation (p), glycosylation (Y) and interactions with membrane lipids. Taken from Takahashi *et al.* (1987) with permission.

The full amino acid sequence of the α_1 subunit has been deduced from the nucleotide sequence of cloned DNA (Tanabe *et al.*, 1987). There are very striking similarities between the α_1 subunit of the calcium channel and the large subunit of the sodium channel. The α_1 protein contains 1873 amino acids with 29% identity of sequence with the sodium channel protein. Furthermore, the similarity between the α_1 subunit and the Na^+ channel protein extends to its proposed transmembrane topology, containing four internal repeat structures each with five hydrophobic segments and one positively charged segment (S4) (cf. Fig. 5.5). It is likely therefore, that the α_1 subunit of the Ca^{2+} channel complex forms the ion conducting pore of the channel. Amino acid sequence data are also available for the α_2 subunit (Ellis *et al.*, 1988). This protein is highly hydrophilic and contains only three possible transmembrane domains. It is therefore more likely to play a regulatory role than a role in channel formation.

5.3.4. *Reconstitution*

Although a central role for the α_1 channel subunit in channel formation has been proposed, the identification of four other polypeptides which are closely associated with 1,4-dihydropyridine receptor activity in purification studies, raises questions concerning the functional significance of these additional components. To answer these questions Ca^{2+} channels purified on the basis of 1,4-dihydropyridine binding activity have been reconstituted into artificial lipid bilayers for electrophysiological recording. Channel preparations containing both the α subunits, the β subunit and at least one of the γ or δ subunits reconstitute calcium conducting channels with a single channel conductance similar to the L-type channel *in vivo* (Flockerzi *et al.*, 1986). These reconstituted channels were also sensitive to calcium channel antagonists, and to cAMP-dependent phosphorylation, consistent with the reincorporation of complete functional Ca^{2+} channel complexes.

To dissect the functional role of each of the Ca^{2+} channel polypeptides it will be necessary to reconstitute individual subunits or defined mixtures of subunits. Preliminary reports suggest that the α_1 subunit of the rabbit skeletal muscle 1,4-dihydropyridine receptor can reconstitute the large Ca^{2+} conductance channel alone, as one would expect from its sequence similarity with the Na^+ channel protein (Hofmann *et al.*, 1987). However, the kinetics of the reconstituted subunit are different to the channel *in vivo*. This result implies that while the α_1 subunit may constitute the voltage sensor and/or calcium channel pore, the other subunits of the 1,4-dihydropyridine receptor complex play an important role in determining the overall properties of the L-type Ca^{2+} channel. Consistent with this, functional Ca^{2+} channels are obtained by expression, in oocytes, of mRNA derived from cDNA sequence of the α_1 subunit (Mikami *et al.*, 1989). Interestingly, higher Ca^{2+} channel activity is seen when mRNA specific for the α_2 subunit is co-injected.

It has been suggested that the absence of Ca^{2+} current and excitation — contraction coupling in skeletal muscle myocytes from mice with muscular dysgenesis is due to the absence of functional Ca^{2+} channel proteins. Microinjection of an expression plasmid carrying a cDNA encoding the α_1 subunit has been shown to restore both dihydropyridine-sensitive Ca^{2+} conductances and excitation — contraction coupling to these cells (Tanabe *et al.*, 1988). These results also implicate strongly the α_1 polypeptide as a functional Ca^{2+} channel component, but do not resolve the role of the other putative subunits.

5.4. Characterisation and purification of potassium channels

Voltage-sensitive K^+ channels are essential in the control of cell excitability, and play a pivotal role in the determination of the duration of action potentials, the firing patterns of neurones and the amount of transmitter released at nerve terminals. Attempts to subdivide K^+ channels into discrete classes reveal a very wide range of channel types with conductances ranging between 2 and 200 pS (Table 5.4) (Rudy, 1988). The 'classical' K^+ channel is the 'delayed rectifier'. This class of channel opens in response to membrane depolarisation and is responsible for repolarisation of the cell membrane during the later phase of the action potential. Repolarising K^+ current can also be carried by Ca^{2+}-activated

Table 5.4.   Classification of potassium channels (see Rudy, 1988)

Channel class	Properties
Delayed rectifier	Voltage-dependent, slow inactivation
A	Voltage-dependent, fast transient current
Inward rectifier	Activated by membrane hyperpolarisation
Ca^{2+} activated	Activated by rises in intracellular Ca^{2+} concentration
Regulated	Activity regulated by neurotransmitter control of second messenger systems or metabolites

K^+ channels. These channels are activated by membrane depolarisation but only in the presence of intracellular Ca^{2+}. At least two different Ca^{2+}-activated K^+ channels have been described with high (100–200 pS) and low (10–20 pS) conductivities, respectively. Further subdivision, at least in the small conductance class, has been made on the basis of their sensitivity to the bee venom polypeptide, apamin.

A further depolarising current can be measured in cells which fire repetitive action potentials. The channels responsible for this current, known as A channels, serve to dampen the electrical activity of the neurone membrane between successive action potentials. In contrast, some K^+ channels open in response to hyperpolarisation. Known as inward rectifiers, these channels carry K^+ current when the membrane is hyperpolarised and inactivate on depolarisation. Subdivision of K^+ channels can also be made on the basis of their regulation. In addition to K^+ channels that are activated in the presence of Ca^{2+} a variety of other K^+ channels have been shown which are regulated by binding of transmitters, GTP binding proteins, cyclic AMP-dependent kinases, protein kinase C, intracellular ATP concentration and putative second messengers arising from arachidonic acid metabolism.

Comparison of kinetic properties and single-channel conductances within the loosely defined groups above allows yet further subdivision of K^+ channels and serves to illustrate the wide diversity of K^+ channel types compared to those for Na^+ and Ca^{2+}. How many of this large family of K^+ channels are present at the neuromuscular junction remains to be demonstrated. However, there is no doubt that a delayed rectifier is present at the presynaptic nerve terminal which is important for repolarisation following an action potential.

5.4.1. *Structural studies of K^+ channels*

As seen for the Na^+ and Ca^{2+} channels, characterisation of the molecular structures responsible for specific cation fluxes using conventional protein biochemistry depends on either naturally occurring neurotoxic molecules or pharmaceutical agents which bind to and modulate channel function with high affinity. Until recently there were few suitable probes for labelling K^+ channels but in the last few years several neurotoxins have been identified that bind to some of the K^+ channel subtypes. The chapter by Dolly describes the use of dendrotoxin and β-bungarotoxin for the characterisation and purification of the A-type K^+ channel protein, and summarises the use of several other toxins (e.g. apamin, noxiustoxin) which bind to Ca^{2+}-activated channels.

A third K^+ channel which is beginning to be studied is the ATP-sensitive channel. A tritiated, photoaffinity reagent, $[^3H]$-glibenclamide, has identified possible components in the Islets of Langerhans and in the brain (Kramer *et al.*, 1988; Bernardi *et al.*, 1988). A polypeptide of Mr 140,000–150,000 is labelled specifically and has been purified by affinity chromatography.

For each of the K^+ channels, progress in their structural characterisation using classical protein biochemical approaches has been hindered by the very low levels of these proteins in the tissues studied. Using a recombinant DNA approach, however, multiple A-type K^+ channel components have been identified following cloning of cDNA for the 'Shaker' locus of *Drosophila melanogaster* (Schwarz *et al.*, 1988). At least five different protein products appear to be derived from the Shaker gene by alternative splicing at the messenger RNA level. Although much smaller than the subunit of the voltage-sensitive Na^+ channel, the K^+ channel proteins appear to share structural similarities with both the Na^+ and Ca^{2+} channel proteins (see Dolly, this volume). Alternative splicing of the messenger RNA may generate multiple tissue-specific K^+ channel subtypes with different physiological properties. If more than one protein product is expressed per tissue, heteromultimeric complexes may occur, each differing in tissue distribution, developmental expression and in their physiological properties. These possibilities remain to be established.

5.4.2. *Common design for voltage-sensitive cation channels*

In each case where amino acid sequence data are available the proposed core structures of the voltage-sensitive channels appear to be related. The similarity in the amino acid sequence of the α_1 Ca^{2+} channel protein with that of the α subunit of the voltage-sensitive Na^+ channel suggests that these two proteins have arisen from a common ancestral gene. When these two proteins are compared with the various K^+ channel proteins from *Drosophila*, little overall similarity is seen with respect to primary sequence. Exceptions to this are the S4-like region and seven other residues which are conserved within the hydrophobic segments (see Dolly, this volume). More similarity is seen when the overall structures are compared. At this level one K^+ channel protein would be the equivalent of a single internal repeat in either the Ca^{2+} or Na^+ channel proteins. It is possible, therefore, that all the voltage-sensitive cation channels have arisen from a common ancestral gene. In this case gene duplication would be sufficient to explain the more complex products of the Ca^{2+} and Na^+ channel genes.

While the molecular structure of the channels responsible for stimulating the release of transmitter at the neuromuscular junction remains to be determined, our knowledge from those in other systems gives us much insight into the possible structural organisation of these macromolecules. Information regarding the channels at the neuromuscular junction will probably be derived by comparison with channels in other tissues where biochemical investigation is not so severely hampered by the restricted amount of material available for study.

References

Barhanin, J., Schmid, A., Lombet, A., Wheeler, K. P., Lazdunski, M and Ellory, J. C. (1983) Molecular size of different neurotoxin receptors on the voltage-sensitive Na^+ channel. *J. Biol. Chem.* **258**: 700–702.

Barhanin, J., Meiri, H., Romey, G., Pauron, D. and Lazdunski, M. (1985) A monoclonal immunotoxin acting on the Na^+ channel, with properties similar to those of a scorpion toxin. *Proc. Natl. Acad. Sci, USA* **82**: 1842–1846.

Bernardi, H., Fosset, M. and Lazdunski, M. (1988) Characterisation, purification and affinity labelling of the brain ^{3}H-glibenclamide-binding protein, a putative neuronal ATP-regulated K^+ channel. *Proc. Natl. Acad. Sci. USA* **85**: 9816–9820.

Catterall, W. A. (1980) Neurotoxins that act on voltage-sensitive sodium channels in excitable membranes. *Ann. Rev. Pharm. Toxicol.* **20**: 15–43.

Catterall, W. A. (1986) Molecular properties of voltage-sensitive sodium channels. *Ann. Rev. Biochem.* **55**: 953–985.

Catterall, W. A. (1988) Structure and function of voltage-sensitive ion channels. *Science* **242**: 50–61.

Catterall, W. A., Seager, M. J. and Takahashi, M. (1988) Molecular properties of dihydropyridine-sensitive calcium channels in skeletal muscle. *J. Biol. Chem.*, **263**: 3535–3538.

Ellis, S. B., Williams, M. E., Ways, N. R., Brenner, R., Sharp, A. H., Leung, A. T., Campbell, K. P., Mckenna, E., Koch, W. J., Hui, A., Schwartz, A. and Harpold, M. M. (1988) Sequence and expression of mRNAs encoding the α_1 and α_2 subunits of a DHP-sensitive calcium channel. *Science* **241**: 1661–1664.

Flockerzi, V., Oeken, H.-J., Hofman, F., Pelzer, D., Cavalie, A. and Twautwein, W. (1986) Purified dihydropyridine-binding site from skeletal muscle t-tubules is a functional calcium channel. *Nature* **323**: 66–86.

Glossman, H., Ferry, D. R., Goll, A., Streissnig, J., and Zernig, G. (1985) Calcium channels and calcium channel drugs: recent biochemical and biophysical findings. *Arzneim.-Forsch. Drug Res.* **35**: 1917–1935.

Glossman, H., Ferry, D. R., Streissnig, J., Goll, A. and Moosburger, K. (1987) Resolving the structure of the Ca^{2+} channel by photoaffinity labelling. *Trends Pharmacol. Sci.* **8**: 95–100.

Hille, B. (1984) *Ionic Channels of Excitable Membranes*, Sinnauer, Sunderland, MA.

Hofmann, F., Naistainczk, W., Rohrkasten, A., Schneider, T., and Sieber, M. (1987) Regulation of the L-type calcium channel. *Trends Pharmacol. Sci.* **8**: 393–398.

Kramer, W., Oekonomopulos, R., Punter, J. and Summ, H.-D. (1988) Direct photoaffinity labelling of the putative sulphonylurea receptor in rat β-cell tumor membranes by ^{3}H-glibenclamide. *FEBS Lett.* **299**: 355–359.

McClesky, E. W., Fox, A. P., Feldman, D. and Tsien, R. W. (1986) Different types of calcium channels. *J. Exp. Biol.* **124**: 177–190.

Meiri, H., Goren, E., Bergmann, H., Zeitoun, I., Rosenthal, Y. and Palti, Y. (1986) Specific modulation of sodium channels in mammalian nerve by monoclonal antibodies. *Proc. Nalt. Acad. Sci. USA* **83**: 8385–8389.

Meiri, H., Spira, G., Sammar, M., Namir, M., Schwartz, A., Komunya, A., Kosower, E. M. and Palti, Y. (1987) Mapping a region associated with Na$^+$ channel inactivation using antibodies to a synthetic peptide corresponding to a part of the channel. *Proc. Natl. Acad. Sci. USA* **84**: 5058–5062.

Noda, M., Ikeda, T., Kayano, T., Suzuki, H., Takeshima, H., Kurasaki, M., Takahashi, H. and Numa, S. (1986a) Existence of distinct sodium channel messenger RNAs in rat brain. *Nature* **320**: 188–192.

Noda, M., Ikeda, T., Suzuki, H., Takeshima, H., Takahashi, T., Kuno, M. and Numa, S. (1986b) Expression of functional sodium channels from cloned cDNA. *Nature* **322**: 826–828.

Noda, M., Shimizu, S., Tanabe, T., Takai, T., Kayano, T., Ikeda, T., Takahashi, H., Nakayama, H., Kanaoka, Y., Minamino, N., Kangawa, K., Matsuo, H., Raftery, M. A., Hirose, T., Inayama, S., Hayashida, H., Miyata, T. and Numa, S. (1984) Primary structure of *Electrophorus electricus* sodium channel deduced from cDNA sequence. *Nature* **312**: 121–127.

Mikami, A., Imoto, K., Tanabe, T., Niidome, T., Mori, Y., Takeshima, H., Narumiya, S. and Numa, S. (1989) Primary structure and functional expression of the cardiac dihydropyridine-sensitive calcium channel. *Nature* **340**: 230–233.

Oiki, S., Danho, W. and Montal, M. (1988) Channel protein engineering: synthetic 22-mer peptide from the primary structure of the voltage-sensitive sodium channel forms ionic channels in lipid bilayers. *Proc. Natl. Acad. Sci.* **85**: 2393–2397.

Rudy, B. (1988) Diversity and ubiquity of K$^+$ channels. *Neuroscience* **25**: 729–749.

Schwartz, T. L., Tempel, B. L., Papazian, D. M., Jan, Y. N. and Jan, L. Y. (1988) Multiple potassium-channel components are produced by alternative splicing at the Shaker locus in *Drosophila*. *Nature* **331**: 137–142.

Strichartz, G., Rando, T. and Wang, G. K. (1987) An integrated view of the molecular toxicology of sodium channel gating in excitable cells. *Ann. Rev. Neurosci.* **10**: 237–267.

Stühmer, W., Conti, F., Suzuki, H., Wang, X., Noda, M., Yahagi, N., Kubo, H. and Numa, S. (1989) Structural parts involved in activation and inactivation of the sodium channel. *Nature* **339**: 597–603.

Takahashi, M., Seagar, M. J., Jones, J. F., Bernhard, F. X. R. and Catterall, W. A. (1987). Subunit structure of dihydropyridine-sensitive calcium channels from skeletal muscle. *Proc. Natl. Acad. Sci. USA* **84**: 5478–5482.

Tanabe, T., Takeshima, H., Mikami, A., Flockerzi, V., Takahashi, H., Kangawa, K., Kojima, M., Matsuo, H., Hirose, T. and Numa, S. (1987) Primary structure of the receptor for calcium channel blockers from skeletal muscle. *Nature* **328**: 313–318.

Tanabe, Y., Beam, K. G., Powell, J. A., and Numa, S. (1988) Restoration of excitation-contraction coupling and slow calcium current in dysgenic muscle by dihydropyridine receptor complementary DNA. *Nature* **336**: 134–139.

Tosteson, M. T., Auld, D. S. and Tosteson, D. C. (1989) Voltage-gated channels formed in lipid bilayers by a positively charged segment of the Na$^+$ channel polypeptide. *Proc. Natl. Acad. Sci. USA* **86**: 707–710.

Vassilev, P. M., Scheuer, T. and Catterall, W. A. (1988) Identification of an intracellular peptide segment involved in sodium channel inactivation. *Science* **241**: 1658–1661.

Functional components at nerve terminals revealed by neurotoxins

6.1. Introduction

An astonishing number of different animals and smaller organisms rely on highly specific neurotoxins to paralyse their prey. This chapter and that by Robert Norman detail the actions of some of these toxins and the nature of their targets; in particular they illustrate the way in which their unique specificities can be harnessed to the study of molecular neurobiology.

Over the past few decades electrophysiological analysis has provided an understanding of the overall process of synaptic transmission, and recent biochemical studies have yielded a wealth of information on the struc-tural/functional properties of several of the receptors and ion channels involved (see Beeson and Barnard, and Norman, this volume). On the other hand, insight gained into the molecular mechanism of transmitter release has been minimal (reviewed by Dunant, 1986), due primarily to the paucity of data available on the presynaptic macromolecules involved. In recent years several toxins that perturb neurotransmission in very selective fashions have been identified (for a list of neurotoxins see Table 3.3, in chapter 3); this review highlights progress being made in the biochemical characterisation of the functional components to which they bind. Emphasis will be placed on the microbial proteins, botulinum (BoNT) and tetanus (TETX) toxins, on dendrotoxins (DTX) from the green mamba, and other K^+ channel toxins. BoNT and TETX display unique abilities to inhibit transmitter release intracellularly, whereas DTX modifies sec-retion by blocking K^+ channels that control cell excitability. Both BoNT (Elston, 1988) and blockers or openers of certain K^+ channels are proving to be of therapeutic use (Cook, 1988).

6.2. Clostridial neurotoxins — probes for studying protein transport and transmitter release

6.2.1. *General properties*

BoNT and TETX are large ($M_r \sim 150,000$), highly toxic proteins, produced respectively by *Clostridium botulinum and C. tetani* and responsible for botulism and tetanus. Both toxins are synthesised as single polypeptides

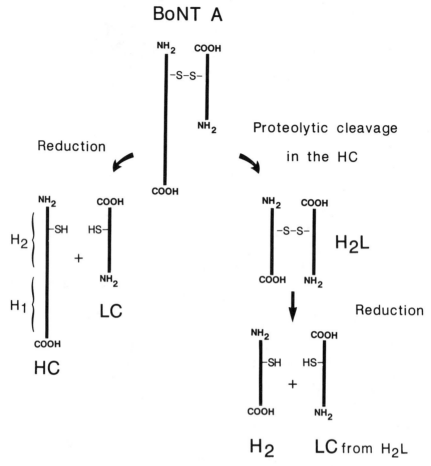

Fig. 6.1. Schematic drawing of the general structure of BoNT, its chains and fragments. Equivalent TETX preparations have been isolated.

and later cleaved by endogenous proteases to yield the fully active 'nicked' forms comprising two disulphide-linked polypeptides with M_r of $\approx 95,000$ (heavy chain, HC) and $\approx 50,000$ (light chain, LC) (reviewed by Dolly *et al.*, 1988; Fig. 6.1). An appreciable degree of homology between BoNT and TETX is apparent when the primary structure of the TETX chains (derived from the cloned nucleotide sequences (Eisel *et al.*, 1986)) are compared with the known partial amino acid sequences of the BoNT chains.

The functional domains of these proteins can be studied by isolation and renaturation of their constituent chains, and of proteolytic fragments (Fig. 6.1). Despite striking similarities in their overall structures and some shared pharmacological properties (outlined later), dramatic differences exist in the clinical effects of these two microbial toxins. Whereas BoNT blocks preferentially acetylcholine (ACh) release from peripheral motor nerves, TETX inhibits transmitter release in certain inhibitory pathways (e.g. glycine) of the central nervous system (CNS); hence, they cause flaccid and spastic paralysis, respectively.

6.2.2. *Comparison of the inhibition of ACh release by BoNT and TETX*

Several types (A–G) of BoNT are produced, respectively, by different strains of *Clostridium botulinum*. All these proteins are approximately the same size and have the general structure depicted in Fig. 6.1. They contain some common epitopes (antibody binding sites) recognised by certain monoclonal antibodies, but can be distinguished by specific antisera. All the toxins produce a near-irreversible (lasting weeks), specific blockade of ACh release from peripheral nerve terminals. The basis of their amazing toxicity (≈ 10 pg kills a mouse) is a remarkably specific reduction in both spontaneous and stimulated quantal release of ACh; no *direct* alteration in any other parameter is detectable although a rapid, partial inhibition by BoNT of the molecular leakage (non-quantal release, see Molenaar, this volume) of ACh from motor nerves has been documented (see Sellin, 1987).

Although treatment of muscle with BoNT A *in vitro* reduces dramatically spontaneous quantal release of ACh (Fig. 6.2; Table 6.1), detected as normal miniature endplate potentials (MEPPs; see chapter 2), a minor species of MEPPs displaying Ca^{2+} insensitivity, slow-rise times and with skewed amplitude distribution, remains unaltered (Dolly *et al.*, 1987a). The same intoxication regime virtually abolishes nerve-stimulated quan-

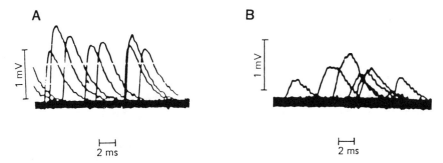

Fig. 6.2 Effect of BoNT A on transmitter release in the mouse diaphragm. MEPPs at a control endplate (**A**); MEPPs after treatment with 10 nM BoNT (**B**). Note the slow rise-times. Many more oscilloscope sweeps were needed since the frequency of MEPPs was markedly reduced. Taken with permission from Dolly *et al.* (1987a).

Table 6.1. Effects of clostridial neurotoxins on spontaneous and nerve-evoked ACh release in triangularis sterni muscle of adult mice

	Spontaneous release frequency (MEPPs/min)	Nerve-evoked release (quanta/pulse)	
		Without 4-AP	With 4-AP
Control	473 ± 24	112 ± 15[a]	728 ± 167[b]
After treatment with	Percentage of control values		
BoNT A	0.3	0.008	1.11
BoNT B	4.0	0.124	0.44
TETX	5.4	0.080	0.35

Values reflect mean ± SE; data were acquired at 37°C.

[a] Value corresponds to the ratio of mean endplate current to the mean miniature endplate current from 17 muscle fibres voltage clamped at −70 mV. Currents were measured using conventional two-electrode voltage clamp techniques.

[b] Value was calculated by scaling the mean number of quanta constituting a normal endplate potential by a factor derived from the ratio of endplate current amplitude in test solution (100 μM 4-AP) to that in control solution ($n = 10$). In these experiments d-tubocurarine (1.5 μM) was present to avoid muscle twitching and to allow the measurement of the relative amplitude of endplate currents in the same muscle fibre under both conditions.

Adapted from Gansel *et al.* (1987).

tal release (Table 6.1). This effect of BoNT A appears to result from a lowering of the Ca^{2+}-sensitivity of the release system. Accordingly, evoked release at endplates treated with BoNT A can be reversed, to variable extents, by raising the intracellular Ca^{2+} concentration: e.g. using high-frequency nerve stimulation, Ca^{2+} ionophores or K^+ channel blockers. An example of the latter, 4-aminopyridine (4-AP), produces a measurable increase in quantal release at treated and untreated endplates but it must be emphasised that the level of release remains minimal relative to that of control muscles not exposed to toxin (Table 6.1).

Curiously, the blockade caused by other types of BoNT (e.g. B) is usually less complete, maintained over a shorter period (reviewed in Sellin, 1987), and responds less well to 4-AP (Table 6.1). Moreover, the asynchronous release produced by high-frequency stimulation of motor nerves treated with B or F toxins (Sellin, 1987) is never seen with BoNT A (Fig. 6.3). Intriguingly, the pattern of inhibition of ACh release produced by TETX (which can also block ACh release at the neuromuscular junction, but with much lower potency than BoNT) was identical to that of BoNT B in terms of blockade of spontaneous or evoked (in the absence or presence of 4-AP) release (Table 6.1), and in causing desynchronisation of stimulated release (Fig. 6.3).

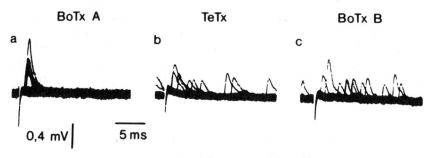

Fig. 6.3. Effects of clostridial neurotoxins on quantal release evoked by 50 Hz nerve stimulation. **a–c**, Superimposed traces in fast time sweep, revealing either synchronous (**a**, 1000 traces) or asynchonous (**b, c**, 100 traces) release of quanta. From Gansel *et al.* (1987).

In summary, the pharmacological effects of TETX and BoNT B (and F) at motor endplates are similar by most criteria (see Gansel *et al.*, 1987), but details of their actions differ significantly from the inhibition produced by type A BoNT. This generalisation is reinforced by experimental results of the 'double-poisoning' of motor nerves with TETX and BoNT A or B (Gansel *et al.*, 1987). The collective findings have been incorporated into a

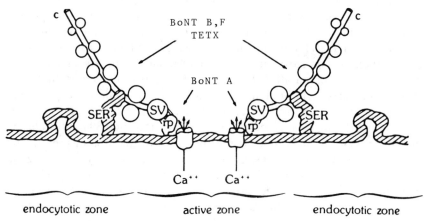

Fig. 6.4. Hypothetical scheme of a motor nerve terminal near an active zone. Synaptic vesicles (SV) arrive at the release sites via the cytoskeletal matrix (c) made up of microtubules, actin and smooth endoplasmic reticulum (SER). Attachment of SV to the cytoskeleton is mediated by proteins including synapsin I (see also Chapter 1). Ca^{2+} enters the nerve terminal through voltage-dependent channels and interacts with a Ca^{2+}-sensitive releasing protein (rp) which facilitates release. The rp may be part of the cytoskeletal matrix or directly associated with the pre-synaptic membrane. Type A BoNT may act on the Ca^{2+} sensitive rp, whereas TETX and BoNT types B and F might act by affecting the availability of vesicles for the release process. Adapted from Sellin (1987).

hypothetical model as depicted in Fig. 6.4. It is envisaged that BoNT A lowers the Ca^{2+}-responsiveness of a macromolecule in the release process whilst TETX, and certain other BoNT types, probably alter the interaction of transmitter vesicles with a component of the cytoskeleton, thereby perturbing synchronised release. The molecular identity of these different target sites remains to be established.

6.2.3. *Internalisation of BoNT at cholinergic nerve endings and the transport of TETX into inhibitory terminals*

In the peripheral nervous system, BoNT blocks primarily transmitter release at nicotinic and muscarinic junctions (Dolly *et al.*, 1988), consistent with the dominant symptoms seen in patients or livestock suffering from botulism. In contrast, inhibition of excitatory noradrenergic transmission in rat anococcygeus muscle, for instance, was not detectable following *in vitro* exposure to BoNT A, except when the preparation was stimulated at low frequency. Consistent with the toxins' cholinergic specificity, electron microscope autoradiographic studies (Dolly *et al.*, 1984a; Black and Dolly, 1986b) showed that ^{125}I-labelled BoNT A and B target to cholinergic nerve terminals in mouse diaphragm muscle and become internalised (Fig. 6.5A). The uptake step, which is temperature-sensitive and energy-dependent (can be prevented by inhibitors of energy production) relies on the presence of saturable binding sites (acceptors) on the plasma membrane (Fig. 6.5B). These acceptors are probably not the pharmacological target of BoNT but play an unknown physiological role; the toxins exploit them to gain entry into the nerve terminals. Similar examination of a mouse ileum preparation labelled with ^{125}I-BoNT showed that only cholinergic nerves can bind and internalise the toxin, unlike peptidergic, purinergic and adrenergic nerve endings. Distinct binding sites exist for types A and B BoNT at respective densities of 150 and $630/m\mu^2$ of plasma membrane, and their location is not restricted to the area of presynaptic membrane from which transmitter release occurs (i.e. the active zone regions, see chapter 1). BoNT acceptors also occur on cholinergic neurones in the CNS, but they are unable to internalise the toxin efficiently (Black and Dolly, 1987); this could explain the negligible central toxicity of BoNT.

Based on these findings, and the numerous demonstrations that BoNT decreases transmitter release from brain neuronal preparations when access *is* achieved (reviewed by Dolly *et al.*, 1988), it can be concluded that acceptor-mediated *uptake* of BoNT by cholinergic nerves in the periphery makes them highly sensitive to these toxins. By analogy, the selectivity of TETX for inhibitory nerve endings could arise from the presence thereon of specific acceptors that mediate efficiently its translocation into the cytoplasm and thereby its local action. This highly specific uptake system

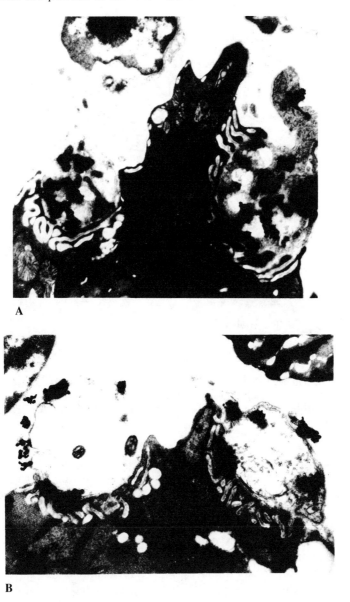

A

B

Fig. 6.5. Electron-microscope autoradiograms of a neuromuscular preparation prelabelled with ^{125}I-BoNT A showing acceptor-mediated targeting and internalisation of the toxin. In (**A**) a discrete deposition of silver grains is seen in the two nerve endings, with a significant proportion of the toxin internalised. Inclusion of an inhibitor of energy production, sodium azide (**B**), prevents the uptake step and reveals the labelled acceptors all around the unmyelinated plasma membrane of the terminals. The complete absence of grains elsewhere demonstrates the remarkable specificity of BoNT. Adapted from Dolly *et al.* (1984a).

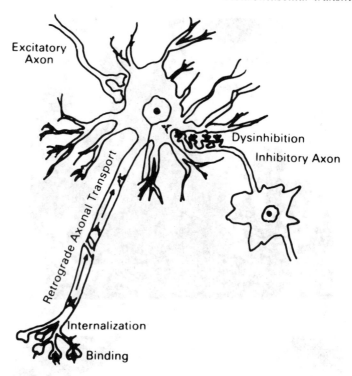

Fig. 6.6. Schematic representation of TETX binding, internalisation, retrograde axonal transport and subsequent selective trans-synaptic transfer from motor neurone dendrites to presynaptic terminals of inhibitory neurones. Taken with permission from Lazarovici *et al.* (1988).

must differ from that involved in the long-distance transport of TETX from the motor nerve terminals of the neuromuscular junction. For the latter, multi-phasic mechanisms are postulated. A hypothetical scheme (see Fig. 6.6) encompassing binding to membrane acceptors on motor nerve terminals, internalisation, retrograde axonal transport and then trans-synaptic transfer into presynaptic inhibitory neurones (via the specific acceptor) where it produces dysinhibition (Lazarovici *et al.*, 1988). Elegant electron microscopic experiments using TETX-collodial gold have clearly demonstrated endocytotic uptake of toxin via coated pits into cultured neurons of mouse spinal cord (Fig. 6.7), probably by means of a high-affinity protein binding site (Critchley *et al.*, 1988).

Even though binding and internalisation steps have been documented for BoNT (see above), and the ^{125}I-labelled BoNT has been demonstrated inside axons (Black and Dolly, 1986c), there is no convincing evidence for retrograde axonal transport *comparable* to that for TETX. As the intracellular inhibitory actions of BoNT and TETX are not transmitter-

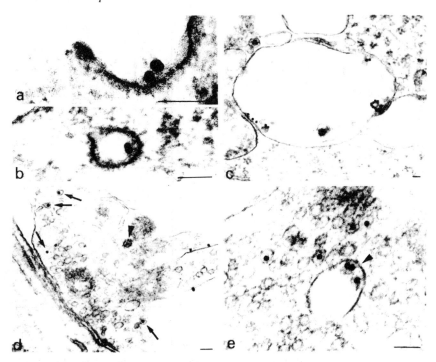

Fig. 6.7. Internalisation of TETX-gold by mouse spinal cord neurones in culture following different incubation conditions. (**a**) 1 h at 4°C, toxin-gold particles are shown inside a coated pit on the surface of the cell body; (**b**) 5 min, 37°C, gold particles are inside an apparent coated vesicle within the cell body; (**c**) 15 min, 37°C, gold particles within a multi-vesicular body; (**d**) 5 min, 37°C; gold particles within a coated vesicle (arrowhead) and in apparent synaptic vesicles in a nerve terminal; (**e**) 15 min, 37°C; gold particles within synaptic vesicles and a larger uncoated vesicle. Bar 0.1 μm. Taken with permission from Critchley *et al.* (1988).

specific (see later), apparent differences in their uptake and translocation could explain (at least so far) why BoNT acts locally at motor nerve endings whereas inhibitory postsynaptic potentials in spinal cord neurones are most susceptible to TETX (Bergey *et al.*, 1987).

6.2.4. *BoNT and TETX inactivate intracellular components concerned with* Ca^{2+}-*induced secretion in a variety of cells*

Direct evidence for an intraneuronal site of action for BoNT was obtained by microinjection of the toxin into the large presynaptic neurones of *Aplysia*, and measurement of changes in quantal transmitter release by recording the response in the postsynaptic neurone (Poulain *et al.*, 1988). Intracellular administration of minute quantities of BoNT A or B (Fig. 6.8)

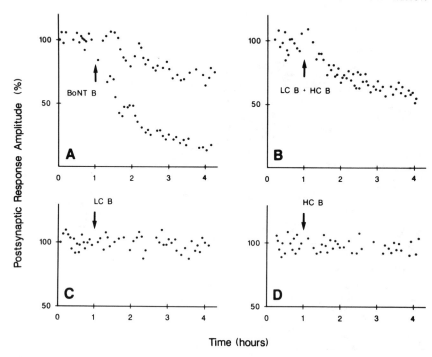

Fig. 6.8.   Decrease in evoked release of ACh by intracellular administration of BoTX or *both* its chains into identified neurones of the buccal ganglion of *Aplysia*. ACh release was evoked by a presynaptic action potential and the amplitude of the postsynaptic response measured before and after (arrow) microinjecting the toxin sample into the presynaptic neurone. The postsynaptic response was plotted against time as a percentage of the control value for that cell. Injection of 1% of the cell volume with 'nicked' BoNT B (0.12 µg/ml, upper and 1.2 µg/ml, lower) gave a time- and concentration-dependent block of quantal release (**A**), as did intraneuronal application of both the separated chains (**B**). In contrast neither the separated renatured LC (**C**) nor HC (**D**) chains were effective. Adapted from Poulain *et al.* (1988) and Maisey *et al.* (1988).

into identified cholinergic neurones in the buccal ganglion diminished nerve-evoked ACh release, without causing any other measurable changes. It was even more striking to find a similar blockade when a non-cholinergic neurone in the cerebral ganglion was treated similarly with BoNT A. In addition, BoNT has been shown to inhibit exocytosis in chromaffin cells (Penner *et al.*, 1986a), and to reduce Ca^{2+}-dependent release of catecholamines from cultured PC12 cells (McInnes *et al.*, 1990) when toxin uptake was facilitated by the use of permeabilisation techniques. These results showed that BoNT acts intracellularly, with similar efficacy, to block release of ACh and the other substances tested. Likewise, TETX has been reported to block exocytosis from chromaffin cells when delivered intracellularly (Penner *et al.*, 1986a; Bittner and Holtz, 1988). Hence, BoNT and TETX may be universal inhibitors of Ca^{2+}-dependent secretion; further experiments in other cells will establish if their targets are truly ubiquitous constituents and could highlight similarities in secretion between neuronal and non-neuronal tissues.

Clearly, the continued use of these unique toxin probes will yield insight into the mechanism and/or control of transmitter release; it will be particularly interesting, in view of their distinct effects (see Fig. 6.4), to determine whether BoNT A and TETX modify different targets or sites. In this regard it is noteworthy that some differences have already emerged in their functional domains. In the case of BoNT A and B (Fig. 6.8), experiments with *Aplysia* neurones have shown that the presence of both chains intracellularly is required for the inhibition of ACh release (Poulain *et al.*, 1988; Maisey *et al.*, 1988) whereas the LC chain of TETX alone is effective (Mochida *et al.*, 1989). The LC of either toxin blocks exocytosis in chromaffin or PC12 cells when the uptake barrier is bypassed (Ahnert-Hilger *et al.*, 1989; McInnes *et al.*, 1990). Further investigations on the intracellular action of the toxins' chains in mammalian motor neurones are required to clarify this discrepancy in the different systems studied. Moreover, comparison of the forthcoming amino acid sequence of BoNT with that available for TETX may shed light on the assignment of structural domains to various roles in the multi-phasic process of intoxication with each toxin.

6.2.5. *Clinical use of BoNT for treating movement disorders*

The cholinergic specificity of BoNT and its selective targeting properties, together with the long duration of paralysis produced by type A (see above), form the basis of its suitability as a therapeutic agent. The original work by Scott (1980) was directed towards the management of strabismus by injecting minute doses of the toxin into single extra-ocular muscles. This has proved in general to have only a temporary effect on the condition, although there are situations in which it has become the treatment of choice (reviewed by Elston, 1988). It is in the treatment of involuntary movement disorders, however, that the use of botulinum toxin is a major therapeutic advance. If such movements are limited to relatively small muscles, or groups of muscles, appropriate doses of the toxin can be used to weaken the fibres without producing a complete palsy. Unwanted movements are thereby abolished for periods of up to 3 months. Examples of conditions treated in this way are blepharospasm, ie. bilateral forceful involuntary eye closure (Fig. 6.9A,B), and hemifacial spasm, in which only the muscles on one side of the face are involved (Fig. 6.9C,D). Other disorders treated with reasonable success include spasmodic torticollis, lateral rectus paresis and external urethral sphincter spasticity (reviewed

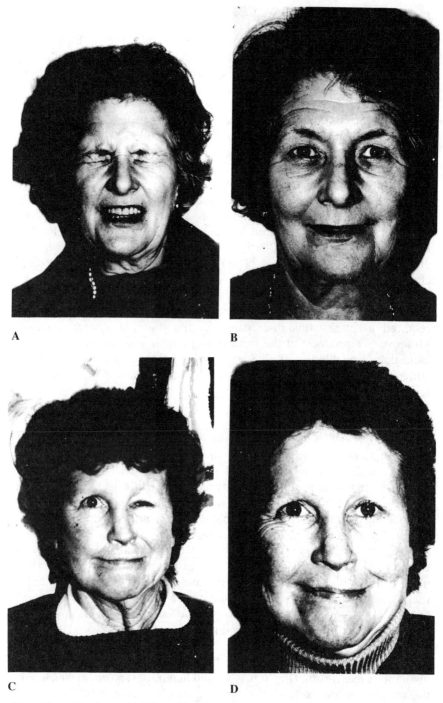

Fig. 6.9. A patient with idiopathic blepharospasm shown before (**A**) and after (**B**) treatment with botulinum toxin injections. Another patient with left hemifacial spasm before (**C**) and after treatment (**D**). These pictures were kindly provided by Dr J. Elston, The National Hospital, Queen Square, and reproduced with permission of the patients.

in Elston, 1988; Sellin, 1987). Apart from the current uses of BoNT in studying secretion, membrane traffic and protein transport, the ability of non-toxic fragments to interact selectively with cholinergic nerves may possibly allow other therapeutic agents to be targeted into diseased neurones.

6.3. Neuronal K^+ channels identified by toxins

K^+ channels are ubiquitous membrane proteins that serve important roles in the nervous system, particularly the control of cell excitability and synaptic transmission. These channels have been categorised into several groups including: voltage-dependent, Ca^{2+}-activated, ATP-sensitive, neurotransmitter and second messenger-operated (reviewed by Castle *et al.*, 1989). This multiplicity of K^+ channels is complicated further by the existence of several variants within each group that show tissue and/or species specificity. A recent awareness of the physiological importance of such channels in different cells, together with the imminent possibility of developing type-specific drugs, has intensified research in this area; the involvement of certain G proteins in modulating some K^+ currents (cf. Miller, 1988) has increased interest even further. However, the lack of agents capable of distinguishing these various K^+ conductances has in the past limited progress. Fortunately, in recent years an array of peptide toxins active on K^+ channels has been discovered (reviewed by Moczydlowski *et al.*, 1988). Their properties will be described here. Together with the successful application of molecular genetics these are affording exciting advances in the characterisation of these important and heterogeneous proteins.

6.3.1. *β-Bungarotoxin, DTX and mast cell degranulating peptide*

Much of the early work on such toxins concerned β-bungarotoxin (β-BuTX) because of its notable toxicity and overall inhibitory action on neuromuscular transmission (reviewed in Dolly *et al.*, 1988). This basic protein, distinct from the α-toxin that blocks postsynaptic AChR (see Beeson and Barnard, this volume), is isolated from the venom of the banded krait and consists of a 7500 M_r polypeptide disulphide-linked to a 13,500 M_r chain that is homologous to Ca^{2+}-activated phospholipase A_2 enzymes. Although other snake venoms possess related toxins with varied structures but containing similar phospholipase A_2 activity, only β-BuTX acts exclusively on the presynaptic membrane at motor end-plates; this unique feature has made it the most attractive of these probes, at least for studies on transmitter release.

Extensive electrophysiological experiments have shown that β-BuTX has a multi-phasic action at the neuromuscular junction. This involves an initial inhibition, then facilitation and finally an irreversible blockade of ACh release. Inhibition of neurotransmission in the CNS was demonstrated by extracellular recording in slices of rodent olfactory cortex, and this was attributed to a preferential (though not exclusive) action on nerve terminal membranes (Halliwell and Dolly, 1982). Accordingly, a ^{3}H-derivative of β-BuTX was found to bind saturably and with high affinity ($K_D \simeq 5 \times 10^{-10}$ M; $B_{max} \simeq 150$ fmol/mg protein) to proteinaceous acceptors on synaptosomal membranes of rat cortex (Othman *et al.*, 1982). Both DTX and toxin I (a close homologue) prevented this binding, consistent with the mutual antagonism between these toxins in their action at the neuromusclar junction (Harvey and Karlsson, 1982) and in synaptosomes (Dolly *et al.*, 1987b).

This pioneering research provided essential clues to the usefulness as probes (Dolly *et al.*, 1984b) of DTX and toxin I, basic single-chain polypeptides from the venom of eastern green and black mambas, containing 59 and 60 residues respectively. Unlike β-BuTX, these smaller toxins lack enzyme activity. Interestingly, both facilitate transmitter release in the peripheral (Harvey and Karlsson, 1982; Harvey *et al.*, 1984) and central (Dolly *et al.*, 1984b, 1987b) nervous systems. Mamba venoms also contain 'fasciculins', inhibitors of ACh esterase, and a novel peptide that may inhibit presynaptic muscarinic AChRs. All these toxic peptides could act synergistically, to increase the postsynaptic effect of ACh, and lead to the intense muscle fasciculations that result in death (Dajas *et al.*, 1988). A basis for the action of DTX and toxin I became apparent when it was discovered (Dolly *et al.*, 1984b; Halliwell *et al.*, 1986) that they inhibit selectively a fast, transient outward K^+ current (A-type) in hippocampal neurones. As such hyperpolarising K^+ conductances are very important in controlling neurone excitability by 'dampening' depolarising inputs, we proposed that their removal by the toxins might explain the convulsive, facilitatory effects observed.

With attention focused on them, these novel K^+ channel probes were subsequently found to inhibit a family of fast, voltage-activated, 4-AP-sensitive K^+ conductances in various peripheral neurones (reviewed in Dolly *et al.*, 1987b; Dolly, 1988). Both toxins are most effective in blocking slowly inactivating variants of this group of K^+ conductances (Fig. 6.10 A) in rat nodose ganglion A cells (Stansfeld *et al.*, 1986, 1987), dorsal root ganglion neurones (Penner *et al.*, 1986b) and at frog node of Ranvier (Benoit and Dubois, 1986). Mast cell degranulating peptide (MCDP) from bee venom also blocks the DTX-sensitive K^+ current in nodose A cells (Stansfeld *et al.*, 1987, Fig. 6.10 A), thus identifying a neuronal target for this toxin that could explain its epileptiform activity (Cherubini *et al.*, 1988) and provide a role for its binding sites in the CNS (Rehm *et al.*, 1988). Curiously, although neurones in superior cervical or dorsal root ganglia and in nodose ganglion C cells possess K^+ current variants with fast

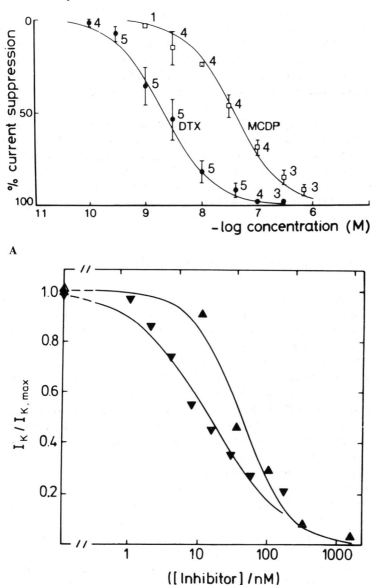

A

B

Fig. 6.10. Dose–response curves for the inhibition by DTX or MCDP of voltage-activated K$^+$ currents in rat sensory neurons (A; ●, DTX; □, MCDP), and in *Xenopus* oocytes (B; ▼, DTX; ▲, MCDP) injected three days previously with cRNA encoding a K$^+$ channel protein from rat brain. The latter was prepared using a rat brain cDNA derived from a cDNA library which had been probed with the *Drosophila* Shaker cDNA for the A-type K$^+$ channel. **A**, from Stansfeld *et al.* (1987); **B**, from Stühmer *et al.* (1988).

inactivation rates, these are virtually insensitive to DTX or 4-AP. Further research is needed to define the relative susceptibility to DTX of the whole spectrum of K^+ current subtypes present in different central and peripheral neurones. Nevertheless, it seems that the slower the inactivation kinetics the greater the sensitivity to both DTX and 4-AP (Dolly *et al.*, 1987b); note that the potency of 4-AP is several orders of magnitude lower and it is less selective.

In view of the appreciable homology in the amino acid sequences of DTX and the smaller chain of β-BuTX, together with the ability of DTX (or toxin I) to prevent β-BuTX binding to its neuronal acceptors (Othman *et al.*, 1982), it is consistent that β-BuTX inhibits a fraction of the voltage-activated K^+ conductance detected at motor nerve terminals (Rowan and Harvey, 1988) and in sensory neurones of dorsal root ganglion (Petersen *et al.*, 1986).

6.3.2. *Use of toxins for identification and localisation of putative K^+ channels*

With electrophysiological evidence available for DTX and β-BuTX as selective ligands it was valid to exploit them in the biochemical character-isation of K^+ channels. Using biologically active ^{125}I-labelled DTX, an apparent homogeneous set of high-affinity binding sites ($K_D \simeq 4 \times 10^{-10}$ M) was detected on synaptosomal membranes of rat cerebral cortex or hippocampus (Dolly *et al.*, 1984b; Black *et al.*, 1986a). However, quantita-tive autoradiographic analysis of rat brain sections labelled with ^{125}I-DTX revealed sites with different affinities in cell layers of cerebellum (Pelchen-Matthews and Dolly, 1989); also, acceptors exhibiting high and low affinity for DTX were detected by binding studies in chick brain (Black and Dolly, 1989) or brain cryostat sections (Pelchen-Matthews and Dolly, demonstrated conclusively by the use of β-BuTX (reviewed in Dolly *et al.*, 1987b, 1988). ^{125}I-β-BuTX binds with high affinity to a subpopulation ($\simeq 25\%$) of the DTX acceptors in rat cerebrocortical synaptosomes (Breeze and Dolly, 1989) or brain cryostat sections (Pelchen-Matthews and Dolly, 1988, 1989) and this is blocked non-competitively by DTX. Additionally, all DTX acceptor subtypes bind β-BuTX, but with low affinity (Black *et al.*, 1988), and interaction at that site seems to underlie the weak ability of β-BuTX to antagonise ^{125}I-DTX binding. Consistent with the relatively low potency of MCDP in inhibiting K^+ conductance, high concentrations of this apian polypeptide were needed to antagonise the binding of both DTX and β-BuTX in the membrane-bound and solubilised states (Stansfeld *et al.*, 1987). Figure 6.11 presents a hypothetical model showing two (though more could exist) acceptor subtypes and the interrelationship of the distinct sites for the numerous toxins. In general support of this scheme, some success has been achieved in using affinity chromatography to isolate,

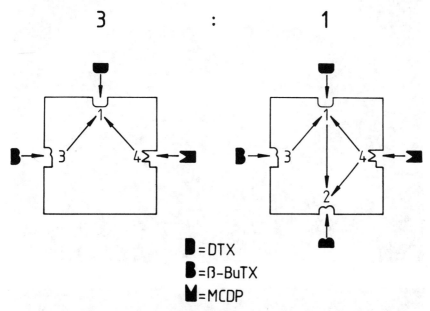

Fig. 6.11. Proposed model of the DTX/β-BuTX/MCDP binding components from rat brain synaptic membranes. One subtype has a high-affinity binding site for β-BuTX (2) as well as the low-affinity site (3) present also on the other. The molar ratio appears to be 1:3. None of the three toxins compete directly with each other. Long arrows represent non-competitive interactions. Adapted from Breeze and Dolly (1989).

from brain synaptic membranes, DTX binding proteins of similar size (Black *et al.*, 1988) that display high or low affinity for β-BuTX (Rehm and Lazdunski, 1988a). Accordingly the acceptors for β-BuTX seem to reside primarily in regions rich in nerve terminals (Fig. 6.12), whilst the DTX sites occur additionally in brain areas containing white matter. These findings indicate that their characteristic locations are adapted to different functions. Hopefully, these acceptor subtypes/K$^+$ channel variants can be discriminated further by new toxins isolated from mamba venom that seem to show differing selectivity for K$^+$ channels (Benishin *et al.*, 1988).

6.3.3. *Structural properties of putative K$^+$ channels*

A subunit of the channel protein ($M_r \simeq 65,000$) was first identified (Mehraban *et al.*, 1984) in rat synaptosomal membranes by cross-linking ^{125}I-DTX to its acceptor, using bifunctional reagents, and analysis by SDS electrophoresis. Experiments performed similarly with chick synaptic membranes yielded a major ($M_r \simeq 75,000$) and a minor ($M_r \simeq 69,000$) polypeptide. As the specific labelling of each with ^{125}I-DTX was reduced

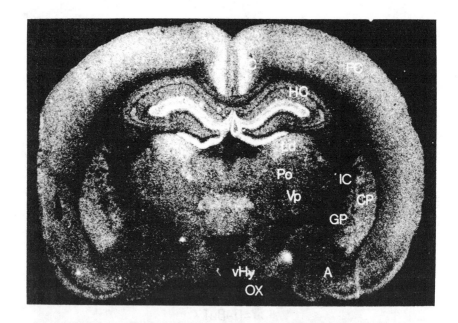

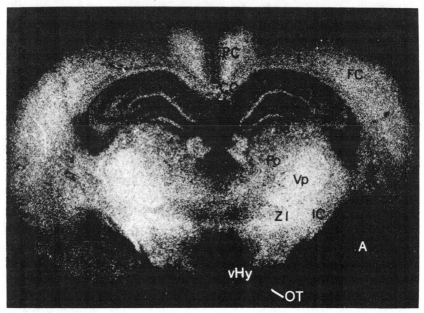

Fig. 6.12. Distribution of ^{125}I-DTX (lower) and ^{125}I-β-BuTx (upper) acceptors/
putative K$^+$ channels in the CNS demonstrated by dark-field images of autoradiograms. In addition to grey matter areas labelled with both toxins, ^{125}I-DTX
appears to bind to white matter regions (e.g. the corpus callosum (CC) and optic
tract (OT)). A, amygdala; FC, frontoparietal cortex; CC, corpus callosum; CP,
caudate putamen; GP, globus pallidus; HC, hippocampal formation; IC, internal
capsule; Ld, laterodorsal thalamic nucleus; OT, optic tract; OX, optic chiasma;
PO, posterior thalamic nuclear group; PC, posterior cingulate cortex; vHY, ventral
hypothalamic area; Vp, ventroposterior thalamic nucleus; Zi, zona incerta.
Adapted from Pelchen-Mathews and Dolly (1988, 1989).

but not abolished by β-BuTX, it was assumed that the two were constituents of both acceptor subtypes (Black and Dolly, 1986b). Cross-linking studies (Rehm *et al.*, 1988) on rat synaptic membranes using ^{125}I-toxin I and ^{125}I-MCDP showed mutually exclusive labelling of a major protein ($M_r \simeq 76,000$), though the possible presence of two non-identical polypeptides was mentioned.

Consistent with discrete sites for the different toxins, each residing on the same acceptor as depicted in the model (Fig. 6.12), the binding activities for DTX, β-BuTX (Black *et al.*, 1988) and MCDP (Rehm *et al.*, 1988) were inseparable following their solubilisation in non-ionic detergent from brain and partial purification by conventional separation methods. Sedimentation analysis of the detergent extracts labelled with ^{125}I-DTX and ^{125}I-β-BuTX gave $S_{20,w} \simeq 13$, and corrected $M_r \simeq 450,000$ (Black *et al.*, 1988). Clearly, therefore, these are oligomeric (multi-subunit) proteins. Complete chromatographic purification of DTX acceptors from rat (Rehm and Lazdunski 1988b) and bovine (Parcej and Dolly, 1989) brain membranes has now been achieved; an affinity for wheat germ lectin indicates that the protein is glycosylated. Both preparations consist of two non-covalently linked subunits with M_r of 37,000 (more intense) and $\simeq$ 75,000, the latter broad band containing the binding sites for DTX and MCDP.

6.3 4. *Sequence of a K$^+$ channel protein predicted from gene cloning*

In a complementary approach to using toxin probes, Shaker mutants (with defective K$^+$ channel) of *Drosophila melanogaster* which exhibit a defective, muscle A-type K$^+$ channel were used to locate and clone the corresponding gene (Schwarz *et al.*, 1988; Pongs *et al.*, 1988). In fact, mRNA for several 'isoforms' of the channel polypeptide occur, ranging in size from 64,000 to 75,000 M_r, due to alternative splicing of a single gene transcript. All the polypeptide products share a common core region that contains several hydrophobic membrane-spanning sequences including the S4-like segment characteristic also of voltage-sensitive Na$^+$ and Ca^{2+} channels; differences are present in N- and C-terminal regions (see also Norman, this volume).

Expression in *Xenopus* oocytes of individual mRNAs gave voltage-dependent, 4-AP-sensitive K$^+$ currents whose kinetics varied with the preparation used (Timpe *et al.*, 1988). Although these resemble an A-type current they are not identical to those detected to date in neuronal membranes; reasons for this anomaly will be discussed below. With the use of the *Drosophila* mRNA sequences as probes, two near-identical genes have been cloned from mouse (Tempel *et al.*, 1988) and rat brain (Baumann *et al.*, 1988); the predicted proteins ($M_r \simeq 56, 400$) show a high degree of homology (>82%; 68% identity) with the fly proteins, particularly in the membrane-spanning regions, and are not dissimilar in size to the larger, toxin-binding subunit of the DTX acceptor (when allowance is made for the attached carbohydrate). The mRNA prepared using the rat brain cDNA has been expressed in oocytes and gave a non-inactivating, tetraethyl-ammonium-sensitive conductance resembling a delayed rectifier K^+ channel (Stühmer *et al.*, 1988).

In view of our work with the toxin acceptors it was reassuring that the K^+ channel was blocked by DTX, MCDP (Fig. 6.10B) or 4-AP but not by β-BuTX. Therefore, it corresponds to the major DTX acceptor subtype (Fig. 6.11) proposed from biochemical studies and is similar to the slowly inactivating K^+ conductance in nodose A cells (Stansfeld *et al.*, 1987). Also these findings, together with the demonstrated inhibition by DTX of a K^+ current in isolated membrane patches of sensory neurones (Stansfeld and Feltz, 1988), show that the toxin acts directly on the channel. The subtle characteristics of the various channel variants are likely (Dolly, 1988) to be created by oligomeric structures of the appropriate subunit composition and stoichiometry; experiments on the expression of *Drosophila* Shaker K^+ channels in oocytes have shown that two distinct mRNAs can contribute to the K^+ current characteristics (Rudy *et al.*, 1988). Moreover, multiple mRNAs have been detected in rat brain using fragments of the cloned K^+ channel as probes (Baumann *et al.*, 1988).

6.3.5. K^+ channels sensitive to other toxins

Noxiustoxin, a 39 residue protein from the Mexican scorpion, was first reported (Carbone *et al.*, 1982) to block selectively and reversibly the delayed rectifier current in squid giant axon. It is two orders of magnitude more potent in stimulating γ-aminobutyrate release from brain synaptosomes and in reducing $^{86}Rb^+$ flux (^{86}Rb is often used for measuring K^+ flux; Sitges *et al.*, 1986). On the other hand, noxiustoxin is a weak blocker of Ca^{2+}-activated, large conductance K^+ channels in skeletal muscle T-tubules, reconsitituted into lipid bilayers (Valdivia *et al.*, 1988). Clearly, this is an interesting toxin whose spectrum of activity on K^+ channel types is still incomplete.

Charybdotoxin, a 37 amino acid basic polypeptide from scorpion venom, blocks the Ca^{2+}-activated, large conductance, voltage-dependent K^+ channels of skeletal muscle T-tubules and other cells (Moczydlowski *et al.*, 1988). It has also been shown to inhibit Ca^{2+}-activated, intermediate conductance K^+ channels in certain cells and a Ca^{2+}-insensitive, voltage-dependent K^+ conductance in lymphocytes (reviewed by Castle *et al.*, 1989). Although charybdotoxin was reported not to affect the delayed rectifier or A-type K^+ channels in *Aplysia* neurones, it does inhibit efficiently two of the three delayed rectifier currents in thymocytes. Also, a K^+ conductance expressed in *Xenopus* oocytes by injecting mRNA encoding for an A-type channel from *Drosophila* was blocked by charybdotoxin (MacKinnon *et al.*, 1988).

Apamin, an 18 residue peptide from the venom of the honey bee, blocks specifically a third type of Ca^{2+}-activated K^+ channel, namely the small-conductance, voltage-insensitive variety (Burgess *et al.*, 1981). In many excitable cells these tetraethylammonium-insensitive channels are involved in the hyperpolarisation that follows an action potential (reviewed by Seager *et al.*, 1988); also, they have been shown to underlie neurotransmitter and hormone-mediated increases in K^+ permeability in several tissues (cf. Castle *et al.*, 1989). Using ^{125}I-labelled apamin, a low content (1–40 fmol/mg protein) of high-affinity binding sites ($K_D \simeq 15$–98 pM) was found in various membrane preparations from CNS and a variety of peripheral tissues (Seager *et al.*, 1988). Although absent from adult innervated skeletal muscle, the apamin-sensitive channel and acceptor sites are detectable in rat fetal muscle, denervated muscle or that from patients with myotonic muscular dystrophy. Photoaffinity labelling studies on neurones and brain synaptic membranes, using an arylazide group attached to different positions on ^{125}I-apamin, yielded polypeptides with M_r of 33,000, 22,000, 86,000 and 59,000. More recently, apamin binding activity in rat brain membranes has been solubilised in detergent and shown to behave as a high molecular weight oligomer (Seager *et al.*, 1988); its complete purification is awaited.

These numerous toxins that act on different K^+ channels should prove invaluable in designing drugs capable of blocking or activating each sub-type in a selective fashion.

Acknowledgements

I thank sincerely all the people in my research group, and collaborators who have contributed to the findings cited herein, particularly those (Drs J. Black, A. Breeze, A. Pelchen-Matthews, B. Poulain and C. Stansfeld) who have prepared figures. Also, I am most grateful to colleagues (Drs, D. Critchley, J. Elston, M. Gansel, P. Lazarovici, L. Sellin and W. Stühmer) for allowing inclusion of illustrations from their publications. My research is supported by Wellcome Trust, MRC, SERC and USAMIIRD (contract no. DAMD-17-88-C-8008).

References

Ahnert-Hilger, G., Weller, U., Dauzenroth, M.-E., Habermann, E. and Gratzl, M. (1989) The tetanus toxin light chain inhibits exocytosis. *FEBS Lett.* **242**: 245–248.
Baumann, A., Grupe, A., Ackermann, A. and Pongs, O. (1988) Structure of the voltage-dependent potassium channel is highly conserved from *Drosophila* to vertebrate central nervous system. *EMBO J.* **7**: 2457–2463.

Benishin, C. G., Sorensen, R. G., Brown, W. E., Krueger, B. K. and Blaustein M. P. (1988) Four polypeptide components of green mamba venom selectively block certain potassium channels in rat brain synaptosomes. *Mol. Pharmacol.* **34**: 152–159.

Benoit, E. and Dubois, J-M. (1986) Toxin I from the snake *Dendroaspis polylepis polylepis*: a highly specific blocker of one type of potassium channel in myelinated nerve fibre. *Brain Res.* **377**: 374–377.

Bergey, G. K., Bigalke, H. and Nelson, P. G. (1987) Differential aspects of tetanus toxin on inhibitory and excitatory synaptic transmission in mammalian spinal cord neurons in culture: a presynaptic locus of action. *J. Neurophysiol.* **57**: 121–131.

Bittner, M. and Holz, R. (1988) Effects of tetanus toxin on catecholamine release from intact and digitonin-permeabilized chromaffin cells. *J. Neurochem.* **51**: 451–456.

Black, A. R., Breeze, A. L., Othman, I. B. and Dolly, J. O. (1986a) Involvement of neuronal acceptors for dendrotoxin in its convulsive action in rat brain. *Biochem. J.* **237**: 397–404.

Black, A. R. and Dolly, J. O. (1986b) Two acceptor sub-types for dendrotoxin in chick synaptic membranes distinguishable by β-bungarotoxin. *Eur. J. Biochem.* **156**: 609–617.

Black, J. D. and Dolly, J. O. (1986c) Interaction of ^{125}I-labelled botulinum neurotoxins with nerve terminals. I. Ultrastructural autoradiographic localization and quantitation of distinct membrane acceptors for types A and B on motor nerves. *J. Cell Biol* **103**: 521–534.

Black, J. D. and Dolly, J. O. (1987) Selective location of acceptors for botulinum neurotoxin A on central and peripheral nerves. *Neuroscience* **23**: 767–779.

Black, A. R., Donegan, C. M., Denny, B. J. and Dolly, J. O. (1988) Solubilisation and physical characterization of acceptors for dendrotoxin and β-bungarotoxin from synaptic membranes of rat brain. *Biochemistry* **27**: 6814–6820.

Breeze, A. L. and Dolly, J. O. (1989) Interactions between discrete neuronal membrane binding sites for the putative K^+ channel ligands β-bungarotoxin, dendrotoxin and mast-cell degranulating peptide. *Eur. J. Biochem.* **178**: 771–778.

Burgess, G. M., Claret, M. and Jenkinson, D. H. (1981) Effect of quinine and apamin on the calcium-dependent potassium permeability of mammalian hepatocytes and red cells. *J. Physiol. (Lond.)* **317**: 67–90.

Carbone, E., Wanke, E., Prestipino, G., Possani, L. D. and Maelicke, A. (1982) Selective blockade of voltage-dependent K^+ channels by a novel scorpion toxin. *Nature* **296**: 90–91.

Castle, N. A., Haylett, D. G. and Jenkinson, D. H. (1989) Toxins in the characterization of potassium channels. *Trends Neurosci.* **12**: 59–65.

Cherubini, E., Neuman, R., Rovira, C. and Ben Ari, Y. (1988) Epileptogenic properties of the mast cell degranulating peptide in CA3 hippocampal neurones. *Brain Res.* **445**: 91–100

Cook, N. S. (1988) The pharmacology of potassium channels and their therapeutic potential. *Trends Pharmacol. Sci.* **9**: 21–28.

Critchley, D. R., Parton, R. G., Davidson, M. D. and Pierce, E. J. (1988) Characterization of tetanus toxin binding and internalisation by neuronal tissue. In: *Neurotoxins in Neurochemistry*, J. O. Dolly, ed., Ellis Horwood, Chichester, pp. 109–122.

Dajas, F., Cervenansky, C., Silveira, R. and Barbeito, L. (1988) Fasciculins: some aspects of their anticholinesterase activity in the central nervous system. In: *Neurotoxins in Neurochemistry*, J. O. Dolly, ed., Ellis Horwood, Chichester, pp.

241–251.

Dolly, J. O. (1988) Potassium channels — what can the protein chemistry contribute? *Trends Neurosci.* **11**: 186–188.

Dolly, J. O., Poulain, B., Maisey, E. A., Breeze, A. L., Wadsworth, J. D., Ashton, A. C. and Tauc, L. (1988) Neurotransmitter release and K^+ channels probed with botulinum neurotoxin and dendrotoxin. In: *Neurotoxins in Neurochemistry*, J. O. Dolly, ed., Ellis Horwood, Chichester, pp. 79–99.

Dolly, J. O., Lande, S. and Wray, D. W. (1987a) The effects of *in vitro* application of purified botulinum neurotoxin at mouse motor nerve terminals. *J. Physiol.* **386**: 475–484.

Dolly. J. O., Stansfeld, C. E., Breeze, A., Pelchen-Matthews, A., Marsh, S. J. and Brown, D. A. (1987b) Neuronal acceptor sub-types for dendrotoxin and their relation to K^+ channels. In: *Neurotoxins and their Pharmacological Implications*, P. Jenner, ed., Raven Press, New York, pp. 81–96.

Dolly, J. O., Black, J., Williams, R. S. and Melling, J. (1984a) Acceptors for botulinum neurotoxin reside on motor nerve terminals and mediate its internalization. *Nature* **307**: 457–460.

Dolly, J. O., Halliwell, J. V., Black, J. D., Williams, R. S., Pelchen-Matthews, A., Breeze, A. L., Mehraban, F., Othman, I. B. and Black, A. R. (1984b) Botulinum neurotoxin and dendrotoxin as probes for studies on transmitter release. *J. Physiol. (Paris)* **79**: 280–303.

Dunant, Y. (1986) On the mechanism of acetylcholine release. Progr. Neurobiol. **26**: 55–92.

Eisel, U., Jarausch, W., Goretzki, K., Henschen, A., Engels, J., Weller, U., Hudel, M., Habermann, E. and Niemann, H. (1986) Tetanus toxin: primary structure, expression in *E. coli*, and homology with botulinum toxins. *EMBO* J. **5**: 2495–2502.

Elston, J. S. (1988) The clinical use of botulinum toxin. *Semin. Ophthalmol.* **3**: 249–260.

Gansel, M., Penner, R. and Dreyer, F. (1987) Distinct sites of action of clostridial neurotoxins revealed by double-poisoning of mouse motor nerve terminals. *Pflügers Arch.* **409**: 533–539.

Halliwell, J. V. and Dolly, J. O. (1982) Preferential action of β-bungarotoxin at nerve terminal regions in the hippocampus. *Neurosci. Lett.* **30**: 321–327.

Halliwell, J, V., Othman, I. B., Pelchen-Matthews, A. and Dolly, J. O. (1986) Central action of dendrotoxin: selective reduction of a transient K^+ conductance in hippocampus and binding to localized acceptors. *Proc. Natl. Acad. Sci. USA* **83**: 493–497.

Harvey, A. L. and Karlsson, E. (1982) Protease inhibitor homologues from mamba venoms: facilitation of acetylcholine release and interactions with prejunctional blocking toxins. *Br. J. Pharmacol.* **77**: 153–161.

Harvey, A. L., Anderson, A. J. and Karlsson, E. (1984) Facilitation of transmitter release by neurotoxins from snake venoms. *J. Physiol. (Paris)* **79**: 222–227.

Lazarovici, P., Yavin, E., Bizzini, B. and Fedinec, A. (1988) Retrograde transport in sciatic nerves of ganglioside-affinity-purified tetanus toxins. In: *Neurotoxins in Neurochemistry*, J. O. Dolly, ed., Ellis Horwood, Chichester, pp. 100–108.

MacKinnon, R., Reinhart, P. H. and White, M. M. (1988) Charybdotoxin block of Shaker K^+ channels suggests that different types of K^+ channels share common structural features. *Neuron* **1**: 997–1001.

Maisey, E. A., Wadsworth, J. D., Poulain, B., Shone, C. C., Melling, J., Gibbs, P., Tauc, L. and Dolly, J. O. (1988) Involvement of the constituent chains of botulinum neurotoxin A and B in the blockade of neurotransmitter release. *Eur. J. Biochem.* **177**: 683–691.

McInnes, C., Edwards, K. and Dolly, J. O. (1990) Ca^{2+}-dependent noradrenaline release from permeabilised PC12 cells is blocked by botulinum neurotoxin A or its light chains. *FEBS Lett.* **261**: 323–326.

Mehraban, F., Breeze, A. L. and Dolly, J. O. (1984) Identification by cross-linking of a neuronal acceptor protein for dendrotoxin, a convulsant polypeptide. *FEBS Lett.* **174**: 116–122.

Miller, R. J. (1988) G proteins flex their muscles. *Trends Neurosci.* **11**: 3–6.

Mochida, S., Poulain, B., Weller, U., Habermann, E. and Tauc, L. (1989) Light chain of tetanus toxin intracellularly inhibits acetylcholine release at neuro-neuronal synapses, and its internatisation is mediated by heavy chain. *FEBS Lett.* **253**: 47–51.

Moczydlowski, E., Lucchesi, K. and Ravindran, A. (1988) An emerging pharmacology of peptide toxins targetted against potassium channels. *J. Membr. Biol.* **105**: 95–111.

Othman, I. B., Spokes, J. W. and Dolly, J. O. (1982) Preparation of neurotoxic ^3H-β-bungarotoxin: demonstration of saturable binding to brain synapses and its inhibition by toxin I. *Eur. J. Biochem.* **128**: 267–276.

Parcej, D. N. and Dolly, J. O. (1989) Dendrotoxin acceptor from bovine synaptic plasma membranes: binding properties, purification and subunit composition of a putative constituent of certain voltage-activated K^+ channels. *Biochem. J.* **257**: 899–903.

Pelchen-Matthews, A. and Dolly, J. O. (1988) Distribution of acceptors for β-bungarotoxin in the central nervous system of the rat. *Brain Res.* **441**: 127–138.

Pelchen-Matthews, A. and Dolly, J. O. (1989) Distribution in the rat central nervous system of acceptor sub-types for dendrotoxin, a K^+ channel probe. *Neuroscience* **29**: 347–361.

Penner, R., Neher, E. and Dreyer, F. (1986a) Intracellularly injected tetanus toxin inhibits exocytosis in bovine adrenal chromaffin cells. *Nature* **324**: 76–78.

Penner, R., Petersen, M., Pierau, F-K. and Dreyer, F. (1986b) Dendrotoxin: a selective blocker of non-inactivating potassium current in guinea-pig dorsal root ganglion neurones. *Pflügers Arch.* **407**: 365–369.

Petersen, M., Penner, R., Pierau, F-K. and Dreyer, F. (1986) β-Bungarotoxin inhibits a non-inactivating potassium current in guinea pig dorsal root ganglion neurones. *Neurosci. Lett.* **68**: 141–145.

Pongs, O., Kecskemethy, N., Müller, R., Krah-Jentgens, I., Baumann, A., Kiltz, H. H., Canal, I., Llamazares, S. and Ferrus, A. (1988) *Shaker* encodes a family of putative potassium channel proteins in the nervous system of *Drosophila*. *EMBO J.* **7**: 1087–1096.

Poulain, B., Tauc, L., Maisey, E. A., Wadsworth, J. D. F., Mohan, P. M. and Dolly, J. O. (1988) Neurotransmitter release is blocked intracellularly by botulinum neurotoxin and this requires uptake of both its polypeptides by a process mediated by the larger chain. *Proc. Natl. Acad. Sci. USA* **85**: 4090–4094.

Rehm, H. and Lazdunski, M. (1988a) Existence of different populations of the dendrotoxin I binding protein associated with neuronal K^+ channels. *Biochem. Biophys. Res. Commun.* **153**: 231–240.

Rehm, H. and Lazdunski, M. (1988b) Purification and subunit structure of a putative K^+-channel protein identified by its binding properties for dendrotoxin I. *Proc. Natl. Acad. Sci. USA* **85**: 4919–4923.

Rehm, H., Bidard, J-N., Schweitz, H. and Lazdunski, M. (1988) The receptor site for the bee venom mast cell degranulating peptide. Affinity labeling and evidence for a common molecular target for mast cell degranulating peptide and dendrotoxin I, a snake toxin active on K^+ channels. *Biochemistry* **27**: 1827–1832.

Rowan, E. G. and Harvey, A. L. (1988) Potassium channel blocking actions of β-bungarotoxin and related toxins on mouse and frog motor nerve terminals. *Br. J. Pharmacol.* **94**: 839–847.

Rudy, B., Hoger, J. H., Lester, H. A. and Davidson, N. (1988) At least two mRNA species contribute to the properties of rat brain A-type potassium channels expressed in *Xenopus* oocytes. *Neuron* **1**: 649–658.

Schwarz, T. L., Tempel, B. L., Papazian, D. M., Jan, Y. N. and Jan, L. Y. (1988) Multiple potassium-channel components are produced by alternative splicing at the *Shaker* locus in *Drosophila. Nature* **331**: 137–142.

Scott, A. B. (1980) Botulinum toxin injection into extraocular muscles as an alternative to strabismus surgery. *Ophthalmology* **87**: 1044–1049.

Seager, M. J., Marqueze, B. and Couraud, F. (1988) Characterization of the apamin-binding protein associated with a Ca^{2+} activated K^+ channel. In: *Neurotoxins in Neurochemistry* J. O. Dolly, ed., Ellis Horwood, Chichester, pp. 178–190.

Sellin, L. C. (1987) Botulinum toxin and the blockade of transmitter release. *Asia Pac. J. Pharmacol.* **2**: 203–222.

Sitges, M., Possani, L. D. and Bayon, A. (1986) Noxiustoxin, a short-chain toxin from the Mexican scorpion *Centruroides noxius*, induces transmitter release by blocking K^+ permeability. *J. Neurosci.* **6**: 1570–1574.

Stansfeld, C. and Feltz, A. (1988) Dendrotoxin-sensitive K^+ channels in dorsal root ganglion cells. *Neurosci. Lett.* **93**: 49–55.

Stansfeld, C. E., Marsh, S. J., Halliwell, J. V. and Brown, D. A. (1986) 4-Aminopyridine and dendrotoxin induce repetitive firing in rat visceral sensory neurones by blocking a slowly inactivating outward current. *Neurosci. Lett.* **64**: 299–304.

Stansfeld, C. E., Marsh, S. J., Parcej, D. N., Dolly, J. O. and Brown, D. A. (1987) Mast cell degranulating peptide and dendrotoxin selectively inhibit a fast-activating potassium current and bind to common neuronal proteins. *Neuroscience* **23**: 893–902.

Stühmer, W., Stocker, M., Sakmann, B., Seeburg, P., Baumann, A., Grupe, A. and Pongs, O. (1988) Potassium channels expressed from rat brain cDNA have delayed rectifier properties. *FEBS Lett.* **242**: 199–206.

Tempel. B. L., Jan, Y. N. and Jan, L. Y. (1988) Cloning of a probable potassium channel gene from mouse brain. *Nature* **332**: 837–839.

Timpe, L. C., Schwarz, T. L., Tempel, B. L., Papazian, D. M., Jan, Y. N. and Jan, L. Y. (1988) Expression of functional potassium channels from *Shaker* cDNA in *Xenopus* oocytes. *Nature* **331**: 143–145.

Valdivia, H. H., Smith, J. S., Martin, B. M., Coronado, R. and Possani, L. D. (1988) Charybdotoxin and noxiustoxin, two homologous peptide inhibitors of the K^+ (Ca^{2+}) channel. *FEBS Lett.* **226**: 280–284.

7 *David Colquhoun*

Agonists, antagonists and synaptic transmission at the neuromuscular junction

7.1. Introduction

The neuromuscular junction is certainly the most-studied, and best-understood synapse. During the past 20 or 30 years the mechanism of synaptic transmission at the neuromuscular junction, and the mode of action of drugs that affect it, have become clear in some detail.

This chapter describes the approaches that can be used to determine exactly how a natural transmitter, its pharmacological analogues, and antagonists interact with the target receptor. A survey of the physiological characteristics of neuromuscular transmission will be given first. This description will be more detailed than that in chapter 2, in order to highlight the biophysical aspects of the electrical properties of the membrane. A number of recent books and reviews deal with the subject-matter in greater detail than is possible here, for example see: Zaimis (1976), Bowman (1980), Peper *et al.* (1982), Colquhoun (1986), Colquhoun *et al.*, 1986, 1987. Much of the present knowledge stems from the work of Bernard Katz and his colleagues: his books *Nerve Muscle and Synapse* (Katz, 1966) and *The Release of Neural Transmitter Substances* (Katz, 1969) remain the ideal introductions to the field.

7.2. The physiology of neuromuscular transmission

7.2.1. *The action of acetylcholine on acetylcholine receptors*

The synthesis, storage and release of transmitter, acetylcholine (ACh), are dealt with elsewhere (Molenaar, this volume), so this description will start from the point where ACh is released from the motor nerve ending and diffuses across the synaptic cleft to the postsynaptic membrane.

The action of ACh on the muscle, and the consequent action potential in the muscle fibre, both involve changes in the permeability of the muscle membrane to sodium and potassium ions. These changes are brought about by the opening of pores or channels in the membrane. It is very important, for the understanding of drug action, to realise that two different regions of the membrane, which contain differing kinds of ion channel, are involved. The endplate area of the muscle, which is directly under the nerve ending and very small (of the order of 50 μm diameter) relative to the length of the fibre, is a highly specialised region of chemically excitable membrane. It is called *chemically excitable* because it contains ion channels which can be caused to open by chemicals such as ACh or suxamethonium. Most of the muscle fibre membrane is quite different from this; it more closely resembles nerve fibre membrane in its properties and it is called an *electrically excitable* membrane. This description arises from the fact that the ion channels in it are caused to open by changes (depolarisation) in the electrical potential difference across the membrane. These channels are, however, not affected by drugs such as ACh or suxamethonium so they are quite unlike those at the endplate. They will be discussed further below.

Let us consider first the release of a single quantum of ACh, which contains 10,000 or so ACh molecules, from the nerve terminal (Kuffler and Yoshikami, 1975). The synaptic cleft is very narrow (around 50 nm) and ACh can diffuse this short distance very rapidly (a few microseconds probably), to reach the endplate membrane. Some of these ACh molecules combine with the ACh receptor molecules in the postsynaptic membrane, but free ACh is rapidly hydrolysed by the acetylcholinesterase that is present in the synaptic cleft, associated with the basement membrane that overlies the endplate. This rapid hydrolysis means that the ACh does not have time to diffuse very far laterally along the cleft, and the action of a quantum is probably confined to a small area, about 2 μm^2, of the endplate membrane (Hartzell *et al.*, 1975).

The ACh receptors are concentrated around the top of the post-junctional folds, and there are about 10,000 or more per μm^2 (of the order of 10^7 ACh receptors per endplate). The number of ACh molecules released is almost enough to saturate all the receptors in the small (2 μm^2) region on which it acts, and a substantial proportion of the released molecules become bound to the receptors (two ACh molecules per receptor). This binding causes most of the ion channels associated with the receptors to open. The ion channels, once open, stay open for a millisecond or so, although the binding to receptors, together with the rapid hydrolysis of ACh, means that the concentration of free ACh in the synaptic cleft falls more rapidly than this (in a few 100 μs) as illustrated diagrammatically in Fig. 7.1(a).

An ACh molecule is unlikely to interact with a receptor more than once before it is hydrolysed or diffuses away. While they are open, the ion channels allow the inflow of sodium ions and efflux of potassium ions. Both ions go through the same channel, which has an electrical conductance of about 50–70 pS (i.e. 50–70 $\times$ 10^{-12} reciprocal ohms) while it is open. Channel opening thus effectively produces a short-circuit across the

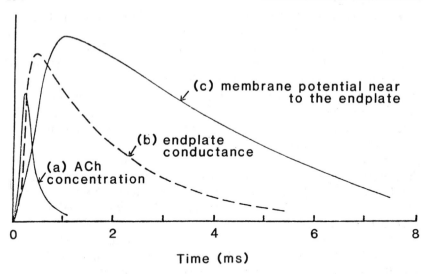

Fig. 7.1. Diagram to illustrate qualitatively the time-course of the effects of ACh released from the muscle fibre. (a) Concentration of ACh in the synaptic cleft below a release site. (b) Conductance of the chemically excitable endplate membrane (directly proportional to the number of nicotinic receptor channels opened by ACh). (c) Change of potential across the endplate membrane, and across the adjacent (electrically excitable) muscle fibre membrane; if this EPP were large enough an action potential (not shown) would be evoked.

membrane, which tends to reduce the normal potential difference across the membrane from its resting value (about -80 mV, inside negative relative to outside) towards a value near zero (the reversal potential for these channels). The opening of a single channel for a millisecond causes a depolarisation of only 0.5 µV or so, too small to be seen directly (the value is found indirectly from fluctuation analysis — see reviews cited in section 7.1). But the effect of one quantum of ACh is to open, almost simultaneously, 1000–2000 channels, producing a total depolarization of 0.5–1.0 mV, the miniature endplate potential (MEPP).

When the nerve is stimulated 50–3000 quanta are released, nearly but not exactly simultaneously. These probably act almost independently of each other, i.e. the area affected by one quantum is so small (see above) that neighbouring quanta are not likely to overlap very much in their effects on the endplate (see also chapter by Engel, this volume). Thus 0.1–0.6 million endplate channels open transiently as illustrated in Fig. 7.1(b), producing a short-circuit conductance of the order of 10 µS, compared with an effective resting conductance of roughly 2 µS (i.e. input resistance of 0.5 MΩ). This is enough to depolarise the endplate almost completely (i.e. to reduce the potential difference across it to nearly zero); this depolarisation is called the endplate potential (EPP). Fig. 7.1(c) shows what the EEP would look like if no action potential were initiated. However, when the EEP reaches a threshold value, -50 mV or so (i.e. around 30 mV depolarised from the resting level), a new sequence of events is initiated in the membrane surrounding the endplate, events that lead to an action potential in the muscle fibre.

7.2.2. *Initiation of an action potential in the electrically excitable muscle membrane*

Before going on to discuss how the events at the endplate influence the rest of the muscle fibre, it will be necessary to digress for a moment to consider the electrical properties of the muscle fibre. It has been stated that ACh opens ion channels in the endplate, short-circuiting it, and producing a depolarisation; it is necessary to know how much of the membrane, apart from the channel itself, is depolarised. If the muscle membrane where a perfect insulator, or the cytoplasm were a perfect conductor, short-circuiting the membrane at one point would depolarise the whole muscle fibre from end to end. But in fact its membrane is leaky and the effect of depolarisation spreads only a few millimetres from the point where the membrane is short-circuited. The maximum depolarisation is at this point, but on each side the extent of depolarisation wanes, falling by half every 1.5 mm (about 25 fibre-diameters) or so along the fibre (see Elmqvist *et al.*, 1960), so ½ cm from the point of the short-circuit, little depolarisation can be seen, as illustrated in Fig. 7.2. This distance may be short compared

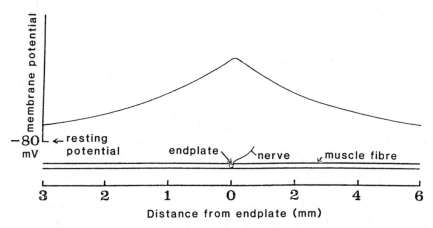

Fig. 7.2. Diagram to illustrate the effect of depolarisation of the (chemically excitable) endplate membrane on the membrane potential of the nearby (electrically excitable) muscle fibre membrane. This illustration is valid only for small depolarisations; once the depolarisation becomes big enough to cause the opening of sodium channels in the electrically excitable membrane their opening would produce further depolarisation and so change the shape of the curve.

with the length of the muscle fibre, but it is long compared with the size of
the endplate, and it is for this reason that the small depolarisations
produced by each open channel, and the larger depolarisations produced
by each quantum, add to one another to produce one big depolarisation. A
second consequence of the passive electrical properties of the muscle fibre
is that the short-circuit does not produce a depolarisation instantaneously.
Several milliseconds mush elapse before the depolarisation is complete
(because the electrical capacitance of the membrane has to be charged as
the voltage changes). For a similar reason, MEPPs and EPPs last substantially longer (around 5 ms) than the underlying conductance change
(compare Figs. 7.1(b) and 7.1(c)).

In the light of the membrane properties discussed above, it will be clear
why a depolarisation at the endplate, the EPP produced by ACh, will also
depolarise a substantial area of the muscle fibre membrane around the
endplate. This is an electrically excitable membrane, rather like that of
nerve fibres. The ion channels in it are opened by the depolarisation
because they are operated by a voltage change (not by agonists as at the
endplate).

There are two quite distinct sorts of voltage-operated ion channels
involved (see also Norman, this volume): (a) sodium channels (which
selectively allow Na^+ to pass when they are open), and (b) potassium
channels (which allow only K^+ to pass when they are open). There are
rather more sodium channels near to the endplate than in the rest of the
muscle fibre (Beam *et al.*, 1985). Potassium is actively pumped into the
cell in exchange for sodium to maintain a steep concentration gradient for
these ions. The effect of opening the channels can be understood, in a
qualitative way, by considering two extreme cases. If the membrane were
permeable to potassium only, the potential across it would be around -100
mV, because of the high potassium concentration inside the cell, relative to
outside it. At the other extreme one can imagine that the cell membrane
was permeable to sodium only; in this case the potential across it would be
about $+50$ mV, in the opposite direction from normal, because of the high
concentration of sodium outside the cell relative to that inside. In fact in
the resting state the membrane is much more permeable to K^+ than to Na^+
and the membrane potential is about -80 to -90 mV. Thus any increase in
Na^+ permeability will tend to move the membrane potential nearer to $+50$
mV.

The behaviour of these channels is illustrated in Fig. 7.3, which shows
how they respond in an artificial experimental situation. The membrane is
suddenly depolarised near to zero by passing current through an electrode
in the fibre, and held depolarised at a fixed level, as shown in Fig. 7.3(a).
This depolarisation causes Na^+ channels to open rapidly as in Fig. 7.3(b),
and it causes the K^+ channels to open too, though more slowly, as shown in
Fig. 7.3(c). The potassium channels stay open as long as the membrane

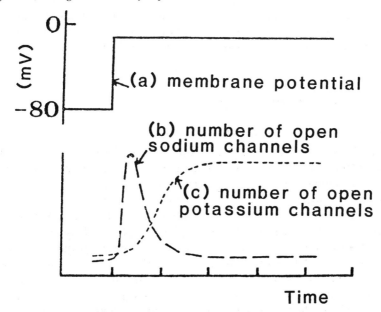

Fig. 7.3. Diagram to illustrate the effect of depolarisation, shown in (**a**), of the electrically excitable membrane in causing the opening of sodium channels (**b**), and of potassium channels (**c**). The step change in membrane potential shown in (**a**) would not occur naturally, but can be produced experimentally by means of a voltage clamp apparatus.

stays depolarised, but the sodium channels behave in a more complicated way, Fig. 7.3(b). Even if the membrane stays depolarised, the sodium channels do not stay open, but shut again quite soon, a phenomenon known as inactivation. Once in this inactivated state, further depolarisation cannot open sodium channels again; they return to normal only after the membrane has been repolarised for a while to reactivate them. While sodium channels are in the inactivated condition, the membrane is refractory and action potentials cannot be triggered.

During transmission the electrically excitable membrane adjacent to the endplate will be depolarised as a result of the EPP that originates at the endplate. This depolarisation causes Na^+ channels to open, and the effect of opening Na^+ channels is to cause still more depolarisation (towards $+50$ mV as above), which in turn causes more Na^+ channels to open, and therefore even more depolarisation and so on. There is therefore a sudden explosive depolarisation (the rate may be 500 V/s or more), and it is this which constitutes the rising phase of an action potential in the fibre. As the sodium channels become inactivated and potassium channels open, the membrane potential falls again towards the resting potential. The action potential, once it has been started, will propagate along the fibre in each direction from the region around the endplate where it started, until it reaches the ends of the fibre. The action potential then causes a contraction of the muscle fibre via a consequent release of calcium from intracellular stores.

7.3. Mechanisms of agonist action

7.3.1. *The structure of the AChR ion channel*

This topic is dealt with in greater detail in the chapter by Beeson and Barnard (this volume). Briefly, mammalian muscle nicotinic acetylcholine receptor/channels are pentameric macromolecules with a subunit structure $\alpha_2\beta\gamma\delta$, as in *Torpedo* electric tissue. However, there are two forms of AChRs in muscle, a junctional or adult type and an extrajunctional or embryonic type (see chapter 1). For bovine receptor, at least, these forms differ at a single subunit, the γ subunit being replaced in the adult by an ε subunit which has a different sequence (Mishina *et al.*, 1986). There is one binding site for ACh (and for tubocurarine and toxins such as α-bungarotoxin) on the extracellular part of each of the two α-subunits. This confirms earlier electrophysiological evidence that the binding of two ACh molecules per channel is needed for efficient opening of the channel. The five subunits appear to be arranged around a central ion channel which, when ACh is bound, can change conformation to an 'open' state which allows the passage of ions. The presence of agonists also induces, more slowly, one or more desensitised conformations of the receptor/ channel molecule (see also chapter 2); these are 'shut', i.e. they do not allow passage of ions, and they are also refractory, i.e. agonists do not cause them to open.

The primary amino acid sequence is now known, from cloning studies, for the receptors from many species. However, little is known so far about the secondary or tertiary structures of the resting receptor, or about the changes in them that occur when the channel opens or becomes desensitized (see chapter 2).

7.3.2. *Rates of drug action*

The synapse works so rapidly that there is no time for the released ACh to reach equilibrium with the receptors. Furthermore when a neuromuscular blocking agent is present, although it may have reached equilibrium with the receptors in their resting state, this equilibrium will be perturbed by the release of ACh from the motor nerve, and therefore neither ACh nor blocking agent will be at equilibrium with the receptors during synaptic transmission. Thus, in order to understand how antagonists and agonists work under physiological conditions it is not enough simply to know their equilibrium affinities (and efficacies); we must also know how fast these ligands associate with, and dissociate from, the receptors.

The main methods for measuring rates of drug action at the endplate are: (1) noise (or fluctuation) analysis, (2) voltage jump relaxations and (3) single-ion channel recording. For events that are sufficiently slow (e.g. some forms of desensitisation) it is also possible to use concentration jump relaxation, i.e. one changes the drug concentration and observes the rate of re-equilibration; this method is limited by the fact that concentration can be changed only relatively slowly, because of diffusion problems (except in the case of outside-out membrane patches — see below).

There have been several reviews of these methods, for example by Neher and Stevens (1977), Colquhoun (1981, 1985). Rather than measuring changes in membrane potential, we measure the flow of current through the membrane which is clamped at a fixed potential set by the experimenter (see chapter 3). This is essential to prevent the distortion of the time-course of events by the membrane capacitance, as discussed above and illustrated in Fig. 7.1. For example, nerve stimulation produces an inward current, the endplate current (EPC), when the membrane potential is clamped, rather than a depolarisation (the EPP). Similarly , release of a single packet of ACh produces a miniature endplate current (MEPC) in clamped fibres. The time-course of the EPC or MEPC shows directly the time-course of the conductance change produced by ACh (see Fig. 7.1), i.e. the current is directly proportional to the number of ion channels open at any instant.

Noise analysis and relaxation analysis provide, in principle, similar information about the rates of the underlying reactions (see, for example, Colquhoun and Hawkes, 1977). Noise analysis provides, in addition, an estimate of the current that flows through a single open ion channel, despite the fact that individual single-channel currents are usually not resolvable in such experiments (though such estimates have not always proved very reliable; e.g. Gardner *et al.*, 1984). Single-channel recording shows more directly the characteristics of individual channel openings, and this method allows resolution of faster events than the other methods. However, because we are looking at the behaviour of a single molecule, the length of individual openings and shuttings varies in a random way (as illustrated in Fig. 7.5). This means that many measurements must be made in order to make inferences about the smooth, average behaviour of the system (which is what would be seen automatically when measuring from a system, such as a whole endplate, that contains many molecules).

7.3.3. *Characteristics of channel openings*

The decay of the EPC is usually well-described by a simple exponential time-course, as shown in Fig. 7.4. Exponential time-courses are commonly

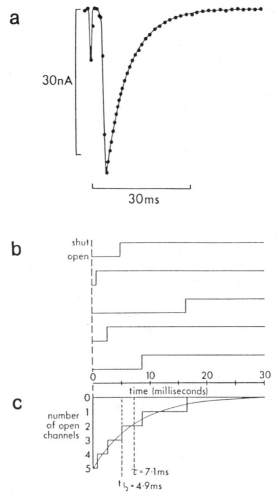

Fig. 7.4. (a) Endplate current (EPC) evoked by stimulation of the motor nerve (mean of seven). Recorded near the endplate of a frog muscle fibre (with membrane potential clamped to −13 mV). The continuous line fitted to the decay phase is a simple exponential curve (with a time constant of 7.1 ms). Inward current is plotted downwards. About 9000 channels were open at the peak (the current is about 3.9 pA per channel). (b) Simulated behaviour of five individual ion channels that were opened, almost simultaneously, by released ACh (opening plotted as a downwards reflection). Each channel stays open for a random (exponentially distributed) length of time, the *mean* length of an opening being (in this example) 7.1 ms. Once a channel shuts it will rarely be re-opened, because of the rapid fall in free ACh concentration. (c) The sum of the five records shown in (b). The exponential form of the decay (with time constant 7.1 ms) is seen to result from the (exponential) distribution of channel lifetimes (mean 7.1 ms). The half-time for the decay corresponds to the median channel lifetime. Reproduced from Colquhoun (1981).

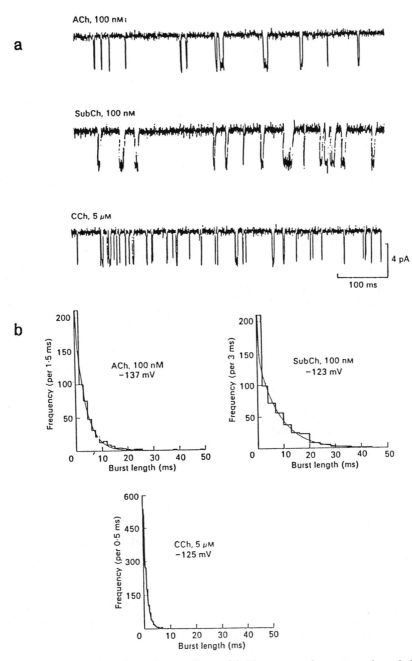

Fig. 7.5. Single ion channel recordings. (a) The traces show examples of the currents that flow through individual endplate channels when they are caused to open by low concentrations of ACh (top) suberyldicholine (middle) and carbachol (bottom). (b) Histograms showing the variability of the durations of individual activations of channel ('burst lengths') produced by the three agonists illustrated in (a). The main (slower) component of distributions such as these gave a mean length of 4.2 ms for ACh, 7.4 ms for suberyldicholine and 1.8 ms for carbachol. Reproduced from Colquhoun and Sakmann, 1985).

observed in whole cells because the variability of the duration of individual openings is usually described by an exponential probability density function (or a mixture of several such distributions) as illustrated in Fig. 7.4. For more details see, for example, Anderson and Stevens (1973), Colquhoun and Hawkes (1983), Colquhoun (1981).

The mean duration of channel opening varies considerably from one agonist to another. For example, as shown in Fig. 7.5, activations of endplate ion channels (in the frog) by ACh last, on average, 3.2 times longer than those produced by carbachol, but are only 56% of the length of those produced by suberyldicholine (a longer chain analogue of suxamethonium) (Colquhoun and Sakmann, 1985), However, the amplitude of openings is the same for all agonists (e.g. Gardner *et al.*, 1984). While the channel is open a current of about 2.7 pA flows through it into the cell, whichever agonist caused it to open (at −90 mV membrane potential in frog at 10°C; in mammals at 37°C the current would be bigger — probably 6–8 pA). Of those channels that are exposed to ACh released from the nerve ending quite a large proportion are opened, despite the presence of acetylcholinesterase. Evidently ACh is a rather effective agonist, but it is only recently (see below) that attempts have been made to measure the affinity of ACh binding to shut channels, and its efficacy in opening channels once bound. The terms affinity and efficacy are used here almost, but not quite, in the classical way defined by Stephenson in 1956 (see Colquhoun, 1987). More surprisingly, it is even more recently that good estimates have been made of the equilibrium concentration–response curve for channel opening.

7.3.4. *Agonists at equilibrium*

It is only by use of single-channel methods (see Sakmann *et al.*, 1980) that it has been possible to obtain adequate estimates of the efficacy of ACh by measurements of the fraction of non-desensitised channels that are open over a wide range of agonist concentrations (other methods have not allowed adequate correction for the profound effects of desensitisation and, at high concentrations, channel block, which is referred to below). This has been done, for example, with adult frog muscle receptors (Ogden and Colquhoun, 1985; Colquhoun and Ogden, 1988) as well as for some cultured tissues (e.g. Sine and Steinbach, 1987), and most recently for adult rat muscle (Mulrine and Ogden, 1988).

In each case the method has been to turn the intense desensitisation shown by nicotinic receptors (see Fig. 7.6a) from being the problem to being the solution. In single-channel records obtained with high agonist concentrations, many channels are open simultaneously at first. After a while, however, desensitisation ensures that there will rarely be more than one channel open at a time. There are long silent periods when all of the

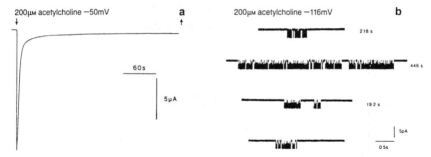

Fig. 7.6. (a) Current through a frog muscle endplate (in a Vaseline-gap voltage clamp) evoked by application of acetylcholine (200 μM). Membrane potential −50 mV, $T = 4°C$. Reproduced from Cachelin, A. B. (1987) (Ph. D. thesis, University of London). (b) Single-channel currents evoked by acetylcholine (200 μM) in frog muscle endplate. The traces shown are parts of a continuous record, the length of the silent period between successive traces being shown at the end of each record. Reporduced from Colquhoun and Ogden (1988).

channels are desensitised, but every now and then one channel will emerge from desensitisation, and a cluster of openings will occur, the openings occurring in rapid succession (because of the high agonist concentration). This is illustrated in Fig. 7.6b. The desensitised periods can be removed from the record, and the response, i.e. fraction of time for which the channel is open (the probability of being open, denoted P_{open}), can be measured during the cluster of openings, i.e. during the time when the channel is not desensitized.

It seems that there are no gross differences in the equilibrium behaviour of frog and rat adult muscle receptors. In both cases ACh is an efficacious agonist in the sense that it is capable of opening most of the ion channels before desensitisation sets in (see also Brett *et al.*, 1986). In both cases ACh itself can block the channel at high concentrations ($K = 0.5–1.5$ mM at negative potentials) leading to reduced P_{open} (see below for further discussion), and in both cases 50% of channels are opened at a concentration (the EC_{50}) of about 15–20 μM at negative potentials, as shown in Fig. 7.7.

During an EPP the concentration of ACh in the synaptic cleft, below the release sites, has been estimated to be 300–1000 μM (though for a very short time only), which is much higher than the EC_{50}. To get a more detailed description of agonist action we need to know more about the rate of action of agonists, as well as their equilibrium behaviour.

7.3.5. *The rate of action of agonists*

The earliest knowledge of rates stemmed from noise analysis (Katz and Miledi, 1972; Anderson and Stevens, 1973). This method gave an estimate

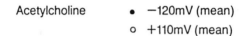

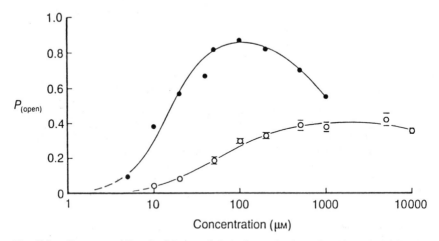

Fig. 7.7.   Response (P_{open}) of frog endplate channels plotted against acetylcholine concentration (log scale) at two different ranges of membrane potentials; upper curve, −95 to −130 mV; lower curve, +85 to +120 mV. Depolarisation reduces the mean length of time for which a channel stays open, and hence the agonist efficacy. Therefore a higher concentration of ACh is required for a given response at +85–120 mV. On the other hand there is less channel block at more depolarised potentials.

of the mean duration of a single activation of the ion channel. This quantity was usually referred to as the 'mean open time' of the channel. For the physiological purpose of understanding synaptic transmission this is an entirely adequate description. For the purposes of understanding mechanisms, however, it is not an adequate description; it entails the assumption that each activation of the channel results in only one opening of the channel. However, recent evidence suggests that several openings occur during activation of the channel by ACh as a result of oscillation of the channel between open and shut forms while ACh (two molecules) remains bound. Such multiple openings are expected if agonist binding and the subsequent conformation change both proceed at comparable rates. Single openings would be seen only if the binding and unbinding of the agonist to the shut channel are much faster than subsequent open–shut isomerisation of the channel (in which case most bindings would be ineffective in producing openings). This was originally suggested, as a working hypothesis, by Anderson and Stevens (1973).

Close examination of the individual activations of the channel shown in Fig. 7.8 shows that they indeed appear to consist of two or three openings

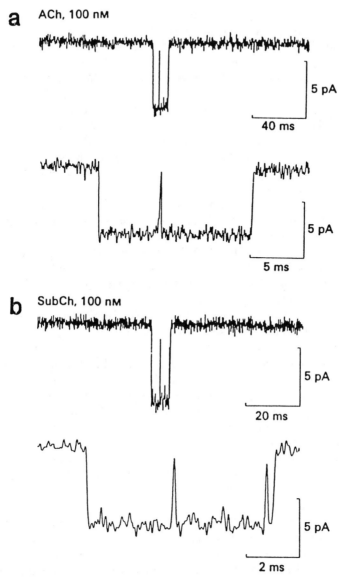

Fig. 7.8. Examples of individual channel activations by two different agonists. (a) Single-channel current activated by ACh, shown at low- and high-time resolution. The upper, low-time resolution trace shows that the activations are well separated in time from adjacent currents. The average frequency of occurrence of activations in this recording was less than one per second. At high-time resolution (lower trace) it is seen that this activation consists of two resolved channel openings separated by a short closure. (b) Single-channel current activated by suberyldicholine. This activation consists of three resolved channel openings separated by two short channel closures. Reproduced from Colquhoun and Sakmann (1985).

in quick succession. These observations of multiple openings allow estimates not only of the channel shutting rate (i.e. its true mean open time) but also of the opening rate of the doubly liganded receptor and the dissociation rate of the agonist from it. Estimates made in this way in adult frog muscle at 10°C suggest that the affinity for acetylcholine binding is quite low (dissociation rate constant about 8×10^3 s^{-1}, equilibrium constant about 80 μM), and is not dependent on membrane potential. Thus the ACh can dissociate rapidly following an opening. The opening rate constant for the doubly occupied channel is very fast ($20-40 \times 10^3$ s^{-1}) compared with the shutting rate constant (about 700 s^{-1} ; mean open time about 1.4 ms), so the equilibrium between open and shut channels (both with two ACh molecules bound) is well over towards the open state, i.e. ACh is an agonist with high efficacy. This is why the EC$_{50}$ is considerably less than the equilibrium constant for the binding reaction (see Colquhoun, 1985, for further explanation).

The high concentration of ACh below a release site ensures rapid binding of ACh, and the fast opening rate constant ensures rapid subsequent channel opening; together they account for the fact that an MEPC takes only about 100 μs to reach its peak (Madsen *et al.*, 1984; Colquhoun and Sakmann 1981, 1983, 1985). Qualitatively similar conclusions apply to mammalian adult-type receptors.

Other agonists that have been tested in this way include carbachol, suxamethonium (succinyldicholine), suberyldicholine, and all of these agonists appear to have reasonably high efficacy: if it were not for desensitisation and channel block they would all be able to open a large fraction of the ion channels when applied in a sufficient concentration. An analysis similar to that described above suggests that the 20-fold lower potency of carbachol relative to ACh is accounted for largely by a 10-fold lower affinity of carbachol for the (shut) receptors, the remaining factor of two results from the lower efficacy of carbachol (i.e. its lower effectiveness in opening channels once bound).

All of these agonists (in concentrations that produce a given degree of activation) are more effective than ACh in blocking the ion channels which they themselves open. Self-block thus limits the maximum response that can be obtained with these other agonists to a greater extent than it does with ACh. Decamethonium, in frog muscle, can open a small fraction (a few per cent at most) of ion channels; however its self-block is so powerful that it is impossible to be sure whether this small maximum response is a result solely of self-block, or whether decamethonium is also a genuine partial agonist, as originally proposed by Del Castillo and Katz (1957) (Adams and Sakmann, 1978; Marshall *et al.*, 1991). Decamethonium may be more effective in the cat (Zaimis and Head, 1976), but comparable experiments on self-block have not yet been done on mammals.

7.3.6. Summary of the mode of action of agonists

Plausible estimates for the rate of binding, and of channel opening, have been made for ACh and other agonists. Most recently, complete equilibrium concentration–response curves, corrected for desensitisation, have been obtained. It has been found that all agonists tested can block the ion channels which they themselves open, but ACh produces less block (for a given degree of channel activation) than other agonists. Channel block by ACh is unlikely to be important under physiological conditions of synaptic transmission, but suxamethonium, and especially decamethonium, produce more potent channel block.

7.4. Mechanisms of antagonistic action

Until recently, neuromuscular blocking agents were classified as either competitive or depolarising blocking drugs. More recently it has been

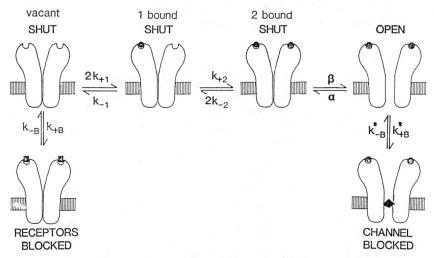

Fig. 7.9. Reaction scheme for activation and block. The two agonist-binding subunits and lipid membrane (shaded) are shown in diagrammatic cross-section. The activation of the channel is thought to be produced primarily by two sequential bindings of agonist molecules followed by isomerisation to the open conformation (top row). The open channel may then be plugged by an antagonist (or by the agonist itself), as illustrated on the bottom right. Alternatively (or in addition) an antagonist may combine with the agonist binding sites (or otherwise exclude the agonist from binding), so producing competitive block (bottom left). Notice that species with one competitive blocker molecule bound (with or without agonist on the other binding site) would be expected to exist too, and are important for understanding the kinetics of competitive block, but are not shown on the diagram, for the sake of simplicity.

found that drugs in both of these categories (and indeed virtually every positively charged molecule that has been tested, as well as many neutral ones) cause block of the open ion channel in addition to their other actions. This block can occur only if the channel is first opened by agonist. None of these agents is known to have ion channel block as its main mode of action on muscle endplate receptors. However, many clinically used agents have yet to be tested by methods that would allow firm conclusions as to the extent to which channel block is important in their actions (see, for example, Colquhoun, 1986). A simplified reaction scheme that shows both competitive and open-channel block is shown in Fig. 7.9.

7.4.1. *Non-depolarising antagonists*

A few agents have been shown to have a primarily competitive mode of action under clinical conditions; for example this is almost certainly the case for tubocurarine and gallamine. Under experimental conditions they also show prominent channel blocking actions but such action is, primarily at least, on the open channel and so will be most prominent in the maintained presence of higher concentrations of agonist.

7.4.1.1. *Channel block.* Acetylcholine is present for a very short time under physiological conditions and, with usual antagonist concentrations, the rate of channel block is not sufficient to block many of the channels during the short time for which they are open (even under conditions where the equilibrium extent of channel block, with a maintained ACh concentration, would actually be quite high).

For example (Colquhoun *et al.* 1979) tubocurarine (at -90 mV, $10°C$ in frog) has an equilibrium constant for open channel block of about 0.06 µM, i.e. a substantially higher affinity than for the competitive action ($K = 0.34$ µM). The high affinity for channel block results from slow dissociation from the open channel (mean blockage duration 1.6 s); the association rate constant, about 1.0×10^7 M^{-1} s^{-1}, is not particularly fast. Thus, at a tubocurarine concentration of 3 µM, which would produce considerable competitive block (90% occupancy at equilibrium), there would be 30 blockages per second of channel open time. If, during normal transmission, channels open once for 1 ms on average, and about 20% of the channels that are exposed to ACh are opened, then only about 0.6% (i.e. 30 $s^{-1} \times 0.001$ s $\times 20\%$) of these channels will be blocked during synaptic transmission (whereas 98% of open channels would be blocked at equilibrium). Furthermore, channel block by all charged compounds will be reduced by the depolarisation which will, of course, occur under physiological conditions. This argument shows that it is not surprising that channel block appears to be unimportant under physiological conditions, even at high stimulation rate (Magleby *et al.*, 1981).

The argument above also underlines the very limited usefulness of arguments based on equilibrium binding for prediction of effects on synaptic transmission. It is necessary, as emphasised above, to know about the rates of interaction with receptors.

7.4.1.2. Competitive antagonists. Although rate constants are known for the channel blocking action of a few antagonists (and would be fairly easy to determine for others), the rate constants for competitive effects (binding to, and dissociation from, the agonist sites) are still unknown for all antagonists. Although this was one of the first quantitative pharmacological questions ever addressed (Hill, 1909), it has proved astonishingly intractable, mainly because of the problem of diffusion which prevents sufficiently rapid changes in antagonist concetration (concentration jumps) being done, and because the lack of dependence of the competitive effect on membrane potential also precludes the use of the voltage jump method.

Recently an attempt has been made to solve this problem by looking for additional shut periods induced by tubocurarine in single-channel recordings made in the presence of high ACh concentrations (N. K. Mulrine and D. C. Ogden, unpublished results). They found little effect of tubocurarine on the fraction of time that a channel appeared to be open; this presumably means that tubocurarine produces relatively few, but rather long, shut periods in the record, so that these shut periods cannot be distinguished from desensitised (or channel-blocked) periods. The observation that shut periods produced by tubocurarine are long may seem surprising in the light of other evidence (see, for example, Colquhoun, 1986), which suggests that tubocurarine equilibrates fairly rapidly. However, simulations show that even if equilibration is fairly rapid, it would nevertheless be expected that quite long shut periods would be produced in the single-channel record, as a result of (rapid) oscillations between several different shut states (each with a different number of agonist or antagonist molecules bound to them). The rates are still not known.

In addition to the lack of knowledge concerning receptor binding rates for competitive antagonists, there are additional problems in understanding their actions in a quantitative way under physiological conditions. These result from the fact that the ACh concentration not only varies with time but is also spatially non-uniform. Furthermore, the volume of the synaptic cleft is very small compared with the number of binding sites that it contains. A relatively small decrease in receptor occupancy by tubocurarine, such as would occur when ACh is released and competes for the same receptor sites, will produce a large (though transient) increase in the free tubocurarine concentration in the synaptic cleft. This will oppose the dissociation of the antagonist and make a reversible antagonist tend to behave as though it were irreversible. This, and related topics, have been well-described by Pennefather and Quastel (1981).

The physiological effect of either competitive block or channel block will be to reduce, in a graded fashion, the size of the depolarisation (the EPP) produced by released ACh. When, on any individual muscle fibre, the EPP is reduced so much that the threshold for action potential generation is not reached, this fibre will fire no action potential and produce no contraction on nerve stimulation. If the threshold *is* reached then the action potential and contraction will be normal. The gradual reduction of muscle tension results from the differences, from fibre to fibre, in the amount of receptor block needed to prevent attainment of the firing threshold. In fact the margin of safety in transmission (the safety factor, see chapter 2) is quite high in most species (Paton and Waud, 1967).

7.4.1.3. Effect of anticholinesterase drugs on non-depolarising block. It is well known that inhibitors of acetylcholinesterase can reverse neuromuscular block produced by non-depolarizing antagonists. ACh persists for a (2–5-fold) longer time in the synaptic cleft when its hydrolysis is inhibited and it must escape by diffusion. Repeated ACh binding to receptors will slow down diffusion (though this effect would be reduced by the presence of a competitive agent that occupies the binding sites). The ACh molecules in each quantum will be able to diffuse laterally, so quanta will overlap in their effects; this will result in a disproportionately large increase in the effectiveness of ACh because of the cooperative shape of the concentration–response curve (Hartzell *et al.*, 1975; Magleby and Terrar, 1975). In the presence of a competitive blocker (even if it is behaving irreversibly — see above) the EPP will become larger following inhibition of acetylcholinesterase, so the threshold for action potential generation is reached in a larger proportion of fibres and contraction strength will increase. This underlies its clinical use in myasthenia gravis, in which there is a reduction in the number of functioning AChRs (see Vincent, this volume).

The effect of channel block should also be reversed by anticholinesterases, especially for slow blockers which produce little block during the brief rising phase of the EPC: at the other extreme, even a channel blocker that was fast enough to come to equilibrium with released ACh should be antagonised to some extent, though the equilibrium concentration–response curve for ACh has a depressed maximum in the presence of the blocker.

Any discussions of anticholinesterase agents must take into consideration the fact that many of them have recently been found to have both agonist and channel-blocking actions themselves, as well as inhibiting acetylcholinesterase (see, for example, Shaw *et al.*, 1985; Bradley *et al.*, 1986).

7.4.2. *Depolarising blocking drugs*

7.4.2.1. Acetylcholine-like action and channel block. It is clear that the most important depolarising blocking drug, suxamethonium (succiny-ldicholine) is an agonist much like any other. In frog muscle it would be capable of opening most of the postsynaptic ion channels at a sufficiently-hig concentration (i.e. it is a full agonist), if it were not for the effects of channel block and desensitisation (Marshall *et al.*, 1990). Its channel blocking effect is more pronounced than that of ACh (equilibrium constant for channel block about 270 μM at −120 mV, compared with 1300 μM for ACh), and this effect limits the maximum equilibrium response that can be attained to about 36% of channels open. Nevertheless, suxamethonium can open more than enough channels to depolarise well beyond threshold (which requires opening of the order of 1% of channels present) and, in any case, the block would be considerably weaker in the depolarised cell. Unfortunately similar experiments have yet to be done in mammalian muscle, although it is clear that large depolarisations can also be produced in cat muscle by micromolar concentrations of suxamethonium (Zaimis and Head, 1976). Thus it seems likely that the blocking action of suxamethonium, which is not hydrolysed by AChE, under physiological conditions is like the action of ACh itself in the presence of anticholinester-ase (Wray, 1981; W.-Wray, 1988). This was originally suggested by the

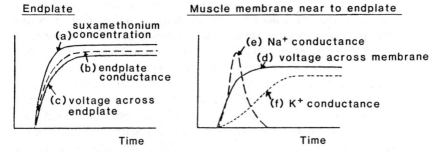

Fig. 7.10. Diagrammatic illustration of effect of suxamethonium or other depolarising neuromuscular blockers during block by prolonged depolarisation. The time-scale is much slower than in Figs. 7.1 and 7.3, the rate of events being controlled by the rate at which suxamethonium reaches the endplate. Left-hand panel shows events at the endplate: as the suxamethonium concentration rises (**a**), endplate channels open increasing its conductance (**b**), and so causing maintained depolarisation of the endplate (**c**); this depolarisation spreads (see Fig. 7.2) to the neighbouring electrically excitable muscle membrane (**d**), the behaviour of which is illustrated in the right-hand panel (compare with Fig. 7.3). The depolarisation of this membrane opens sodium channels transiently (**e**), which may initiate a few action potentials (not shown), but soon the sodium channels inactivate, and potassium channels are held open (**f**), so no further action potentials can be produced, and the membrane near the endplate has become inexcitable.

work of Burns and Paton (1951): prolonged depolarisation of the endplate region, resulting from the prolonged presence of suxamethonium, at first initiates some action potentials, but soon most of the sodium channels within a few millimetres of the endplate become inactivated. However, the potassium channels remain open, as illustrated in Fig. 7.10. Thus the perijunctional membrane becomes electrically inexcitable and the depolarisation can no longer initiate action potentials, so no muscle contraction ensues.

Del Castillo and Katz (1957) suggested that decamethonium might be a partial agonist, and consequently might be expected to reduce the response to high acetylcholine concentrations, as discussed above. In the frog, channel block by decamethonium is more prominent that with suxamethonium, but even the 1–2% cent of channels that are openable by decamethonium would be enough to produce a large depolarisation. Channel block by decamethonium has not been studied in detail in mammals, but it is known that it can produce a large depolarisation in cat muscle (Zaimis and Head, 1976). The work of Burns and Paton (1951) and of Wray (1981) makes it likely that in cat muscle the main mode of action of decamethonium under physiological conditions is prolonged depolarisation, as described above. Such block would, of course, be expected to be exacerbated by anticholinesterase drugs, which is what is observed to happen, at least in the early stages.

7.4.2.2. *Other actions of depolarising antagonists.* It has been proposed at various times that these agents might work by a number of mechanisms other than prolonged depolarisation. For example, the following mechanisms have all been suggested: (1) desensitisation, (2) changes in intracellular ion concentration and/or activation of the sodium pump, (3) reduction in the depolarising effect of ACh release as a result of the increased endplate conductance caused by the depolarising agent, (4) a partial agonist action of the depolarizing agent which will result in competitive-like inhibition of the response to high ACh concentrations, and, most recently, (5) open channel block by the depolarising antagonist. All of these will occur to a greater of lesser extent with all agonists, except for the partial agonist effect which has been shown to be negligible for suxamethonium (in frog muscle), and has yet to be demonstrated in other species and with other agents.

It is unlikely, as discussed above, that any ot these mechanisms is of primary importance under physiological conditions, at least in the early stages of block (see, for example, Colquhoun, 1986, for a more detailed discussion). After neuromuscular block by depolarising agents has been established for some time, it has been observed to change its characteristics: the block may be reversed, rather than aggravated, by anticholinesterase drugs, but will be aggravated by tubocurarine. There has been a good deal of discussion of this 'dual-block' phenomenon in the literature (e.g. Zaimis and Head, 1976). Sometimes it has been said that 'the block changes with time from depolarising block to competitive block', but this sort of statement is clearly, from the point of view of mechanism, nonsensical. A drug cannot be an agonist one minute and an antagonist the next. The mechanism of the dual-block phenomenon is still uncertain. One simple explanation was proposed by Colquhoun (1986). The observed phenomena seem to be quite explicable, in principle, if the depolarising blocking drug were simply a good agonist producing prolonged depolarisation. After it has been present for a long time, however, the endplate (and therefore the surrounding muscle membrane) would be likely to repolarise gradually as a result of desensitisation, redistribution of ions (and possible consequent activation of an electrogenic sodium pump), and, perhaps, ion channel block. When repolarisation occurs, regardless of its mechanism, the inactivation of the sodium channels in the periaxonal membrane will be removed and the electrical excitability of the muscle membrane will be restored. It might be supposed that this would be of no help in restoring transmission if, for example, many receptors were desensitised, and so were unavailable for activation by released transmitter. However, a small fraction only of the total number of receptors need to be activated to produce a depolarisation beyond threshold in many species, so even if many are unavailable it is still possible to get efficient transmission, especially if the proportion of the available receptors that is activated is increased by inhibition of acetylcholinesterase (see Colquhoun, 1986, for more detailed arguments).

7.4.3. *Summary of the mode of action of neuromuscular blocking drugs*

In the past few years all the competitive blocking drugs, as well as all agonists (and thus all depolarising blocking drugs), have been found to block open ion channels in addition to their other actions. Much is known about the rates of channel block, but little is known, even now, about the rates of competitive antagonist binding. Many agents, however, have not yet been tested by appropriate methods to investigate such actions. Channel blocking actions may be very prominent under experimental conditions. Nevertheless the evidence that is available at present suggests that under physiological conditions non-depolarising blocking drugs are effective largely as a result of their competitive effects, as has always been supposed. Likewise depolarising blocking drugs work largely by prolonged depolarisation causing electrical inexcitability of the perijunctional muscle membrane; the change in the characteristics of block that may occur after long exposure to them may result simply from repolarisation of the muscle membrane consequent on desensitisation, ion concentration shifts, electrogenic sodium pump activation or channel block.

References

Adams, P. R. (1981) Acetylcholine receptor kinetics. *J. Membrane Biol.* **58**: 161–174.

Adams, P. R. and Sakmann, B. (1978) Decamethonium both opens and blocks end-plate channels. *Proc. Natl. Acad. Sci. USA* **75**: 2994–2998.

Anderson, C. R. and Stevens, C. F. (1973) Voltage clamp analysis of acetylcholine produced end-plate current fluctuations at frog neuromuscular junction. *J. Physiol.* **235**: 655–691.

Beam, K. G., Caldwell, J. H. and Campbell, D. T. (1985) Na channels in skeletal muscle concentrated near the neuromuscular junction. *Nature* **313**: 588–590.

Bowman, W. C. (1980) *Pharmacology of Neuromuscular Function*. Wright, Bristol.

Bradley, T. J., Sterz, R. and Peper, K. (1986) Agonist and inhibitory effects of pyridostigmine at the neuromuscular junction. *Brain Res.* **376**: 199–203.

Brett, R. S., Dilger, J. P., Adams, P. R. and Lancaster, B. (1986) A method for the rapid exchange of solutions bathing excised membrane patches. *Biophys. J.* **50**: 987–992.

Burns, B. D. and Paton, W. D. M. (1951) Depolarization of the motor end-plate by decamethonium and acetylcholine. *J. Physiol.* **115**: 41–73.

Colquhoun, D. (1978) Farmacologia dei farmaci miorilassanti. In: *Farmacologia Clinica e Terapia*, Vol. 1, A. Bertelli, ed., C. G. Edizione Medico Scientifiche, Torino, pp. 453–472.

Colquhoun, D. (1981) How fast do drugs work? *Trends Pharmacol. Sci.* **2**: 212–217.

Colquhoun, D. (1985) Imprecision in presentation of binding studies. *Trends Pharmacol. Sci.* **6**: 197.

Colquhoun, D. (1986) On the principles of postsynaptic action of neuromuscular blocking agents. In: *New Neuromuscular Blocking Agents, Handbook of Experimental Pharmacology*, D. A. Kharkevich, ed., Springer-Verlag, Berlin, pp. 59–113.

Colquhoun, D. (1987) Affinity, efficacy and receptor classification: is the classical theory still useful? In: *New Perspectives on Hormone Receptor Classification*, J. W. Black, D. H. Jenkinson and V. P. Gerskowitch, eds Alan Liss; New York, pp. 103–114.

Colquhoun, D. and Hawkes, A. G. (1977) Relaxation and fluctuations of membrane currents that flow through drug-operated ion channels. *Proc. Roy. Soc. B* **199**: 231–262.

Colquhoun, D. and Hawkes, A. G. (1983). The principles of the stochastic interpretation of ion channel mechanisms. In: *Single Channel Recording*, B. Sakmann and E. Neher, eds, Plenum Press, New York, pp. 135–175.

Colquhoun, D. and Ogden, D. C. (1988) Activation of ion channels in the frog end-plate by high concentrations of acetylcholine. *J. Physiol.* **395**: 131–159.

Colquhoun. D. and Sakmann, B. (1981) Fluctuations in the microsecond time range of the current through single acetylcholine receptor ion channels. *Nature* **294**: 464–466.

Colquhoun, D. and Sakmann, B. (1983) Bursts of openings in transmitter-activated ion channels. In: *Single Channel Recording*, B. Sakmann and E. Neher, eds, Plenum Press, New York, pp. 345–364.

Colquhoun, D. and Sakmann, B. (1985) Fast events in single-channel currents activated by acetylcholine and its analogues at the frog muscle end-plate. *J. Physiol.* **369**: 501–557.

Colquhoun, D., Dreyer, F. and Sheridan, R. E. (1979) The actions of tubocurarine at the frog neuromuscular junction. *J. Physiol.* **293**: 247–284.

Colquhoun, D., Ogden, D. C. and Cachelin, A. B. (1986) Mode of action of agonists on nicotinic receptors. In: *Ionic Channels in Neural Membranes*, J. M. Ritchie, ed., Liss; New York, pp. 255–273.

Colquhoun, D., Ogden D. C. and Mathie, A. (1987) Nicotinic acetylcholine receptors of nerve and muscle: functional aspects. *Trends Pharmacol. Sci.* **8**: 465–472.

Del Castillo, J. and Katz, B. (1957) Interaction at end-plate receptors between different choline derivatives. *Proc. Roy. Soc. B* **146**: 369–381.

Elmqvist, D., Johns, T. R. and Thesleff, S. (1960) A study of some electrophysiological properties of human intercostal muscle. *J. Physiol.* **154**: 602–607.

Gardner, P., Ogden, D. C. and Colquhoun, D. (1984) Conductances of single ion channels opened by nicotinic agonists are indistinguishable. *Nature* **309**: 160–162.

Hartzell, H.C., Kuffler, S. W. and Yoshikami, D. (1975) Post-synaptic potentiation: interaction between quanta of acetylcholine at the skeletal neuromuscular synapse. *J. Physiol.* **251**: 427–463.

Head, S. D. (1983). Temperature and end-plate currents in rat diaphragm. *J. Physiol.* **334**: 441–459.

Hill, A. V. (1909) The mode of action of nicotine and curari determined by the form of the contraction curve and the method of temperature coefficients. *J. Physiol.* **39**: 361–373.

Katz, B. (1966). *Nerve, Muscle and Synapse*, McGraw-Hill, New York.

Katz, B. (1969). *The Release of Neural Transmitter Substances*, Liverpool University Press, Liverpool.

Katz, B. and Miledi, R. (1972) The statistical nature of the acetylcholine potential and its molecular components. *J. Physiol.* **224**: 665–699.

Kuffler, S. W. and Yoshikami, D. (1975) The number of transmitter molecules in a quantum: an estimate from iontophoretic application of acetylcholine at the neuromuscular synapse. *J. Physiol.* **251**: 465–482.

Madsen, B. W., Edeson, R. O., Lam, H. S. and Milne, R. K. (1984). Numerical simulation of miniature endplate currents. *Neurosci. Lett.* **48**: 67–74.

Magleby, K. L. and Terrar, D. A. (1975) Factors affecting the time course of decay of end-plate currents: a possible cooperative action of acetylcholine on receptors at the frog neuromuscular junction. *J. Physiol.* **244**: 467–495.

Magleby, K. L., Pallotta, B. S. and Terrar, D. A. (1981) The effect of (+)-tubocurarine on neuromuscular transmission during repetitive stimulation in the rat, mouse, and frog. *J. Physiol.* **312**: 97–113.

Marshall, C. G., Ogden, D. C. and Colquhoun, D. (1990). The actions of suxamethonium (succinyldicholine) as an agonist and channel blocker at the nicotinic receptor of frog muscle. *J. Physiol.* **428**: 154–174.

Marshall, C. G., Ogden, D. C. and Colquhoun, D. (1991). Activation of ion channels in the frog end-plate by several analogues of acetylcholine. *J. Physiol.* (In press).

Mishina, M., Takai, T., Imoto, K., Noda, M., Takahashi, T., Numa, S., Methfessel, C. and Sakmann, B. (1986) Molecular distinction between fetal and adult forms of msucle acetylcholine receptor. *Nature* **321**: 406–411.

Mulrine, N. K. and Ogden, D. C. (1988) The equilibrium open probability of nicotinic ion channels at the rat neuromuscular junction. *J. Physiol.*

Neher, E. and Stevens, C. F. (1977) Conductance fluctuations and ionic pores in membranes. *Annu. Rev. Biophys. Bioeng.* **6**: 345–381.

Ogden, D. C. and Colquhoun, D. (1985). Ion channel block by acetylcholine, carbachol and suberyldicholine at the frog neuromuscular junction. *Proc. Roy.*

Soc. B **225**: 329–355.

Paton, W. D. M. and Waud, D. R. (1967) The margin of safety of neuromuscular transmission. *J. Physiol.* **191**: 59–90.

Pennefather, P. and Quastel, D. M. J. (1981) Relation between subsynaptic receptor blockade and response to quantal transmitter at the mouse neuromuscular junction. *J. Gen. Physiol.* **78**: 313–344.

Peper, K., Bradley, R. J. and Dreyer, F. (1982) The acetylcholine receptor at the neuromuscular junction. *Physiol. Rev.* **62**: 1271–1340.

Sakmann, B., Patlak, J. and Neher, E. (1980) Single acetylcholine-activated channels show burst-kinetics in presence of desensitizing concentrations of agonist. *Nature* **286**: 71–73.

Shaw, K. P., Aracava, Y., Akaike, A., Daly, J. W., Rickett, D. L. and Albuquerque, E. X. (1985) The reversible cholinesterase inhibitor physostigmine has channel-blocking and agonist effects on the acetylcholine receptor–ion channel complex. *Mol. Pharmacol.* **28**: 572–538.

Sine, S. M. and Steinbach, J. H. (1987) Activation of acetylcholine receptors on clonal mammalian BC3H-1 cells by high concentrations of agonist. *J. Physiol.* **385**: 325–359.

Stephenson, R. P. (1956) A modification of receptor theory. *Br. J. Pharmacol.* **11**: 379–393.

Wray, D. (1980). Noise analysis and channels at the postsynaptic membrane of skeletal muscle. *Progr. Drug Res.* **24**: 9–56.

Wray, D. (1981). Prolonged exposure to acetylcholine: noise analysis and channel inactivation in cat tenuissimus muscle. *J. Physiol.* **310**: 37–56.

W.-Wray, D. (1988) Neuromuscular transmission In: *Disorders* of *Voluntary Muscle*, J. Walton, ed., Churchill Livingstone, London, pp. 74–108.

Zaimis, E. (1976) *Neuromuscular Junction. Handbook of Edxperimental Pharmacology*, Vol. 42, E. Zaimis, ed., Springer, Berlin.

Zaimis, E. and Head, S. (1976) Depolarizing neuromuscular blocking agents. In: *Neuromuscular Junction, Handbook of Experimental Pharmacology*, Vol. 42, E. Zaimis, ed., Springer, Berlin, pp. 365–419.

Acetylcholine receptors at the neuromuscular junction

Ever since the demonstration by Dale *et al.* (1936) that a stimulated nerve–muscle preparation produced acetylcholine (ACh), and that this substance could cause contractures in muscle preparations, it has been clear that an ACh 'receptor' must be present at the neuromuscular junction. This concept became even stronger when electrophysiologists began to map the response to ACh applied through iontophoretic pipettes. However, the ability to define the nature of the receptor awaited the discovery of high-affinity labels, in particular the α-neurotoxins, the development of techniques for purifying and characterising membrane proteins, and the eventual cloning of their genes. This chapter summarises the main approaches that were used, and our present knowledge concerning the structure and developmental regulation of the AChR at the neuromuscular junction. More detailed reviews are available, for instance Maelicke (1986) and Claudio (1989).

8.1. Characterisation and purification of acetylcholine receptors

8.1.1. *Distribution of AChRs*

The distribution of AChRs in muscle was originally determined by measuring 'ACh sensitivity' (see Chapter 2). It was found that the AChR was present only at the neuromuscular junction in normal muscle, but when the nerve to a muscle was cut or damaged ACh sensitivity appeared, over 1 or 2 weeks. throughout the muscle fibre (Axelsson and Thesleff, 1959; Miledi, 1960). A little later, Lee and his colleagues (see Lee, 1972) discovered that a polypeptide from the venom of the banded krait, *Bungarus multicinctus*, blocked neuromuscular transmission irreversibly. That this toxin, named α-bungarotoxin (α-BuTX), bound to the AChRs was confirmed by the fact that the distribution of ^{125}I-α-BuTX binding sites mirrored that of ACh sensitivity in normal and denervated muscle, and that binding was inhibited by cholinergic agonists and antagonists.

The amount of AChR in normal mammalian muscle is low, about 0.1 μg/g of tissue, although it increases 10–50-fold after denervation. However, the electric organs of various rays and eels are embryonically derived

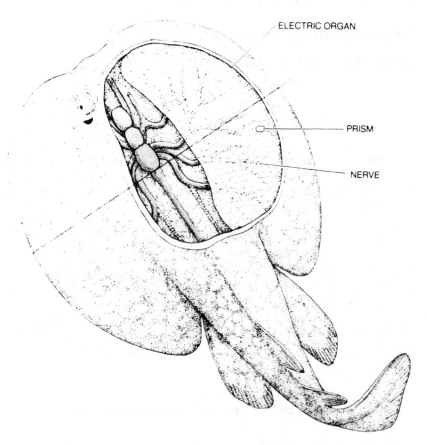

Fig. 8.1. (a) Drawing of the electric fish *Torpedo marmorata*, demonstrating the
electric organ (taken with permission from Dunant and Israël, 1985). (b) An
electron micrograph of a negatively stained fragment of AChR-rich membrane
from the electric organ of *Torpedo marmorata*. The AChRs are seen as ring-like or
pentameric structures protruding from the membrane. Taken with permission from
Giersig *et al.*, 1986.

from muscle and are much more richly innervated. Indeed, about 50% of
the postsynaptic surface has a high density of AChRs providing a total of
about 100 µg/g. Thus the electroplax of *Torpedo* and *Electrophorus*
provided an ideal starting point for purification of receptors (Fig. 8.1).

8.1.2. *Purification*

The AChR was purified by affinity chromatography, mainly using
α-cobratoxin-sepharose columns, after extraction of membrane proteins in

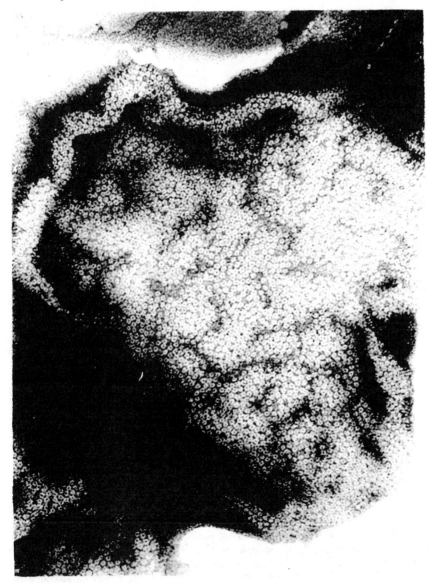

Fig. 8.1 **(b)**

detergent (see Chapter 3). The purified material was a glycoprotein (it bound to lectin columns) which behaved on gel filtration and sucrose density gradients as a macromolecule of about 300 kD. However, when subjected to polyacrylamide gel electrophoresis (PAGE) it separated into four distinct subunits, α, β, γ and δ (Fig. 8.2).

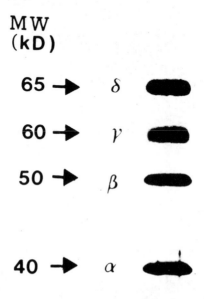

Fig. 8.2. SDS/PAGE analysis of AChR purified from *Torpedo marmorata*. The gel has been stained with Coomassie brilliant blue. The AChR complex can be purified from solubilised membranes by α-toxin-sepharose chromatography, and is found to be composed of four subunits designated α, β, γ and δ. Taken with permission from Sumikawa *et al.*, 1981.

The purified electroplax receptor protein in detergent displayed many of the pharmacological characteristics of the AChR in the native state i.e. it bound ACh, α-tubocurarine and other cholinergic ligands with appropriate affinity (see Heidmann and Changeux, 1978). Moreover, antisera from rabbits immunised with the purified protein inhibited the ACh response of the electric organ (Patrick and Lindstrom, 1973), and of rabbit neuro-muscular preparations. In addition, the protein could be reincorporated into lipid bilayers, by dialysis to remove the detergent, and shown to mediate agonist-induced cation fluxes (see McNamee and Ochoa, 1982). Thus, the pure protein was indeed the AChR.

In 1980 the first 50 or so amino acids were sequenced from the NH_2 termini of each of the AChR subunits. It was found that there was significant homology between them, and a stoichiometry of α_2, β, γ, δ (Raftery *et al.*, 1980; Conti-Tronconi *et al.*, 1982). The N-terminal amino acid sequences enabled several groups to devise oligonucleotides with which to probe cDNA libraries from electric organ. In this way the cDNAs for each of the *Torpedo* subunits were cloned and eventually sequenced, allowing the full amino acid sequences to be determined. The cross-hybridisation of the *Torpedo* cDNAs, to cDNA or genomic clones coding for the muscle AChR, has subsequently enabled the AChR amino acid sequences to be determined for other species.

8.1.3. *General features of the AChR*

What information about AChRs can be obtained from the sequences of the cDNA and genomic clones, and how does it add to what is already known? It is well established that the nicotinic AChR of the electric organ of *Torpedo* is a membrane-bound glycoprotein that contains four homologous subunits. The stoichiometry of α_2, β, γ, δ, initially deduced from N-terminal amino acid sequencing (Raftery *et al.*, 1980), is also well established. Moreover, in the case of the *Torpedo* AChR the arrangement of the subunits around the central ion channel can be visualised (see Lindstrom, Fig. 8.2). There are conflicting reports about the observed stoichiometry of the muscle AChR. cDNA cloning showed that each of the *Torpedo* subunit polypeptides was the product of a distinct gene (Numa *et al.*, 1983). The presence of analogous genes in those species which have been subjected to AChR cDNA cloning, i.e. calf, rat, mouse, chicken and now human (see later), and their subsequent expression in *Xenopus* oocytes, strongly suggests they have a similar structure to that of the *Torpedo* AChR (reviewed in Claudio, 1989). Thus, the pentameric arrangement of four homologous subunits in stoichiometry α_2, β, γ, δ around a central ion channel is likely to be the case in general for muscle AChRs.

The existence of isoforms of a given subunit may lead to some of the variance in reports of subunit stoichiometry. Isolation of cDNAs for calf AChR revealed an isoform of the γ subunit (Takai *et al.* 1985), termed the ϵ-subunit, that replaces the γ subunit during maturation of the neuro-muscular junction (see below and Chapter 1). The presence of the ϵ subunit has now also been established in rat, mouse and man (Criado *et al.*,

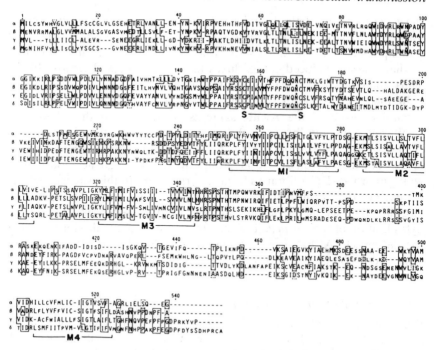

Fig. 8.3. Alignment of the amino acid sequences of the four subunit precursors of the *Torpedo californica* AChR. Gaps (–) have been inserted to achieve maximum homology. The positions in the aligned sequences including gaps are numbered beginning with the initiating methionine. The positions of the putative disulphide bridge (S–S) and the putative transmembrane segments (M1–M4) are shown. The asparagine residues as possible sites of glycosylation are indicated by asterisks. Taken with permission from Numa *et al.*, 1983.

1988; Buonanno *et al.*, 1989; Beeson, unpublished data). Hence, in these species the oligomeric structure in mature muscle is α, β, δ, ε.

Once the nucleotide sequence for either cDNA or genomic clones has been obtained then the amino acid sequence can be deduced. A comparison of the amino acid sequences shows the five subunits to be clearly related, with about 40% amino acid identity between them in any given species (Fig. 8.3). However, each subunit is much more strongly conserved between species with about 80–90% or more identity between vertebrate muscle AChRs (Fig. 8.4). This homology is not uniform along the polypeptide chain; as illustrated in Fig. 8.3 and 8.4 the greatest homology is found in those regions termed M1, M2 and M3. It is predominantly these regions that have been used as probes in the cross-hybridisation between species.

What other characteristics of AChRs can be identified by examination and analysis of the primary amino acid sequence? The sequences derived

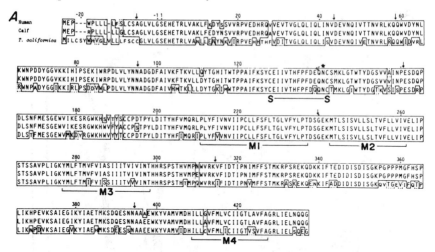

Fig. 8.4. Alignment of the amino acid sequences of the human, calf and *Torpedo californica* AChR α subunit precursors. The high level of homology suggests that structural features have been conserved through evolution. The sequences were obtained from cDNA clones (calf and *Torpedo californica*) and genomic clones (human) and are shown by the one-letter amino acid notation. Gaps (−) have been inserted in the prepeptide region to achieve maximum homology. Amino acid residues are numbered beginning with the amino-terminal residue of the mature α subunit. Taken with permission from Noda *et al.*, 1983.

from cDNAs begin with a stretch of hydrophobic amino acids that are not found in the mature protein. These 'leader' sequences, characteristic of secreted proteins and some membrane proteins, indicate that the NH_2 terminus has been inserted through the membrane into the lumen of the endoplasmic reticulum during synthesis and will therefore end up on the extracellular surface. Limited proteolytic digestion indicates the N-terminals of all of the subunits are extracellular. In addition, the first 210 amino acids (*Torpedo* AChR numbering) are predominantly hydrophilic; consequently most models have assigned this region as being the main extracellular domain. Within it, universally and exclusively on the α-subunit, are adjacent cysteine residues at positions 192 and 193. Affinity alkylation using agonist-like reagents such as bromoacetylcholine has shown that the high-affinity ACh binding site is adjacent to these cysteines, which are bridged (Kao and Karlin, 1986). It is now common to define an AChR α subunit by the presence of the double cysteine residues at 192 and 193 (see also Lindstrom, this volume).

The α neurotoxin binding site is also on the α subunit (Fig. 8.5a), and can be shown to bind both to synthetic and to recombinant peptides that include the sequence 185–196 (containing the adjacent cysteine residues). However, there is also evidence that other low-affinity agonist sites exist on

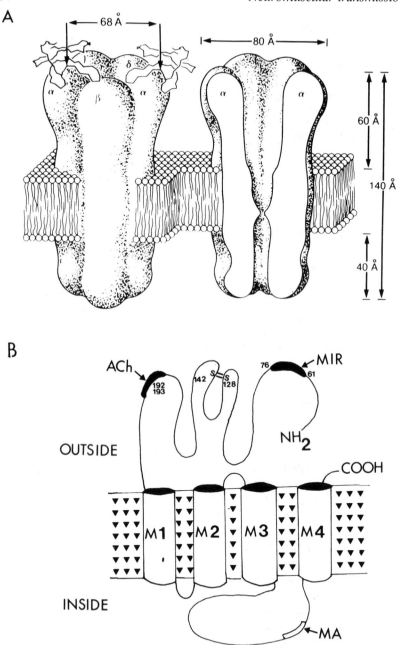

Fig. 8.5. (a) A model of the AChR showing the subunits within the membrane and the positions of bound α-toxin molecules. Taken with permission from Taylor *et al.* 1986. (b) Minimal model of the topology of the α subunit across the membrane.

the other subunits, and there is still uncertainty as to the location at which agonists actually bind to open the channel. As illustrated in the chapter by Lindstrom (this volume), both the binding of α-BuTX and of antibodies directed against the main immunogenic region can be visualised by electron microscopic image analysis, and is seen to be on the tops of the two α subunits.

All of the AChR subunits cloned so far, including several neuronal types (see Lindstrom, this volume) also contain cysteine residues at positions corresponding to 128 and 142 of the *Torpedo* α subunit. These cysteines are thought to be involved in the correct folding of the AChR. Experiments using site-directed mutagenesis (Mishina *et al.*, 1986), in which either one of these two cysteines was changed to a serine, led to the loss of AChR function. This extracellular region also contains an asparagine residue at position 141 available for *N*-glycosylation (*N*-glycoprotein linkage occurs at sequences Asn–X–Ser or Asn–X–Thr) which, along with the cysteines at 128 and 142, is conserved in all four subunits.

A minimal model, therefore, of the topology of α subunit within the membrane has an extracellular region followed by the highly conserved hydrophobic transmembrane regions M1, M2 and M3, then a cytoplasmic loop containing a region that could form an amphipathic helix (MA) found between M3 and M4 in all subunits. The sequence of MA does not show the same degree of homology as M1, M2 and M3, and its significance, as yet, is unknown. Finally, there is the less well conserved hydrophobic M4 crossing the membrane, thus placing the C-terminus in the extracellular space (see Fig. 8.5b). However, as discussed in more detail by Lindstrom, there is still uncertainty about the tertiary structure of each subunit.

8.2. Relating structure to function

It may be seen from the previous section that knowledge of the primary amino acid sequence, as obtained from cDNAs, does not provide many answers with respect to the structure/function relationship of AChRs, but rather provides a framework for detailed predictive models. What experiments can be used to test these models? The main problem of studying the function of the AChR is that by definition it must be within a membrane to act as a ligand-gated ion channel, and once a membrane has been disrupted function can no longer be recorded. One method used to overcome this problem is microinjection of *Xenopus* oocytes. *Xenopus* oocytes have been shown to faithfully synthesise and assemble a variety of biologically active neurotransmitter receptors after injection with exogenous mRNA (reviewed in Barnard and Bilbe, 1987). The SP6 system enables RNA to be made from cloned cDNAs. Consequently, it is possible to microinject RNAs for the AChR into oocytes which synthesise AChRs and enable electrophysiological recordings of function to be made; thus providing an isolated system in which the powerful techniques of molecular biology and electrophysiology may be combined.

The synthesis of mRNA from the respective subunit cDNAs of *Torpedo* followed by the expression of fully functional channels in oocytes was the first definitive proof that all the information necessary for the formation of an ion channel was contained within the subunit mRNA nucleotide sequences (Mishina *et al.*, 1984). Therefore, provided cDNAs containing the full coding region are available, site-directed mutagenesis can be used to make single amino acid changes, and the effect of these on function can be measured in *Xenopus* oocytes. The first experiments using these techniques (Mishina *et al.*, 1986) were not conclusive in that they could not establish whether alterations of physiological responses were due to changes in functionally important or structurally important regions of the α subunit. One means of overcoming this problem was to use different combinations of subunit RNAs for injections, in particular the use of hybrid AChRs, in which the subunit RNAs from different species are co-injected.

The most conclusive experiment with different subunit combinations was the demonstration of the role of the ε-subunit (Mishina *et al.*, 1985). In electrophysiological studies of mammalian muscles, two types of AChR have been detected, an adult type with a brief channel open time (~2 ms at room temperature) and a higher conductance, and an embryonic type with about four-fold the adult channel open time and a channel conductance of only about 70% of that of the adult type. A novel subunit, the ε subunit, had been cloned from calf muscle (Takai *et al.*, 1985). Microinjection of

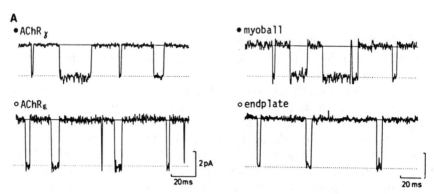

Fig. 8.6. Single channel openings of AChR-γ and AChR-ε channels expressed after the microinjection of synthetic AChR mRNA into *Xenopus* oocytes (left column) compared with those of native AChR channels measured in fetal (myoball) and adult (endplate) bovine muscle (right column). The longer channel open time associated with the presence of the γ subunit is seen in contrast to the shorter channel open-time recorded when the ε subunit is present. Taken with premission form Methfessel, 1986.

Xenopus oocytes with cDNA-derived mRNAs for the α, β, γ and δ subunits of the calf AChR gave AChRs in the oocytes membrane with the characteristics of those found in fetal calf muscle, whereas injection of mRNAs for the α, β, ε and δ subunits gave AChRs in the oocyte membrane characteristic of mature bovine muscle (see Fig. 8.6). It was also demonstrated that mRNA for the ε subunit is present in adult muscle, replacing the γ subunit, which is present in embryonic muscle.

By using hybrid AChRs, made by combining subunits from different species, or chimaeric AChRs, in which small segments of a single subunit are replaced by an analogous segment from another species, it is possible to look for changes in AChR function characteristic of the substituted subunit or segment. Typically each of the *Torpedo* AChR subunits is replaced in turn by its bovine homologue. When the *Torpedo* δ subunit was replaced by the calf δ subunit single-channel open times similar to the calf rather than the parental *Torpedo* AChR were observed. In this way it could be shown that the structural features giving rise to ion channel conductance characteristics reside mainly on the δ subunit (White *et al.*, 1985; Imoto *et al.*,1986). By using chimaeras between the *Torpedo* and bovine δ subunits Imoto *et al.* (1986) showed that the α helix M2 and the amino acids connecting M2 and M3 influence conductance. Further investigations (Imoto *et al.*, 1988), using point mutations to alter charged residues between the M1 and M2, and M2 and M3 regions for all four subunits of *Torpedo*, indicated that these charged residues were important determinants of ionic conductance. Interestingly the *Torpedo* γ subunit is equivalent to the ε subunit rather than the γ subunit of mammalian muscle with respect to these charged amino acids. Similar experiments (Leonard *et al.*, 1988) showed that changing polar residues within M2 could also influence ionic conductance.

The conclusions from these experiments support the structural model of the AChR in which M1, M2, and M3 from each subunit are transmembrane domains participating in the formation of the ion channel, and in which the M2 region from each of the subunits lines the pore. Further support comes from some non-competitive antagonists which are thought to bind within the pore and so block the channel. Some radiolabelled non-competitive antagonists (chlorpromazine and triphenylmethylphosphonium) may be attached covalently to their site of action by photoactivation with UV light. Subsequent enzymatic digestion and peptide analysis of the AChR showed the site of binding to be a serine residue at position 262 of the δ chain (Giraudat *et al.*, 1986; Hucho *et al.*, 1986) and at homologous positions on the α and β subunits; all of these lie within the M2 hydrophobic segment.

Despite these complex experiments which point to M2 lining the ion channel and rings of negatively charged groups near or at the ends of M2 involved in gating and conductance, the overall topology and opening mechanism remains uncertain. What is likely is that other members of the AChR gene superfamily will have a very similar ion channel structure, even though some are anion rather than cation selective (for review see Unwin, 1989).

8.3. Receptor types in different muscle types

As noted above, and discussed further by D. Colquhoun in this volume, the mammalian embryonic type of AChR contains the γ subunit and in the adult type this is replaced by the ε subunit. No difference has been found in the channel properties of the AChRs on fast-twitch or slow-twitch mammalian muscles. Slow-twitch muscles tend to have a low but measurable density of extrajunctional receptors even in the adult, innervated state, but these are predominantly of the adult type, as is true at their endplates.

In amphibian and snake adult twitch muscle endplates a higher conductance channel with a mean open time of several milliseconds is found (roughly equivalent to that of mammalian muscles) while in their slow, tonic muscle endplates there is both the latter, and an 's-channel' of lower conductance with a two-component open time distribution (Colquhoun and Sakmann, 1985). The s-channel is not the same as the low-conductance embryonic AChR type of mammals, since this also exists in amphibian muscle. In birds the situation is again different. In chicken muscle it has been shown that there is no developmental change in the AChR lifetime or conductance (Schuetz, 1980). The structural basis of these species differences is not as yet known, though interestingly two distict genes coding for two forms of the amphibian α subunit have recently been cloned (Hartman and Claudio, 1990).

8.4. The human AChR

The studies summarised above enable us to learn much about the AChR of *Torpedo* and vertebrate muscle. However, for the investigation of human disorders such as myasthenia gravis or inherited myasthenia it is advantageous to use clones for the human AChR genes. Genomic clones for the human muscle α and δ subunits (Noda *et al.*, 1983; Shibahara *et al.*, 1985) and cDNAs for the human α, β, γ and δ subunits (Schoepfer *et al.*, 1988; Luther *et al.*, 1989; Beeson *et al.*, 1989b) have now been isolated. As expected, the sequences show a high degree of homology with the equivalent subunits of other mammalian species, typically around 97% for the α subunit and 90% for the others.

However, analysis of subunit clones from a human muscle cDNA library led to the unexpected discovery of two α subunit isoforms (Beeson *et al.*, 1990b). One was as predicted from the genomic sequence (Noda *et al.*, 1983) and confirmed in a cDNA clone (Schoepfer *et al.*, 1988), whereas the

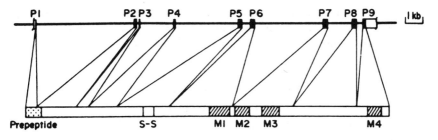

a

b

Fig. 8.7. The genomic structure of the human AChR α subunit gene. (a) The coding sequence for the α subunit gene was thought to be made up of nine exons (protein-coding sequences) separated by eight introns (non-coding sequences). The exons (P1–P9) are shown on the upper line, with the corresponding regions of the protein shown below. Taken with permissin from Noda *et al.*, 1983. (b) Structure of the human α subunit gene showing the position of the novel exon P3A within the gene. Restriction sites for the exzymes BamHI, BglII and EcoRI are shown (Beeson *et al.*, 1990b).

second form contained an insert of an extra 25 amino acids located between residues 58 and 59. The genomic structure of the human α subunit (Noda *et al.*, 1983) divides the gene into nine exons (P1–P9) divided by eight introns, with each exon being analogous to the homologous sequence of the calf α subunit cDNA (Fig. 8.7a). Analysis of a freshly isolated genomic clone showed that the sequence of the 25 amino acid insert was present, located between exons P3 and P4 (Fig. 8.7b), and so was termed P3A. Moreover, analysis of mRNA isolated from muscle indicated that the two types of α subunit mRNA (ie. both with and without P3A) are found in approximately equal amounts. The most likely explanation of this finding is that alternate splicing of exons generates two forms of the α subunit mRNA, and correspondingly two isoforms of the human muscle AChR α subunit. The presence of similar isoforms in other species could not be detected; moreover the new exon, P3A, is in the extracellular coding region (exons P1–P4) whose genomic structure is conserved in all AChR genes so far cloned (reviewed in Buonanno *et al.*, 1989) apart from the *Drosophila* ARD gene.

The functional significance of the two isoforms has yet to be determined.

However, this finding raises the possibility of alternate exon splicing in other AChR genes, and may give clues as to the cause of differing AChR channel properties in some muscle types (see above)

8.4.1. *The human AChR α-BuTX binding site*

One region of interest is the main binding site for α-BuTX. The human amino acid sequence in this region, amino acids 185–196, contains three or four differences from *Torpedo*, mouse or calf AChR. In particular there is a substitution of a serine residue for the tryptophan residue found for all other species at position 187. This substitution is thought to underlie the relatively weak binding of ^{125}I-α-BuTx to the human sequence (Neumann *et al.*, 1986). However, the binding affinity for the native AChR is only slightly lower than that for *Torpedo* AChR, presumably due to the contribution of other regions of the AChR in determining overall binding affinity (A. Vincent, unpublished). The absence of Trp 187 might explain the observation that humans bitten by sea snakes do not show pathological evidence of postsynaptic poisoning in contrast to other mammals. These hydroelapidae venoms contain 'short' α neurotoxins rather than the 'long' α neurotoxins such as α-BuTX, and short neurotoxins do not appear to bind to the human amino acid sequence 179–191 (Low and Corfield, 1987) and bind with only low affinity to native human AChR (A. Vincent, unpublished)

8.4.2. *Chromosomal localisation of AChRs*

Although the homology between the AChR subunits indicates that each has been derived from a common ancestral gene, studies in mouse have shown the subunit genes to be located on three different chromosomes. We have recently localised the human muscle AChR genes, showing that three

Table 8.1. Chromosomal localisation of human AChR subunits
Methods:
(A) Chromosomal localisation — Southern blotting of human–rodent somatic cell hybrids.
(B) Regional localisation — *in situ* hybridisation to metaphase chromosome spreads.

	Human		Mouse* chromosome
	Chromosome	*Localisation*	
α subunit	2	2q24–2q32	17
β subunit	17	17p11–17p12	11
γ subunit	2	2q33–2q35	1
δ subunit	2	2q33–2q35	1

*Heidmann *et al.*, 1986.

of them are on chromosome 2 (Beeson *et al.*, 1990a) (Table 8.1). In fact the α subunit is located close to the γ and δ genes, which in mouse, chicken and man are known to be tightly linked. The β subunit is located in an analogous region between mouse chromosome 11 and human chromosome 17, which is highly conserved.

8.4.3. *The use of the human AChR genes in the study of human disorders*

As described elsewhere (Engel, this volume) there are several congenital forms of myasthenic syndromes which appear to affect AChR number and function, some of which may be due to the abnormalities in the control of AChR expression and others to a genetic defect in the AChR itself. The presence of abnormalities in the AChR genes, or of closely linked control sequences, can be investigated by Southern blotting, using AChR subunit cDNAs as probes, and then carrying out family linkage studies on any observed RFLPs (see Chapter 3). AChR genes from normal individuals or patients with myasthenia gravis show some polymorphisms (Lobos *et al.*, 1989) though these are all thought to be within intron (i.e. non-coding) sequences. The screening of around 20 inherited myasthenia cases (Harrison *et al.*, unpublished) again revealed a number of RFLPs (Fig. 8.8), though none of these have been linked to a defect. These results, perhaps not surprisingly, indicate that the genetic defects, if they are within the AChR coding genes, are not gross deletions or insertions. Small changes in the sequence, such as point mutations, would not necessarily be detected by RFLP studies. The studies described in the section relating structure to function suggest that cases of the 'slow channel syndrome' (see Engel, this volume) might easily be caused by as little as a single amino acid change. The technique of gene amplification using PCR (see Chapter 3) will greatly facilitate the search for single base pair changes, though the screening of five genes for each patient means this is still a considerable undertaking.

In myasthenia gravis autoantibodies directed at determinants on the human AChR cause a loss of functional AChR and a defect in neuromuscular transmission. Although many of the antibodies derived in experimental studies are directed against the main immunogenic region on the two α subunits (see Lindstrom, this volume), and these include the sequence α67–76 (Barkas *et al.*, 1988; Tzartos *et al.*, 1988), it appears that not all the autoantibodies bind to this region (see Vincent, this volume).

More detailed studies of both antibody binding sites and T cell epitopes (sequences that are responsible for T cell proliferation and thereby turning on of antibody production) have been restricted by the low level of AChR in normal innervated human muscle (<2 pmol/g). The rhabdomyosarcoma cell line TE 671 (McAllister *et al.*, 1977) has been shown to express muscle AChRs, but only at levels broadly similar to those found in denervated

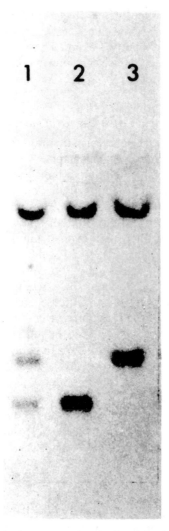

Fig. 8.8. An RFLP for the human α subunit. Southern botting of genomic DNA digested with the restriction enzyme PvuII, and probed with a ^{32}P-labelled α subunit cDNA, demonstrates heterozygous (lane 1) and the two homozygous (lanes 2 and 3) allelic forms of the gene (Harrison *et al.*, unpublished).

human leg muscle (up to 4 pmol/g). As a means of producing up to milligram quantities of each subunit, cDNAs have been introduced into either prokaryotic or eukaryotic expression systems. In general prokaryotic systems, though they may produce large quantities, are unable to synthesise complicated transmembrane proteins in native conformation; whereas eukaryotic systems, though they have the capacity to synthesise

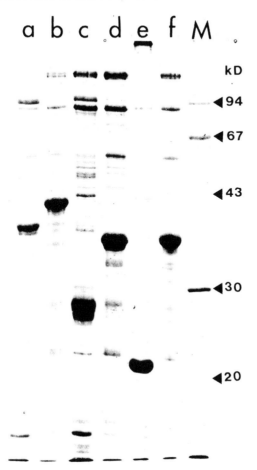

Fig. 8.9. Expression of human α subunit polypeptides in *E. coli*. Inclusion body preparations of expressed α subunit polypeptides analysed by SDS/PAGE on a 12.5% (w/v) polyacrylamide slab gel and stained with Coomassie blue. The α subunit polypeptides, ranging in size from the almost full-length (b) (amino acids 37–429) to the smaller fragment (e) (amino acids 37–181), constitute the major protein present and are seen as the heavily stained bands. (Taken with permission from Beeson *et al.*, 1989a).

and correctly assemble a multi-subunit ion channel, tend to generate the gene products at far lower levels.

Relatively large quantities of full-length and shorter fragments of the human α subunit have been produced in *Escherichia coli* (Fig. 8.9) (Beeson *et al.*, 1989a), and after purification using preparative polyacrylamide gel electrophoresis these polypeptides have been used to stimulate and clone T cells from myasthenia gravis patients (see Vincent, this volume). Although still at an early stage, this approach holds considerable promise as a means of characterising the T cell responses which underlie antibody production in this disease.

The synthesised polypeptides do not, unfortunately, bind with high affinity or specificity either monoclonal antibodies raised against native human AChR or patient's autoantibodies, presumably because the extracellular domain of the isolated α subunit chain does not assume the correct conformation. A eukaryotic expression system may overcome this problem. The reconstitution of functional *Torpedo* AChR from cDNAs stably integrated into the genome of mouse fibroblast L cells has been reported (Claudio *et al.*, 1989). The next step will be to try to achieve the functional expression of human AChR in a similar system.

8.5. Regulation of subunit mRNA levels

As summarised in chapter 1, the AChR goes through a series of stages during embryonic development which result in changes in its amount, distribution, turnover and electrophysiological characteristics. An under-

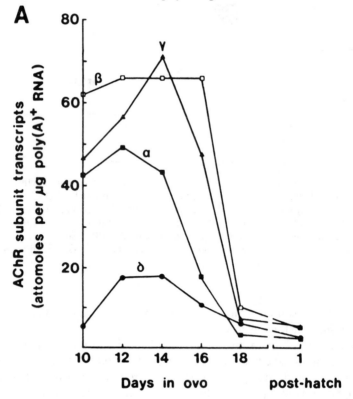

Fig. 8.10   (a)

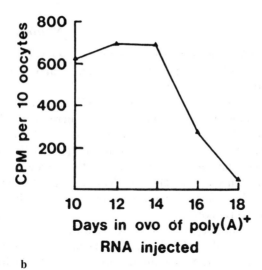

b

c

Fig. 8.10. AChR levels in the developing chick embryo: correlation of steady-state mRNA levels with AChR synthesis and AChR present in muscle. (a) Profile of the steady-state levels of the four subunit transcripts, obtained by densitometric scanning of the bands seen on Northern blots of mRNA isolated at different stages of embryo development. (b) Expression of AChR in *Xenopus* oocytes after microinjection of poly(A)$^+$RNA isolated at stages of embryo development. AChR synthesis was measured by the level of ^{125}I α-bungarotoxin found in extracts from batches of 10 oocytes. (c) AChR protein levels found in muscle extracts taken at stages in embryo development. AChR was measured by ^{125}I α-bungarotoxin binding, and the level calculated per milligram of protein extract. Taken with permission from Moss *et al.*, 1989.

standing of what controls these changes, at the level of gene expression, as well as of considerable fundamental interest, may give insight into some inherited forms of myasthenia.

In the chick embryo an increase in AChR protein in pectoral muscle during development is paralleled by an increase in the total receptor mRNA available for translation and a coordinate increase in the steady-state levels of each subunit transcript (Fig. 8.10). The levels peak at around 12–14 days *in ovo* and there is then a similar coordinate sharp decrease in transcript levels and AChR content. The results strongly suggest that the availability of the subunit mRNAs plays a regulatory role in receptor expression.

The steady-state levels of mRNA are affected both by the rate of gene transcription and the mRNA stability. Buonanno and Merlie (1986) have shown for the α and δ subunits of mouse that the AChR increase which occurs upon myoblast fusion is due to an increase in the rate of subunit gene transcription. Confirmation that this is the case for other subunits and other species depends upon information on the half-life of individual mRNAs. However, if one considers the mRNA levels when the α subunit is at its maximum. the ratios are 1:1.3:1.2:0.4 respectively for α, β, γ and δ. Since this is very different to the stoichiometry of α_2, β, γ, δ of the assembled protein, then it is likely that either levels of transcripts of α or δ, or both α and δ, are limiting the assembly process.

The possibility of a mRNA limiting AChR synthesis is consistent with finding that this mRNA can be selectively upregulated. Fischbach and co-workers (Harris *et al.*, 1988) have found a brain-derived regulatory protein, 'ARIA', which specifically elevates AChR α subunit mRNA in cultured chick myotubes. Further the α subunit mRNA is also augmented, albeit to a more modest extent, by calcitonin-gene-related-peptide (CGRP) in cultured chick myoblasts (Laufer and Changeux, 1987). Further studies have shown this to be selective for the α subunit mRNA out of the four AChR mRNAs.

In the case of the δ subunit mRNA, not only is the level low but a higher molecular weight transcript persists both in the development of chick muscle (Moss *et al.*, 1989) and calf muscle (Mishina *et al.*, 1985). The persistence of the unspliced form may indicate that the regulation of the processing of the δ RNA transcript to form mRNA is a limiting factor.

Information gained from studies of mRNA levels shows that they correlate with the observed increase and decrease in AChR protein levels in muscle. The long time span of around 20–30 mim (Merlie *et al.*, 1983, see Lindstrom, Fig. 9.1) between the initiation of α subunit synthesis and the formation of an intact functional AChR molecule in the membrane would allow for some post-translational control over AChR assembly and location in the membrane, but it is clear that the primary control of AChR synthesis is at the transcriptional level. Goldman *et al.* (1988) have shown that direct electrical stimulation of denervated rat soleus muscles suppresses the normallly observed increase in the steady-state mRNA levels down to or below these detected in innervated muscle. The connection between electrical stimulation and control of gene transcription has yet to be worked out, but its resolution will be an important step in our understanding of synaptogenesis and the formation of the neuromuscular junction.

V Acetylcholinesterase (AChE) of the neuromuscular junction

In vertebrate skeletal muscle, AChE is of great importance for the rapid termination of the impulse transmission by its destruction of ACh. A number of forms of AChE are found which are either globular or behave on density gradients as very large, asymmetric molecules. The largest of the latter has a sedimentation constant of about 16 S in mammals and 20 S in birds. An analogous form in *Electrophorus* electric organ contains twelve identical AChE catalytic subunits, linked by disulfides to a collagenous tail (Massoulié and Bon, 1982). In *Torpedo* electric organ the

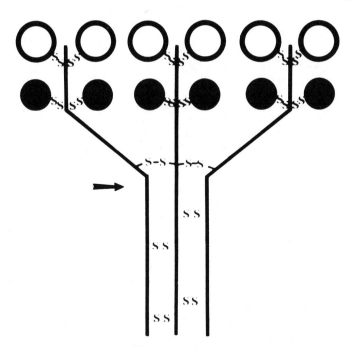

Fig. 8.11. Proposed model for the 20S asymmetric chick AChE. Catalytic subunits are AChE (○) or BuChE (●). The lines represent the tail filaments, shown as containing a triple helical structure, contiguous with a noncollagenous terminal region within the same 58kD subunit. A minimum set of disulphide bridges (SS) is shown. The arrow shows the site for collagenase digestion. (Tsim *et al.*, 1988. Reproduced with permission.)

structure of the catalytic subunit (65 kDa) has been established by cDNA cloning (Schumacher *et al.*, 1986). The collagen tail is believed to anchor this 16–20 S form to the basal lamina at the neuromuscular junction, by non-covalent interactions with heparan sulphate proteoglycan (McMahan *et al.*, 1978; Inestrosa *et al.*, 1982). Further, a cholinesterase of different specificity, termed pseudocholinesterase or butyrylchyolinesterase (Bu-ChE) exists in skeletal and cardiac muscles. The two catalytic subunits of AChE and BuChE, are homologous but derive from different genes.

The endplate (asymmetric) form of AChE, which has a molecular weight of the order of 1 million, is difficult to purify, but recently this was done from young chick twitch muscle by affinity chromatography and its composition was determined (Tsim *et al.*, 1989). It turned out that it contains 6 catalytic units of AChE and 6 of BuChE in a hybrid structure, linked convalently by a triple-stranded collagen tail (Fig. 8.11). This is the form in embryonic and early post-hatch chick muscles. A similar hybrid form has been found in mammalian muscle at embryonic stages only (Tsim and Barnard, in preparation). In adult muscle from birds and mammals, however, the BuChE subunits are all replaced by AChE subunits.

References

Axelsson, J. and Thesleff, all S. (1959) A study of supersensitivity in denervated mammalian skeletal muscle. *J. Physiol.* (*Lond.*) **147**: 178–193.

Barkas, T., Gabriel, J-M., Mauron, A., Hughes, J., Roth, B., Alliod, C., Tzartos, S. and Ballivet, M. (1988) Localisation of the main immunogenic region of the nicotinic acetylcholine recepter. *J. Biol. Chem.* **263**: 5916–5920.

Barnard, E. A. and Bilbe, G. (1987) Functional expression in the *Xenopus* oocyte of mRNAs for receptors and ion channels. In: *Neurochemistry: A Practical Approach*, Turner, A. J. and Bachelard, H., eds, IRL Press, Oxford, pp. 243–270.

Beeson, D., Brydson, M., Wood, H., Vincent, A. and Newsom-Davis, J. (1989a) Human muscle AChR: cloning and expression in *E. coli* of cDNA for the alpha subunit. *Biochem. Soc. Trans.* **17**: 219–220.

Beeson, D., Brydson, M. and Newsom-Davis, J. (1989b) Nucleotide sequence of human muscle AChR beta subunit. *Nucleic Acids Res.* **17**: 4391.

Beeson, D., Jeremiah, S., West, L., Povey, S. and Newsom-Davis, J. (1990) Assignment of the human nAChR genes: the alpha & delta subunit genes to chromosome 2 and the beta subunit gene to chromosome 17. *Ann. Hum. Genet.* **54**: 199–208.

Beeson, D., Morris, A., Vincent, A. and Newsom-Davis, J. (1990) The human muscle mcotivic acetylcholine receptor α-subunit exists as two isoforms: a norel exon. *EMBO J.* **9**: 2101–2106.

Buonanno, A. and Merlie, J. (1986) Transcription regulation of the nicotinic acetylcholine receptor genes during muscle development. *J. Biol. Chem.* **261**: 11452–11455.

Buonanno, A., Mudd, J. and Merlie, J. (1989) Isolation and characterisation of the beta and epsilon subunit genes of mouse muscle AChR. *J. Biol. Chem.* **264**: 7611–7616.

Claudio, T. (1989) Molecular genetics of acetylcholine receptor channels. In:

Frontiers in Molecular Biology, Molecular Neurobiology, Glover, D. and Hames, D., eds, IRL Press, Oxford, pp. 63–126.

Claudio, T., Paulson, H., Green, W., Ross, A., Hartman, D. and Hayden, D. (1989) Fibroblasts transfected with *Tropedo* AChR beta, gamma, and delta subunit cDNAs express functional receptor when infected with a retroviral alpha recombinant. *J. Cell. Biol.* **108**: 2277–2290.

Colquhoun, D. and Sakmann, B. (1985) Fast events in single-channel currents activated by acetylcholine and its analogues at the frog muscle endplate. *J. Physiol.*, **369**: 501–557.

Conti-Tronconi, B. M., Gotti, C., Hunkapillar, M. and Raftery, M. A. (1982) Mammalian muscle acetylcholine receptor: A supramolecular structure formed by four related proteins. *Science* **218**: 1227–1229.

Criado, M., Witzemann, V., Koenen, M. and Sakmann, B. (1988) Nucleotide sequence of the rat muscle AChR epsilon subunit. *Nuclein Acids Res.* **16**: 10920.

Dale, H., Feldberg, W. and Vogt, M. (1936) Release of acetylcholine at voluntary motor nerve endings. *J. Physiol. (Lond.)* **86**: 353–380.

Dunant, Y. and Israël, M. (1985) The release of acetylcholine. *Sci. Am.* **252**: 40–46.

Giersing, M., Kunath, W., Sack-Kongehl, H. and Hucho, F. (1986) Ultrastructural analysis of the native AChR. In: *Nicotinic Acetylcholine Receptor: Structure and Function* Maelicke, A., ed., NATO ASI series, Vol. 3, Springer-Verlag, Berlin, pp. 7–17.

Giraudat, J., Dennis, M., Heidmann, T., Chang, J-Y. and Changeux, J-P. (1986) Structure of the high-affinity binding site for noncompetitive blockers of the acetylcholine receptor: serine-262 of the delta subunit is labelled by [^{3}H]chlorpromazine. *Proc. Natl. Acad. Sci. USA* **83**: 2719–2723.

Goldman, D., Brenner, H. and Heinemann, S. (1988) Acetylcholine receptor alpha, beta, gamma and delta subunit mRNA levels are regulated by muscle activity. *Neuron* **1**: 329–333.

Harris, D., Falls, D., Dill-Devor, R. and Fischbach, G. (1988) Acetylcholine receptor-inducing factor from chick brain increases the level of mRNA encoding the receptor alpha subunit. *Proc. Natl. Acad. Sci. USA* **85**: 1983–1987.

Hartman, D. and Claudio, T. (1990) Coexpression of two distinct muscle acetylcholine receptor alpha subunits during development. *Nature* **343**: 372–375.

Heidmann, T. and Changeux, J.-P. (1978) Structural and functional properties of the acetylcholine receptor protein in its purified and membrane-bound states. *Annu. Rev. Biochem.* **47**: 317–357.

Heidmann, O., Buonanno, A., Geoffroy, B., Robert, B., Guenet, J.-L., Merlie, J. and Changeux, J-P. (1986) Chromosomal localisation of muscle nicotinic acetylcholine receptor genes in the mouse. *Science* **234**: 866–868.

Hucho, F., Oberthur, W. and Lottspeich, F. (1986) The ion channel of the nicotinic acetylcholine receptor is formed by the homologous helices M2 of the receptor subunits. *FEBS Lett.* **205**: 137–142.

Imoto, K., Methfessel, C., Sakmann, B., Mishina, M., Mori, Y., Konno, T., Fukada, K., Kurasaki, M., Bujo, H., Fujita, Y. and Numa, S. (1986) Location of a delta subunit region determining ion transport through the membrane. *Nature* **324**: 670–674.

Imoto, K., Busch, C., Sakmann, B., Mishina, M., Konno, T., Nakai, J., Bujo, H., Mori, Y., Fukada, K. and Numa, S. (1988) Rings of negatively charged amino acids determine the acetylcholine receptor channel conductance. *Nature* **335**: 645–648.

Inestrosa, N., Silberstein, L. and Hall, Z. (1982) Association of the synaptic form of acetylcholinesterase with extracellular matrix in cultured mouse muscle cells.

Cell **29**: 71–79.

Kao, P. and Karlin, A. (1986) Acetylcholine receptor binding site contains a disulphide cross-link between adjacent half-cysteinyl residues. *J. Biol. Chem.* **261**: 8085–8088.

Laufer, R. and Changeux, J-P. (1987) Calcitonin gene-related peptide elevates cyclic AMP levels in chick skeletal muscle: possible neurotrophic role a coexisting neuronal messenger. *EMBO J.* **6**: 901–906.

Lee, C. Y. (1972) Chemistry and pharmacology of polypeptide toxins in snake venoms. *Annu. Rev. Pharmacol.* **12**: 265–280.

Leonard, R., Labarca, C., Charnet, P., Davidson, N. and Lester, H. (1988) Evidence that the M2 membrane-spanning region lines the ion-channel pore of the nicotinic receptor. *Science* **242**: 1578–1581.

Lobos, E., Rudnick, C., Watson, M. and Isenberg, K. (1989) Linkage disequilibrium study of RFLPs detected at the human muscle nicotinic acetylcholine receptor subunit genes. *Am. J. Genet.* **44**: 522–533.

Low, B. and Corfield, P. (1987) AChR: alpha toxin binding site-theoretical and model studies. *Asia Pacific J. Pharmacol.* **2**: 115–127.

Luther, M., Schoepfer, R., Whiting, P., Casey, B., Blatt, Y., Montal, M. and Lindstrom, J. (1989) A muscle AChR is expressed in the human cerebellar medulloblastoma cell line TE 671. *J. Neurosci.*, **9**: 1082–1096.

McMahan, U., Sanes, J. and Marshall, L. (1978) Cholinesterase is associated with the basal lamina at the neuromuscular junction. *Nature* **271**: 172–178.

McNamee, M. and Ochoa, E. (1982) Reconstitution of acetylcholine receptor function in model membrane. *Neuroscience* **7**: 2305–2319.

Maelicke, A. (ed.) (1986) *Nicotinic Acetylcholine Receptor: Structure and Function*, NATO ASI series, Vol. 3, Springer-Verlag, Berlin.

Massoulié, J. and Bon, S. (1982) The molecular forms of cholinesterase and acetylcholine esterase in vertebrates. *Annu. Rev. Neurosci.* **5**: 57–106.

McAllister, R., Isaacs, H., Rongey, R., Peer, M., Au, W., Sonkup, S. and Gardner, M. (1977) Establishment of a human medulloblastoma cell line. *Int. J. Cancer.* **20**: 206–212.

Merlie, J., Sebbane, R., Gardner, S., Olsen, E. and Lindstrom, J. (1983) The regulation of acetylcholine receptor expression in mammalian muscle. *Cold. Spring Harbor Symp. Quant. Biol.* **48**: 135–146.

Methfessel, C. (1986) Molecular electrophysiology of cloned AChR channels expressed in *Xenopus* oocytes. In: *Nicotinic Acetylcholine Receptor: Structure and Function*, Maelicke, A., ed., Springer-Verlag, berlin, pp. 263–273.

Miledi, R. (1960) The acetylcholine sensitivity of frog muscle fibres after complete or partial denervation. *J. Physiol (Lond)* **151**: 1–23.

Mishina, M., Kurosaki, T., Tobimatsu, T., Morimoto, Y., Noda, M., Yamomoto, T., Tereo, M., Lindstrom, J., Takashi, T., Kuno, M. and Numa. S. (1984) Expression of functional acetylcholine receptors from cloned cDNAs. *Nature* **307**: 604–608.

Mishina, N., Tobimatsu, T., Imoto, K., Tanaka, K., Fujita, Y., Fukada, K., Kinasaki, M., Takahashi, H., Mormoto, Y., Hirose, T., Inayama, S., Takahashi, T., Kuno, M. and Numa, S. (1985) Location of functional regions of the acetylcholine receptor alpha subunit by site-directed mutagenesis. *Nature* **313**: 364–369.

Mishina, M., Takai, T., Imoto, K., Noda, M., Takahashi, T., Numa, S., Methfessel, C. and Sakmann, B. (1986) Molecular distinction between fetal and adult forms of muscle acetylcholine receptor. *Nature* **321**: 406–411.

Moss, S., Darlison, M., Beeson, D. and Barnard, E. (1989) Developmental expression of the genes encoding the four subunits of the chicken muscle acetylcholine receptor. *J. Biol. Chem.* **264**: 20199–20205.

Neumann, D., Dora, B., Fridkin, M. and Fuchs, S. (1986) Analysis of ligand binding to the synthetic dodecapeptide 185–96 of the acetylcholine receptor alpha subunit. *Proc. Natl, Acad. Sci. USA* **83**: 9250–9253.

Noda, M., Furutani, Y., Takahashi, H., Toyosato, M., Tanabe, T., Schimitzu, S., Kikyotani, S., Kayano, T., Hirose, T., Inayama, S. and Numa, S. (1983) Cloning and sequence analysis of calf cDNA and human genomic DNA encoding alpha subunit precursor of muscle acetylcholine receptor. *Nature* **305**: 818–823.

Numa, S., Noda, M., Takahashi, H., Tanabe, T., Toyosato, M., Furutani, Y. and Kikyotani, S. (1983) Molecular structure of the nicotinic acetylcholine receptor. *Cold Spring Harbor Symp. Quant. Biol.* **48**: 57–70.

Patrick, J. and Lindstrom, J. (1973) Autoimmune response to acetylcholine receptor. *Science* **180**: 871–872.

Raftery, M., Hunkapillar, M., Strader, C. and Hood, L. (1980) Acetylcholine receptor: complex of homologous subunits. *Science* **208**: 1454–1457.

Schoepfer, R., Luther, M. and Lindstrom, J. (1988) The human medulloblastoma cell line TE 671 expresses a muscle-like acetylcholine receptor. *FEBS Lett.* **226**: 235–240.

Schuetz, S. M. (1980) The acetylcholine channel open time in chick muscle is not decreased following innervation. *J. Physiol. (Lond.)* **303**: 111–124.

Schumacher, M., Camp, S., Maulet, Y., Newton, M., MacPhee-Quigley, K., Taylor, S., Friedmann, T. and Taylor, P. (1986) Primary structure of *Torpedo californica* acetylcholinesterase deduced from its cDNA sequence. *Nature* **319**: 407–409.

Shibahara, S., Kubo, T., Perski, H., Takahashi, H., Noda, M. and Numa, S. (1985) Cloning and sequence analysis of human genomic DNA encoding the gamma subunit precursor of muscle acetylcholine receptor. *Eur. J. Biochem.* **146**: 15–22.

Sumikawa, K., Houghton, M., Emtage, S., Richards, B. and Barnard, E. (1981) Active multi-subunit AChR assembled by translation of heterologous mRNA in *Xenopus* oocytes. *Nature* **292**: 862–864.

Takai, T., Noda, M., Mishina, M., Shimizu, S., Furutani, Y., Kayano, T., Ikeda, T., Kubo, T., Takahashi, H., Takahashi, T., Kuno, M. and Numa, S. (1985) Cloning, sequencing and expression of cDNA for a novel subunit of AChR from calf muscle. *Nature* **315**: 761–764.

Taylor, P., Herz, J., Johnson, D. and Brown. R. (1986) Topography of the acetylcholine receptor as revealed by fluorescence energy transfer. In: *Nicotinic Acetycholine Receptor: Structure and Function*, Maelicke, A., ed., NATO ASI series, Vol. 3, Springer-Verlag, Berlin, pp. 61–74.

Tsim, K., Randall, W. and Barnard, E. (1988) An asymmetric form of muscle acetylcholinesterase contains three subunit types and two enzymic activities in one molecule. *Proc. Natl. Acad. Sci. USA* **85**: 1262–1266.

Tsim, K., Randall, W. and Barnard, E. (1989) Synaptic acetylcholinesterase of chicken muscle changes during development from a hybrid to a homogeneous enzyme. *EMBO J.* **7**: 2451–2456.

Tzartos, S., Kokla, A., Walgrave, S. and Conti-Tronconi, B. (1988) Localisation of the main immunogenic region of human muscle acetylcholine receptor to residues 67–76 of the alpha subunit. *Proc. Natl. Acad. Sci. USA* **85**: 2899–2903.

Unwin, N. (1989) The structure of ion channels in membranes of excitable cells. *Neuron* **3**: 665–676.

White, M., Mayne, K., Lester, H. and Davidson, N. (1985) Mouse–*Torpedo* hybrid acetylcholine receptors: Functional homology does not equal sequence homology. *Proc. Natl. Acad. Sci. USA* **82**: 4852–4856.

Monoclonal antibodies in the study of acetylcholine receptors

9.1. Introduction

Most of the membrane proteins described in this book have been purified and characterised by virtue of their specificity for certain pharmacological ligands or neurotoxins, for example α-bungarotoxin (α-BuTX) for the acetylcholine receptor (AChR), tetrodotoxin for the sodium channel and di-hydropyridines for the calcium channel. Once the protein has been isolated, however, one needs a more extensive array of probes for different parts of the molecule. Monoclonal antibodies (mAbs) can be raised against the whole molecule, the isolated subunits, or synthetic sequences and used in a wide variety of studies, as will be illustrated in this chapter.

9.1.1. *Monoclonal antibodies*

Monoclonal antibodies are immunoglobulins (usually IgG or IgM) of single specificity made by fusing a plasma cell with an immortal myeloma cell line. The resulting hybrids can be cloned to yield individual cell lines each secreting large amounts of an antibody of unique specificity. There are two good reasons for using monoclonal antibodies (mAbs) to study acetylcholine receptors (AChRs): (1) as mentioned above, they are useful probes for AChR proteins, and (2) they are model autoantibodies for the study of myasthenia gravis (MG), an autoimmune disease in which autoantibodies to AChRs impair neuromuscular transmission (see Vincent, this volume). Of course, polyclonal antisera to purified AChRs, to their subunits, and to synthetic AChR peptides are also very useful. Antisera are easier to make than mAbs and they contain a range of antibody specifications and immunoglobulin types (which may be a flaw or a virtue, depending on the application); but antisera are limited in quantity and limited in specificity by the purity of the immunogen. mAbs of exquisite specificity can be made in basically unlimited amounts and are easily purified.

A third reason for using antibodies to study AChRs is historical. Biochemical studies of AChRs usually use the electric organs of electric eels or rays because the organs contain relatively prodigious amounts of AChR: 50 mg batches of AChR can routinely be affinity-purified on a cobra toxin column from ½ kg of electric organ, and a large *Torpedo califorica* may have 3–4 kg of electric organ. Electric organ cells evolved from skeletal muscle cells with the loss of contractile proteins and the gain of 1000-fold or more in AChR concentration, permitting the basic processes of neuromuscular transmission to produce large currents at high voltage. In 1973, when we first affinity-purified what we thought were AChRs from the electric organ of *Electrophorus electricus*, we wanted to prove that the protein really was AChR (Patrick and Lindstrom, 1973). So we immunized rabbits with the protein in order to test if antisera would block the function of AChRs in electric organ cells. It did! Better still, the rabbits died of muscle weakness that resembled MG. Soon these studies of 'experimental autoimmune myasthenia gravis' (EAMG) led to the realisation that the muscular weakness in both EAMG and MG is caused by an antibody-mediated autoimmune response to AChRs, as will be detailed in later chapters (De Baets, Vincent, this volume). Since then, studies of AChRs, anti-AChR antibodies, EAMG, and MG have synergistically co-evolved.

AChRs are a focus of interest here, both for their intrinsic role in neuromuscular transmission and as a model ligand-gated ion channel neurotransmitter receptor. mAbs directed at various targets on the molecule provide useful tools for localising AChRs in muscle and neuronal tissue, purifying AChR proteins, studying their subunit composition, localising subunits within the macromolecule, and amino acid sequences within the subunits, and studying the synthesis and assembly of AChR subunits. They have also helped to elucidate the antigenic structure of the AChR and the role of antibodies in the pathogenesis of myasthenia gravis.

The purpose of this chapter is to provide an illustrated overview of the ways in which mAbs have been used. For more detailed discussions and extensive references, several recent reviews provide a convenient entry to the literature on the use of mAbs for studying AChRs and other receptors (Lindstrom, 1985), the biochemical structure of muscle-type AChRs (Maelicke, 1987), MG (Lindstrom *et al.*, 1988), and neuronal nicotinic AChRs (Lindstrom *et al.*, 1987).

9.2. Synthesis of acetylcholine receptors

It is of considerable interest to learn how the subunits of a complex macromolecule such as the AChR (see Beeson and Barnard, this volume) are synthesised and brought together to form the final protein. The synthesis and assembly of AChR subunits has been studied in native muscle cells in culture (Merlie *et al.*, 1983), in yeast (Fujita *et al.*, 1986) and fibroblasts transfected with α subunit cDNAs (Blount and Merlie, 1988), and in frog oocytes injected with cloned subunit cDNAs, mutant cDNAs or native mRNAs (Mishina *et al.*, 1985). These techniques are described briefly elsewhere (Chapter 3). In all of these systems, mAbs have been

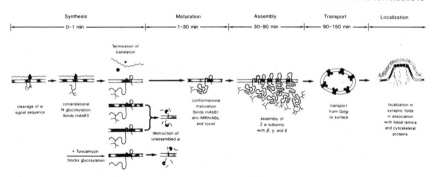

Fig. 9.1. The synthesis of AChRs in muscle cells in culture can be studied by pulse-labelling the nascent subunits with ^{35}S-methionine and using mAbs to precipitate them. This figure illustrates the different stages. The nascent chains bind mAb 61 before translation is completed. After further maturation they also bind mAb 35 (anti-MIR) and α-bungarotoxin. The assembly of the five subunits, and their transport to the cell surface, takes place after maturation of the individual subunits. For details see Merlie *et al.*, 1983.

used to identify subunit proteins and to detect their conformational maturation and assembly. Of particular use have been mAb 61, which recognises denatured α subunits, and mAb 35 which binds to a region on the extracellular surface of the native molecule which has been termed the main immunogenic region or MIR.

Figure 9.1 summarises work from the laboratory of John Merlie on synthesis of AChRs by a mouse muscle cell line. Nascent α subunits pulse-labelled with ^{35}S-methionine could be recognised by immune precipitation with mAb 61. During the first 30 min after synthesis, the α subunits underwent conformational maturation. The MIR then took on a nearly native conformation which allowed the α subunits to be recognised by mAb 35. At this time the ACh binding site achieved a more active conformation and bound α-BuTX with moderate affinity, but it did not bind small cholinergic ligands with high affinity. Assembly of subunits into mature AChRs occurred between 30 and 90 min after synthesis, and was detected by the ability of a mAb to a single subunit to precipitate intact AChRs.

Cloned *Torpedo* electric organ α subunits expressed in yeast cells appear to go through some conformational maturation and appear on the cell surface. However, conformational maturation may be aberrant because mAb binding indicated that part of the sequence which is on the cytoplasmic surface in native AChRs is on the extracellular surface in yeast (Fujita *et al.*, 1986). By contrast, cloned mouse muscle α subunits expressed in fibroblasts appear to mature normally and have oriented correctly in the membrane (Blount and Merlie, 1988).

In studies of AChRs using *in vitro* mutagenesis and expression of cloned subunit cDNAs in oocytes, mAbs are essential aids to determine whether the altered subunits are properly synthesised and assembled (Mishina *et al.*, 1985).

9.3. Subunit association within the AChR

Several lines of evidence suggest that AChR subunits in the native molecule are oriented like barrel staves around a central cation channel whose opening is regulated by binding of acetylcholine to the α subunits. A low-resolution three-dimensional structure of the AChR has been obtained by Nigel Unwin and co-workers (Brisson and Unwin, 1985). They found that AChR-rich membrane fragments of electric organ spontaneously formed tubular structures in which the AChRs were arranged in crystalline arrays. Optical diffraction analysis of electron micrographs of these arrays resulted in electron density maps that have produced a rather detailed

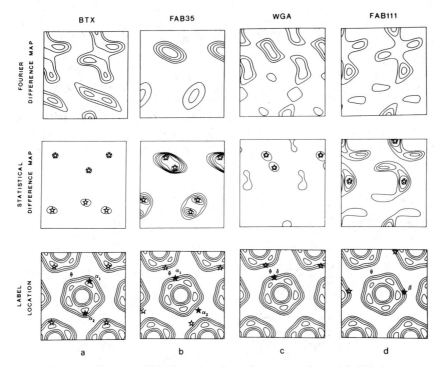

Fig. 9.2. Localisation of binding sites for α-bungarotoxin, mAb Fab fragments directed at α and β subunits, and wheat germ agglutinin by optical diffraction analysis of two-dimensional crystalline arrays of *Torpedo* electric organ membranes. Stars in the bottom panel indicate the position of the various labels derived from the difference between the electron density maps shown above (see Kubalek *et al.*, 1987).

image of AChR. Viewed from above, AChRs look like pentagonal doughnuts (see bottom panel for Fig. 9.2).

In order to determine which subunits corresponded to the five-electron density peaks around the AChR, probes specific for the α, β and γ subunits were used as labels (Kubalek *et al.*, 1987). Diffraction patterns of labelled and unlabelled arrays were then determined (see Fig. 9.2, upper panel), and the difference between the electron density maps was plotted to localise the labels (Fig. 9.2, middle panel). The ACh binding site was localised by α-BuTX to the top of the α subunits. Because it has a molecular weight of only 8000, α-BuTX could be localised fairly precisely, although its relatively small size made it difficult to detect the changed pattern. Monovalent Fab fragments (molecular weight 50,000) of mAb 35 were also used to localise the MIR to the outer surface of the α subunits; β subunits were located using an Fab of mAb 111 and δ subunits were located using the lectin, wheat germ agglutinin. In *Torpedo* electric organ, adjacent AChRs are linked into dimers by a disulfide bond between their δ subunits. This, therefore, limited the positions of the subunits in the crystalline array. Based on these findings the subunits would appear to be organised around the cation channel in the order shown in Fig. 9.2, lower panel.

9.4. **Polypeptide chain orientation within subunits**

The AChR subunits have sequence homologies throughout their length as a consequence of their evolution by gene duplication from a common ancestor (Noda *et al.*, 1983a; see also Beeson and Barnard, this volume).

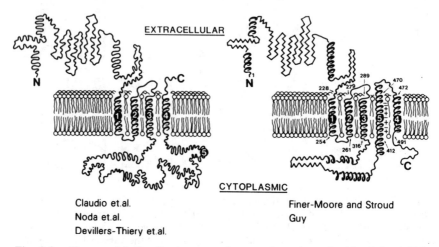

Fig. 9.3. Two models for the transmembrane orientation of each of the AChR polypeptide chains. For references see text (9.4).

Therefore, one expects the same basic transmembrane orientation of the polypeptide chain in each of the subunits. Various models were proposed (Fig. 9.3) based on inspection of the amino acid sequence.

Several lines of evidence suggest that much of the N-terminal half of AChR subunits is extracellular and rather rigidly conformed. The first 200 or so amino acids are thought to be extracellular because this sequence contains the glycosylation site at asparagine 141, and the MIR (Barkas *et al.*, 1987), and affinity labelling experiments show that the ACh binding site on the α subunits is near cysteines at positions 192 and 193 (Kao *et al.*, 1984). In contrast, much of the C-terminal half of AChR subunits is on the cytoplasmic surface and this part is less rigid and much of it is recognised by mAbs to denatured subunits (see below).

Three groups initially noticed four stretches of at least 20 hydrophobic amino acids and proposed that these might form transmembrane helices in contact with the hydrophobic core of the lipid bilayer (Fig. 9.3; Noda *et al.*, 1983a; Devillers-Thiery *et al.*, 1983; Claudio *et al.*, 1983). Later, two other groups proposed that a fifth, amphipathic helix (i.e. with a hydrophobic side and a hydrophilic side), was the barrel stave contributed by each subunit to the lining of the cation channel (Fig. 9.3; Guy, 1983; Finer-Moore and Stroud, 1984).

One approach to resolve the problem of the number and position of transmembrane domains is to use mAbs to locate peptide sequences on one side or other of the membrane, but these studies have provided data inconsistent with both of the models shown in Fig. 9.3. The binding sites for antisera and mAbs specific for the C-terminal 10 amino acids of several subunits have been localised to the cytoplasmic surface (Lindstrom *et al.*, 1984; Ratnam and Lindstrom, 1984; Ratnam *et al.*, 1986a; Young *et al.*, 1985) but, assuming that the N-terminal is outside, these data are inconsistent with the four transmembrane-domain model. However, other experiments in which the disulphide bond between the penultimate (C-terminal) residues of δ subunits was reduced (by an impermeable reagent) have suggested that these cysteines must be on the extracellular surface (McCrea *et al.*, 1987).

To try to resolve these questions the binding sites for mAbs were first mapped to amino acid sequences on the α subunit by testing their ability to immune precipitate ^{125}I-labelled synthetic peptide fragments as shown in Fig. 9.4 (Ratnam *et al.*, 1986b). These mAbs were then used to determine the transmembrane orientation of these sequences by immunoelectron microscopy, as shown in Fig. 9.5 (Ratnam *et al.*, 1986a): AChR-rich membrane fragments were permeabilised by osmotic shock and then labelled with the mAb; bound mAbs were localised using a double layer of rabbit anti-rat Ig followed by protein A conjugated with small colloidal gold particles. Reference mAbs for the extracellular surface (mAb 35 to the MIR) or the cytoplasmic surface (mAb 111 to a site on β subunits

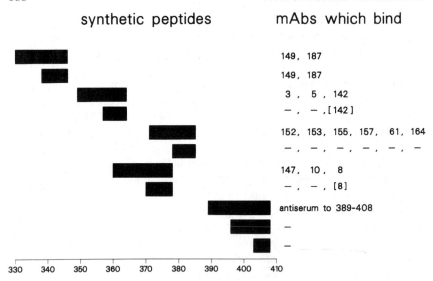

Fig. 9.4. Mapping the binding sites of mAbs to AChR α subunits by their ability to precipitate ^{125}I-labelled synthetic peptides representing the sequence between 330 and 408 of the α subunit. From Ratnam *et al.*, 1986a.

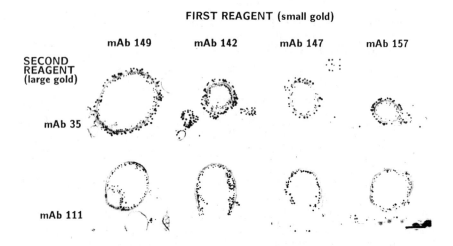

Fig. 9.5. Determining the transmembrane orientation of sequences of the AChR α subunits by locating the binding of sequence-specific mAbs to AChR-rich membrane vesicles. The mAbs were localised by using an anti-rat Ig followed by protein A covalently attached to either large or small colloidal gold particles. mAb 35 binds to the MIR and therefore indicates the extracellular surface of the AChR; mAb 111 binds to the cytoplasmic surface of the β subunit. MAbs 142, 147, and 157 clearly all bind to the cytoplasmic surface. From Ratnam *et al.*, 1986a.

known to be on the cytoplasmic surface of AChRs in muscle) were then applied and localised similarly with large collodial gold particles. These results showed that mAbs specific for sequences from 339–378 bound on the cytoplasmic surface. This indicates that the putative amphipathic transmembrane domain is actually on the cytoplasmic surface and suggests that the putative hydrophobic transmembrane domain M4 may not cross the membrane as depicted in the model.

Thus there is still controversy concerning the transmembrane orientation of the polypeptide chains. A major problem of using sequence-specific mAbs and immunoelectron microscopy is that, even though one may be able to get antibodies to a particular synthetic peptide of interest, these antibodies frequently do not react with native AChR, because in the native AChR the sequence is buried, or in an unrecognisable conformation (Ralston *et al.*, 1987).

High resolution X-ray crystallography of three-dimensional AChR crystals will ultimately precisely determine the orientation of the AChR subunit polypeptide chains. Several laboratories are now working on obtaining suitable crystals. Meanwhile, it is well to bear in mind that the four hydrophobic stretches that were initially proposed to form transmembrane helices are among the most conserved sequences in subunits of AChRs from various tissues and species, and in other members of this gene family (see Fig. 9.8). This no doubt means that these sequences are structurally important, probably not simply as helices surrounded by the lipid core of the membrane, but as critical interfaces between polypeptide chain segments within and especially between subunits. The conserved feature of the ligand-gated ion channel gene family which include nicotinic AChRs from muscles and nerves (reviewed in Lindstrom *et al.*, 1987), GABA receptors (Schofield *et al.*, 1987), and glycine receptors (Grenningloh *et al.*, 1987), may be the ability to form an ion channel via the specific ordered association of similar subunits around a central channel.

9.5. Antigenic structure

9.5.1. *Antibody binding sites*

One characteristic feature of the AChR, which must reflect some conserved structural organisation, is the presence of a main immunogenic region (MIR) (Tzartos and Lindstrom, 1980; Tzartos *et al.*, 1981, 1983); many of the mAbs made to native AChRs compete with each other for binding, and any one of these mAbs can inhibit the binding of half or more of serum antibodies to native AChRs. Moreover, rat mAbs to the MIR can, on average, inhibit the binding of half or more of MG patients' serum autoantibodies to AChRs (Tzartos *et al.*, 1982; see also Vincent, this volume). For this reason, in particular, there is considerable interest in developing techniques by which to identify the exact amino acid sequences recognised by antibodies raised against the native structure.

Antibodies to the MIR have high affinity for native (i.e. structurally intact AChR), but bind only very weakly to denatured subunits. Because of the low affinity of MIR mAbs for denatured subunit, precise mapping of the MIR by binding to small synthetic peptides has been difficult. However, using peptides glutaraldehyde-linked to polylysine-coated microwells as antigen, in ELISA or solid-phase immunoassays (see Chapter 3), several mAbs to the MIR have been shown to bind with low affinity, but high specificity, to α subunit peptides containing the sequence 67–76 (Barkas *et al.*, 1988; Tzartos *et al.*, 1988). Other mAbs to the MIR do not bind under these conditions and their binding may depend absolutely on the native conformation of the AChR.

Antibodies to the MIR are pathologically significant in MG, which can be explained partly by the position of the MIR on the extracellular surface of the native molecule. They do not directly impair AChR function (Blatt *et al.*, 1986) because the MIR faces away from both the ACh binding site and the cation channel (see Fig. 9.2). However, antibodies to the MIR can cause loss of AChR by increasing the rate of AChR internalisation (this is termed antigenic modulation), because (being divalent) they efficiently crosslink AChRs through their MIRs (Conti-Tronconi *et al.*, 1981; Tzartos *et al.*, 1985) on the α subunits of adjacent AChRs (see Fig. 9.2). The MIR mAbs cannot crosslink the two subunits *within* an AChR because the two MIRs are on opposite sides of the molecule and orientated away from each other (Conti-Tronconi *et al.*, 1981). A monovalent Fab fragment of mAb 35 (to the MIR) can protect human muscle in culture from the antigenic modulation of AChR caused by MG patients' autoantibodies (Tzartos *et al.*, 1985; see Vincent, this volume) confirming the importance of both the MIR and divalent antibody in determining antibody-induced AChR modulation. In addition, because the MIR is on the extracellular surface (Tzartos *et al.*, 1987) antibodies to the MIR can also bind to AChRs in living muscle cells and fix complement, causing focal lysis of the postsynaptic membrane.

In contrast to the extracellular region of the AChR the C-terminal third of each subunit appears to be less rigidly structured, and antibodies to the cytoplasmic surface of native AChRs also recognise denatured subunits (McCrea *et al.*, 1987; Souroujon *et al.*, 1986). The binding sites of these mAbs have been mapped as indicated in Figs. 9.6 and 9.7. Figure 9.6 summarises the results of a great number of experiments in which proteolytic fragments of purified *Torpedo* AChR subunits were resolved according to molecular weight by SDS/PAGE and then transferred onto covalently reactive paper (Western blotting, see Chapter 3). Firstly, fragments containing the C-terminus were identified using antibodies to C-terminal decapeptides. These antibodies were then eluted and the

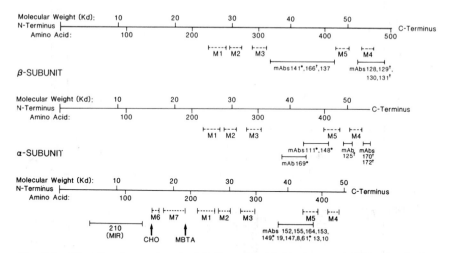

Fig. 9.6. Results of mapping the binding of mAb binding to AChR subunits by the peptide mapping technique (see text). Reproduced from Ratnam *et al.*, 1986b.

sequence recognised by each mAb was determined by the difference in sequence between the smallest C-terminal peptide it did not bind and the next larger C-terminal peptide that it did bind.

Figure 9.7 summarises the results of studies in which immune precipitation of small ^{125}I-labelled synthetic peptides was used to identify the sequences recognised by antisera to AChR and its subunits. Using this method one would only be able to detect in the antisera the presence of antibodies that can also bind to short, synthetic sequences. In addition to prominent epitopes in the C-terminal third, there are several prominent epitopes in the N-terminal half of the α subunits (Fig. 9.7B; Sargent *et al.*, 1983) which are recognised by antisera raised against the isolated subunit, but antibodies to these epitopes do not bind well to native AChRs (Fig. 9.7A).

Although most mAbs to AChRs do not block AChR function (Wan and Lindstrom, 1985), it is possible to make mAbs which do block function either by competing for the ACh binding site or by allosteric mechanisms (Mochly-Rosen and Fuchs, 1985; Mihovilovic and Richman, 1984; Fels *et al.*, 1986; Whiting *et al.*, 1985). MAbs are quite sensitive to subtleties of antigen conformation; although the two α subunits in an AChR appear to have the same sequence, they differ in conformation, perhaps as a result of the different subunits which surround them in the native AChR (see Fig. 9.2). Most mAbs that bind at or near the ACh binding site bind to only one of the two sites (Mihovilovic and Richman, 1984; Fels *et al.*, 1986; Whiting *et al.*, 1985). The ACh binding sites also differ in affinity for curare (Neubig

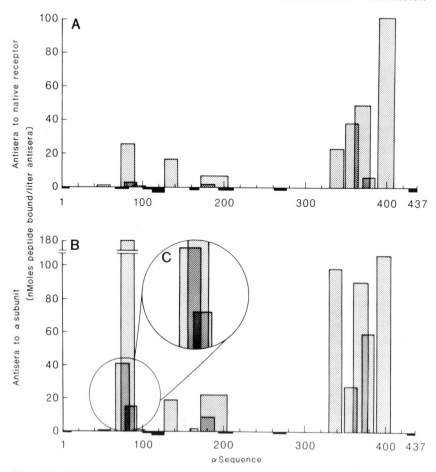

Fig. 9.7. Mapping epitopes which are recognised by serum antibodies directed against native AChR (**A**) or α subunit (**B**). Most of the antibodies raised against the native AChR that can bind to ^{125}I-labelled synthetic peptides only recognise sequences towards the C-terminus (**A**). In contrast antibodies raised against the isolated α subunit also recognise sequences towards the N-terminus (**B**), but these antibodies do not react with native AChR.

and Cohen, 1979; Sine and Taylor, 1980) and in reactivity with the affinity labelling reagent ^{3}H-MBTA (Damle and Karlin, 1978; Wolosin *et al.*, 1980).

MAbs depend for their binding on only a few amino acids of the antigen, and can be quite sensitive to the conformation of these amino acids. For this reason most mAbs to AChRs are quite specific for subunit and species (Tzartos *et al.*, 1986), despite the overall sequence homologies between subunits of an AChR (Noda *et al.*, 1983a) and the even greater sequence homologies of corresponding subunits between species (Noda *et al.*,

1983b). However, some epitopes are rather strongly conserved and, in some cases, extensive crossreaction can be observed. For example, mAb 35 (to the MIR) in chickens reacts with AChRs in muscle, ganglia, and brain (Whiting *et al.*, 1987). In none of these cases does mAb 35 recognise a simple linear sequence of amino acids (mAb 35 did not bind to peptide 67–76). Instead, this mAb recognises the shape of a structural feature which is conserved in these AChRs.

Nevertheless, subtle differences between AChRs can make big differences in crossreaction. For example, mAb 35 does not recognise one of two AChR subtypes from chicken brain; it binds AChR from calf muscle and ganglia but not from calf brain; it recognises AChRs from rat muscle but not rat ganglia or brain; and in humans, mAb 35 recognises AChRs from muscle but not brain (see Lindstrom *et al.*, 1987 for detailed references). Incidentally, these results are also consistent with the idea (reviewed in Lindstrom *et al.*, 1987) that the structure of AChRs in muscle evolved to its contemporary form by the time of elasmobranchs like *Torpedo*, and has changed relatively little since, whereas the evolution of structure of AChRs in neurones has been in more rapid flux.

9.5.2. *T cell epitopes*

The formation of antibodies to AChRs requires T helper lymphocytes as well as B lymphocytes. Therefore, consideration of the antigenic structure of AChRs also involves considering how AChR is recognised by T cells. This has been studied in less detail than has the interaction of antibodies with AChRs. However, a number of generalisations seem to apply (reviewed in Lindstrom *et al.*, 1988). Unlike B cells, which use immunoglobulin to recognise intact antigens, T cells see proteolytic fragments of antigens generated by antigen-presenting cells, and presented on the surface of these cells bound to class II histocompatibility antigens. The binding specificity of the class II molecules on the antigen-presenting cell limits the peptides which can be presented to T cells. The most prominent B cell epitopes depend on the native conformation of the MIR, and for that reason alone differ from prominent T cell epitopes. Thus the same peptide fragments are rarely recognised by both antibodies and T cells (Hohlfeld *et al.*, 1981; Tami *et al.*, 1987; Fujii and Lindstrom, 1988). For example, the synthetic peptides used in Fig. 9.7 were tested for their ability to induce proliferation of T lymphocytes from AChR-primed Lewis rats. Substantial proliferation was obtained only with peptides containing the sequences 73–88 and 101–116.

9.6. Neuronal nicotinic AChRs

Muscle nicotinic AChRs are part of a larger gene family of ligand-gated ion channels which includes nicotinic AChRs in neurones, neuronal α-

Primordial receptor homopolymer

	Muscle AChR	Brain AChR	Ganglion AChR	αBgt-Binding Protein	Glycine R	GABA R	?R
Subunits	α β γ δ (ε)	α β (β')	α β	α β γ δ	α β	α β	?
Ligand	ACh	ACh	ACh	?	glycine	GABA	?
Channel	cation	cation	cation	?	anion	anion	?
Cysteine ≈192,193	in ACh binding subunit	in ACh binding subunit	in ACh binding subunit	in ACh binding subunit	no	no	?
Cysteine ≈128,142	yes	yes	yes	probably	yes	yes	probably
Hydrophobic sequences ~M1,M2,M3,M4	yes	yes	yes	probably	yes	yes	probably

Fig. 9.8. Proteins of the ligand-gated ion channel superfamily. This family contains receptors for several different ligands, with different pharmacological specificities (e.g. muscle and brain AChR), and with different ion-conducting channels. However, there is conservation of hydrophobic sequences and of cysteine residues. These receptors are reviewed in detail in Lindstrom *et al.*, 1987.

bungarotoxin binding protein of unknown function, and receptors for GABA and glycine, as shown in Fig. 9.8 (Lindstrom *et al.*, 1987; Ralston *et al.*, 1987; Schofeld *et al.*, 1987). This family does not include muscarinic receptors, which are part of another family of proteins. These act through GTP binding proteins and include rhodopsin and adrenergic receptors (Kubo *et al.*, 1986).

Neuronal nicotinic AChRs differ from muscle AChRs pharmacologically, in subunit structure and, in some cases, in functional role. Brain nicotinic AChR have μM affinity for nicotine, by contrast with the μM affinity of muscle AChRs; and most neuronal AChRs do not bind α-bungarotoxin (see Lindstrom *et al.*, 1987). Neuronal AChRs have been purified using mAbs, as shown in Fig. 9.9, but there is very little antigenic crossreaction between AChRs of muscle and nerve. For example, MG patients' autoantibodies do not react with AChRs from human brain (Whiting *et al.*, 1987). However, mAb 35 to AChRs from electric eel binds to AChRs in chicken neurones, which could be purified on an mAb 35 affinity column. mAbs to this purified material were then used to purify AChRs from rat brains (Whiting and Lindstrom, 1986) as summarised in Fig. 9.9. These neuronal AChRs consist of only two kinds of subunits, one of which binds ACh and can be affinity labelled by ^{3}H-MBTA, the same reagent which labels α subunits of muscle-type AChRs at cysteines 192, 193 (Kao *et al.*, 1984). In chicken ciliary ganglia, neuronal AChRs have a postsynaptic role basically similar to that of AChRs in muscle. However, in

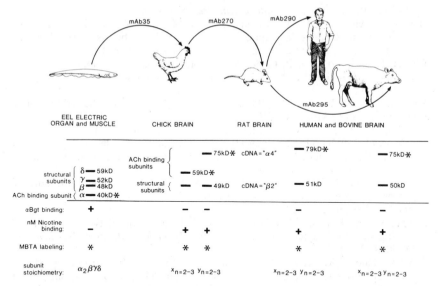

Fig. 9.9. Using mAbs to purify and characterise neuronal nicotinic AChRs from different species. mAbs raised against one AChR could be used to purify receptor from the brain of another species. Reproduced from Lindstrom *et al.*, 1987.

chicken optic tectum or rat superior colliculus, there are AChRs on the projections from retinal ganglion cells which may act in a presynaptic role (Swanson *et al.*, 1987). Studies of neuronal nicotinic AChRs may violate many of our preconceptions about AChRs that are based on knowledge from muscle receptor. On the other hand, they offer a broad perspective for considering the evolution of AChR structure and its functional significance.

Acknowledgements

I thank Maya Spies for secretarial assistance. Work in this laboratory is supported by grants from the NIH, the US Army, the Muscular Dystrophy Association, the Council for Tobacco Research and the Los Angeles and California Chapters of the Myasthenia Gravis Foundation.

References

Barkas, T., Mauron, A., Roth, B., Alliod, C., Tzartos, S., and Ballivet, M. (1987) Mapping the main immunogenic region and toxin binding site of the nicotinic acetylcholine receptor. *Science* 235: 77–80.
Barkas, T., Gabriel, J.–M., Mauron, A., Hughes, G., Roth, B., Alliod, C., Tzartos, W. and Ballivet, M. (1988) Monoclonal antibodies to the main immunogenic region of the nicotinic acetylcholine receptor bind to residues

61–76 of the α subunit. *J. Biol. Chem.* **263**: 5916–5920.

Blatt, Y., Montal, M., Lindstrom, J. and Montal, M. (1986) Monoclonal antibodies directed against epitopes in the β and γ subunits of the *Torpedo* cholinergic receptor affect channel gating. *J. Neurosci.* **6**: 481–486.

Blount, P. and Merlie, J. P. (1988) Native folding of an acetylcholine receptor α subunit expressed in the absence of other receptor subunits. *J. Biol. Chem.*, **263**: 1072–1080.

Brisson, A. and Unwin, N. (1985) Quaternary structure of the acetylcholine receptor. *Nature* **315**: 474–477.

Claudio, T., Ballivet, M., Patrick, J. and Heinemann, S. (1983). *Torpedo californica* acetylcholine receptor 60,000 dalton subunit: nucleotide sequence of cloned cDNA deduced amino acid sequence, subunit structural predictions. *Proc. Natl. Acad. Sci. USA* **80**: 111–115.

Conti-Tronconi, B., Tzartos, S. and Lindstrom, J. (1981) Monoclonal antibodies as probes of acetylcholine receptor structure. II. Binding to native receptor. *Biochemistry* **20**: 2181–2191.

Damle, V. and Karlin, A. (1978) Affinity labelling of one of two a-neuro-toxin binding sites in acetylcholine receptor from *Torpedo californica*. *Biochemistry* **17**: 2039–2045.

Devillers-Thiery, A., Giraudat, J., Bentaboulet, M. and Changeux, J.–P. (1983) Complete mRNA coding sequence of the acetylcholine binding subunit of *Torpedo marmorato* acetylcholine receptor: a model for the transmembrane organization of the polypeptide chain. *Proc. Natl. Acad. Sci. USA* **80**: 2067–2071.

Fels, G., Plumer-Wilk, R., Schreiber, M. and Maelicke, A. (1986) A monoclonal antibody interfering with binding and response of the acetylcholine receptor. *J. Biol. Chem.* **261**: 15746–15754.

Finer-Moore, J. and Stroud, R. (1984) Amphipathic analysis and possible formation of the ion channel in an acetylcholine receptor. *Proc. Natl. Acad. Sci. USA* **81**: 155–159.

Fujii, Y. and Lindstrom, J. (1988) Specificity of the T cell immune response to acetylcholine receptor in experimental autoimmune myasthenia gravis: response to subunits and synthetic peptides. *J. Immunol.* **140**: 1830–1837.

Fujita, N., Nelson, N. Fox, T., Claudio, T., Lindstrom, J., Reizman, H. and Hess, G. (1986) Biosynthesis of the *Torpedo californica* acetylcholine receptor subunit in yeast. *Science* **231**: 1284–1287.

Grenningloh, G., Rienitz, A., Schmitt, B., Methfessel, C., Zensen, M., Beyruther, K., Gudelfinger, E. and Betz, H. (1987) The strychnine binding subunit of the glycine receptor shows homology with nicotinic acetylcholine receptors. *Nature* **328**: 215–220.

Guy, R. (1983). A structural model of the acetylcholine receptor channel based on partition energy and helix packing calculations. *Biophys. J.* **45**: 249–261.

Hohlfeld, R., Kalies, I., Neinz, F., Kalden, J. and Wekerle, H. (1981) Autoimmune rat T lymphocytes nonspecific for acetylcholine receptors: purification and fine specificity. *J. Immunol.* **126**: 1264–1355.

Kao, P., Dwork, A., Kaldany, R., Silver, M., Wideman, J., Stein, S. and Karlin, A. (1984) Identification of the subunit half cysteine specifically labeled by an affinity reagent for the acetylcholine receptor binding site. *J. Biol. Chem.* **259**: 11662–11665.

Kubalek, E., Ralston, S., Lindstrom, J. and Unwin, N. (1987) Location of subunits within the acetylcholine receptor: analysis of tubular crystals from *Torpedo marmorata*. *J. Cell Biol.* **105**: 9–18.

Kubo, T., Fujuda, K., Mikami, A., Maeda, A., Takashi, H., Michina, M., Haga,

T., Haha, K., Ichiyama, A., Kangawa, K., Kojima, M., Matusuo, H., Hirose, T. and Numa, S. (1986) Cloning, sequencing, and expression of complementary DNA encoding the muscarinic acetylcholine receptor. *Nature* **323**: 411–416.

Lindstrom, J. (1985) Nicotinic acetylcholine receptors: use of monoclonal antibodies to study synthesis, structure, function and autoimmune response. In: *Monoclonal and Anti-idiotypic antibodies: Probes for Receptor Structure and Function*, J. Venter, C. Fraser and J. Lindstrom, (eds), Alan R. Liss, New York, pp. 21–57.

Lindstrom, J., Shelton, G. D. and Fujii, Y. (1988) Myasthenia gravis. *Adv. Immunol.* **42**: 233–284.

Lindstrom, J., Schoepfer, R. and Whiting, P. (1987) Molecular studies of the neuronal nicotinic acetylcholine receptor family. *Molec. Neurobiol.*, **1**: 281–337.

Lindstrom, J., Criado, M., Hochschwender, S., Fox, J. L. and Sarin, V. (1984) Immunochemical tests of acetylcholine receptor subunit models. *Nature* **311**: 573–575.

Maelicke, A. (1987) Structure and function of the nicotinic acetylcholine receptor. In: *Handbook of Experimental Pharmacology: The Cholinergic Synapse*, V. P. Whittaker, vol. ed., Springer-Verlag, Berlin, pp. 267–300.

McCrea, P., Popot, J.-L. and Engelman, D. (1987) Transmembrane topography of the nicotinic acetylcholine receptor δ subunit. *EMBO J.* **6**: 3619–3626.

Merlie, J. P., Sebbane, R., Gardner, S., Olsen, E. and Lindstrom, J. (1983) The regulation of acetylcholine receptor expression in mammalian muscle. *Cold Spring Harbor Symp. Quant. Biol.* **XLVIII**: 135–146.

Mihovilovic, M. and Richman, D. (1984) Modification of bungarotoxin and cholinergic ligand binding properties of *Torpedo* acetylcholine receptor by a monoclonal anti-acetylcholine receptor antibody. *J. Biol. Chem.* **259**: 15051–15059.

Mishina, M., Tobimatsu, T., Imoto, K., Tanaka, K., Fujita, Y., Fukuda, K., Kurasaki, M., Takahashi, H., Morimoto, Y., Hirose, T., Inayama, S., Takahashi, T., Kuno, M. and Numa, S. (1985) Location of functional regions of acetylcholine receptor subunit by site-directed mutageneisi. *Nature* **313**: 364–369.

Mochly-Rosen, C. and Fuchs, S. (1981) Monoclonal anti-acetylcholine receptor antibodies directed against the cholinergic binding site. *Biochemistry* **20**: 5920–5924.

Neubig, R. and Cohen, J. B. (1979) Equilibrium binding of ^{3}H-tubocurarine and ^{3}H-acetylcholine by *Torpedo* postsynaptic membranes: stoichiometry and ligand interactions. *Biochemistry* **18**: 5464–5475.

Noda, M., Takahashi, H., Tanabe, T., Toyosato, M., Kikyotani, S., Furutani, Y., Hirose, T., Takashima, H., Inayama, S., Miyata, T. and Numa, S. (1983a) Structural homology of *Torpedo californica* acetylcholine receptor subunits. *Nature* **302**: 528–532.

Noda, M., Furutani, Y., Takahashi, H., Toyosato, M., Tanabe, T., Shimizu, S., Kikyotani, S., Koyano, T., Hirose, T., Inayama, S. and Numa, S. (1983b) Cloning and sequence analysis of calf cDNA and human genomic DNA encoding subunit precursor or muscle acetylcholine receptor. *Nature* **305**: 818–823.

Patrick, J. and Lindstrom, J. (1973) Autoimmune response to acetylcholine receptor. *Science* **180**: 871–872.

Ralston, S., Sarin, V., Thanh, H., Rivier, J., Fox, J. L. and Lindstrom, J. (1987) Synthetic peptides used to locate the bungarotoxin binding site and immunogenic regions on subunits of the nicotinic acetylcholine receptor. *Biochemistry* **26**: 3261–3266.

Ratnam, M. and Lindstrom, J. (1984) Structural features of the nicotinic acetylcholine receptor revealed by antibodies to synthetic peptides. *Biochem. Biophys. Res. Commun.* **122**: 1225–1233.

Ratnam, M., Le Nguyen, D., Rivier, J., Sargent, P. and Lindstrom, J. (1986a) Transmembrane topography of nicotinic acetylcholine receptor: immunochemical tests contradict theoretical predictions based on hydrophobicity profiles. *Biochemistry* **25**: 2633–2643.

Ratnam, M., Sargent, P., Sarin, V., Fox, J. L., Le Nguyen, D., Rivier, J., Criado, M. and Lindstrom, J. (1986b) Location of antigenic determinants on primary sequences of subunits of nicotinic acetylcholine receptor by peptide mapping. *Biochemistry* **25**: 2621–2632.

Sargent, P., Hedges, B., Tsavaler, L., Clemmons, L., Tzartos, S. and Lindstrom, J. (1983) The structure and transmembrane nature of the acetylcholine receptor in amphibian skeletal muscles revealed by crossreacting monoclonal antibodies. *J. Cell Biol.* **98**: 609–618.

Schofield, P., Darlison, M., Fujita, N., Burt, D., Stephenson, A., Rodriguez, H., Rhee, L., Ramachandran, J., Reale, V., Glencorse, T., Seeburg, P. and Barnard, E. (1987) Sequence and functional expression of the $GABA_A$ receptor shows a ligand-gated receptor super-family. *Nature* **328**: 221–227.

Sine, S. and Taylor, P. (1980) The relationship between agonist occupation and the permeability response of the cholinergic receptor revealed by bound cobra a-toxin. *J. Biol. Chem.* **255**: 10144–10156.

Souroujon, M., Neumann, D., Pizzighella, S., Safran, A. and Fuchs, S. (1986) Localisation of a highly immunogenic region on the acetylcholine receptor α subunits. *Biochem. Biophys. Res. Commun.* **135**: 82–89.

Swanson, L., Simmons, D., Whiting, P. and Lindstrom, J. (1987) Immunohistochemical localisation of neuronal nicotinic receptors in the rodent central nervous system. *J. Neurosci.* **7**: 3334–3342.

Tami, J., Urs, O. and Krolick, K. (1987) T cell hybridomas reactive with the acetylcholine receptor and its subunits. *J. Immunol.* **138**: 732–738.

Tzartos, D. and Lindstrom, J. (1980) Monoclonal antibodies used to probe acetylcholine receptor structure; localisation of the main immunogenic region and detection of similarities between subunits. *Proc. Natl. Acad. Sci. USA* **77**: 755–759.

Tzartos, S., Rand, D., Einarson, B. and Lindstrom, J. (1981) Mapping surface structures on electrophorus acetylcholine receptor using monoclonal antibodies. *J. Biol. Chem.* **256**: 8635–8645.

Tzartos, S., Seybold, M. and Lindstrom, J. (1982) Specificity of antibodies to acetylcholine receptors in sera from myasthenia gravis patients measured by monoclonal antibodies. *Proc. Natl. Acad. Sci. USA* **79**: 188–192.

Tzartoz, S., Langeberg, L., Hochschwender, S. and Lindstrom, J. (1983) Demonstration of a main immunogenic region on acetylcholine receptors from human muscle using monoclonal antibodies to human receptor. *FEBS Lett.* **158**: 116–118.

Tzartos, S., Sophianos, D. and Efthimiadis, A. (1985) Role of the main immunogenic region of acetylcholine receptor in myasthenia gravis: an Fab monoclonal antibody protects against antigenic modulation by human sera. *J. Immunol.* **134**: 2343–2349.

Tzartos, S., Hochschwender, S., Vasques, P. and Lindstrom, J. (1987) Passive transfer of experimental autoimmune myasthenia gravis by monoclonal antibodies to the main immunogenic region of the acetylcholine receptor. *J. Neuroimmunol.* **15**: 185–194.

Tzartos, S., Kokla, A., Wlagrave, S. and Conti-Tronconi, B. (1988) Localisation of the main immunogenic region of human muscle acetylcholine receptor to residues 67–76 of the α subunit. *Proc. Natl. Acad. Sci. USA* **85**: 2899–2903.

Tzartos, S., Langeberg, L., Hochschwender, S., Swanson, L. and Lindstrom, J. (1986) Characteristics of monoclonal antibodies to denatured Torpedo and to native calf acetylcholine receptors: species, subunit and region specificity. *J. Neuroimmunol.* **10**: 235–253.

Wan, K. and Lindstrom, J. (1985) Effects of monoclonal antibodies on the function of acetylcholine receptors purified from Torpedo californica and reconstituted into vesicles. *Biochem.* **24**: 1212–1221.

Whiting, P., Vincent, A. and Newsom-Davis, J. (1985) Monoclonal antibodies to Torpedo acetylcholine receptor; characterisation of antigenic determinants within the cholinergic binding site. *Eur. J. Biochem.* **150**: 553.539.

Whiting, P. and Lindstrom, J. (1986) Purification and characterization of a nicotinic acetylcholine receptor from chick brain. *Biochemistry* **25**: 2082–2093.

Whiting, P., Cooper, J. and Lindstrom, J. (1987) Antibodies in patients with myasthenia gravis do not bind to acetylcholine receptors from human brain. *J. Neuroimmuno.* **16**: 205–213.

Wolosin, J., Lyddiatt, A., Dolly, J. and Barnard, E. (1980) Stoichiometry of the ligand-binding sites in the acetylcholine receptor oligomer from muscle and from electric organ. *Eur. J. Biochem.* **109**: 495–505.

Young, E., Ralston, E., Blake, J., Ramachandran, J., Hall, Z. and Stroud, R. (1985) Topological mapping of acetylcholine receptor; evidence for a model with five transmembrane segments and a cytoplasmic COOH-terminal peptide. *Proc. Natl. Acad. Sci. USA* **82**: 626–630.

Congenital myasthenic syndromes

10.1. Introduction

Although uncommon, diseases of the neuromuscular junction (NMJ) have been of unusual interest to students, clinicians and investigators. For students they nicely illustrate how the application of basic science principles can unravel complicated disorders. For clinicians they represent a challenge in diagnosis; and beyond that there is the gratification that comes from being able to remove or improve the symptoms of a disabling illness. For investigators there is satisfaction in discovering the causes of such 'old' diseases as myasthenia gravis or the Lambert–Eaton syndrome, and in recognising new diseases, such as the slow-channel myasthenic syndrome.

The NMJ diseases are acquired or inherited. The acquired ones fall into two major groups, autoimmune and toxic. Some of the toxins that affect neuromuscular transmission are referred to in the chapters by Dolly and by Norman. The chapters by Vincent and Wray deal with the two autoimmune diseases, myasthenia gravis and the Lambert–Eaton syndrome.

This chapter focuses on the congenital myasthenic syndromes (Table 10.1). The study of these disorders demonstrates very aptly the application of a wide range of techniques to investigation of human disease. The last decade or so has led to a much deeper understanding of the pathophysiology of the congenital myasthenic syndromes, and in several cases pin-pointed the probable abnormality at the molecular level. The next decade will doubtless reveal the precise genetic defects in a number of conditions.

10.2. The safety margin of neuromuscular transmission

In each myasthenic syndrome the safety margin of neuromuscular transmission is compromised by one or more specific mechanisms. Although mentioned elsewhere in this book (see Chapter 2 and the chapter by Colquhoun, this volume), a clear understanding of the concept of the safety margin is essential for grasping the pathogenesis of these syndromes, and so the factors that affect the safety margin are discussed further here (see also Magleby, 1986a).

Table 10.1.   Congenital myasthenic syndromes

Well-characterised syndromes
Familial infantile myasthenia*
Paucity of synaptic vesicles and reduced quantal release[†]
Endplate acetylcholinesterase deficiency*
Slow-channel syndrome[‡]
High-conductance fast-channel syndrome[‡]
Endplate AChR deficiency*
Abnormal ACh-AChR interaction[†]

Partially characterised syndromes
AChR deficiency and increased affinity for d-tubocurarine
Possible defect in ACh synthesis, mobilisation or storage
Familial limb-girdle myasthenia*

---

*Autosomal recessive inheritance.
[†]Autosomal recessive inheritance suspected.
[‡]Autosomal dominant inheritance.

The motor endplate consists of a nerve terminal separated from the postsynaptic regions by the synaptic space. Acetylcholine (ACh) is stored in quantal packets (6000–10,000 molecules per packet) in synaptic vesicles in the nerve terminal, and released by exocytosis.

Depolarisation of the nerve terminal by a nerve impulse opens voltage-sensitive calcium channels in the presynaptic membrane. The calcium influx increases the probability of synaptic vesicle exocytosis, and exocytosis of numerous vesicles occurs adjacent to active zones in the presynaptic membrane. There is evidence to indicate that the voltage-sensitive calcium channels are associated with regularly arrayed large membrane particles in the active zones (see also Wray, this volume).

The postsynaptic region contains junctional folds containing on their terminal expansions acetylcholine receptor (AChR) molecules packed at a density of about 10^4 sites per square micrometre. The binding of two ACh molecules to an AChR molecule opens the AChR ion channel. When the ion channel closes, ACh dissociates from the AChR. Acetylcholinesterase (AChE) is distributed throughout the basal lamina of the synaptic space at a density of about 2500 sites per square micrometre.

In the resting state single ACh quanta are randomly released into the synaptic space. The high local ACh concentration saturates all nearby AChE sites so that most ACh molecules can reach postsynaptic AChRs. The AChR packing density is so high that ACh only needs to diffuse about 0.3 μm along the top and 0.3 μm down along the junctional folds before it meets all the AChR it can saturate (see Salpeter, 1987). The opening of the AChR ion channels in response to ACh results in depolarisations of the muscle fibre known as miniature endplate potentials (MEPPs). When the ion channel closes, ACh dissociates from AChR and ACh is hydrolysed by

AChE to choline and acetate. Choline is taken up by the nerve terminal and is reutilised for ACh synthesis.

The MEPP amplitude, therefore, depends on the number of ACh molecules in the quantum, the number of available AChRs, the geometry of the synaptic space, and the average depolarisation generated by the opening of an AChR ion channel. The MEPP duration depends on the average channel open time, the functional state of the AChE which normally curtails the action of ACh, and the cable properties of the muscle fibre surface membrane.

The quanta released by a nerve impulse generate an endplate potential (EPP) the amplitude of which depends on the MEPP amplitude and the number of quanta released by the nerve impulse (m). The value of m depends on the probability of release (p) and the number of quanta readily available for release (n) according to the relationship $m = np$. *The safety margin of meuromuscular transmission is defined as the difference between the actual EPP amplitude and the EPP amplitude required to trigger the muscle fibre action potential.*

Repetitive stimulation results in a frequency dependent depression of the EPP amplitude, and therefore of the safety margin, to a certain plateau. The decrease is mainly due to a decrease in n. Repetitive stimulation also can facilitate transmitter release by increasing p, or n, or both. The temporal profiles of the opposing processes are such that: (1) a defect of neuromuscular transmission is most readily detected by a train of 5–10 stimuli delivered at a low (2–3 Hz) frequency, because under these conditions there is a reduction in n without any facilitation; (2) tetanic stimulation results in transient improvement (facilitation) and then a worsening of the defect as n is decreased.

10.3. Familial infantile myasthenia (FIM)

10.3.1. *Clinical features*

This disease presents in early infancy or childhood. The earliest symptoms are intermittent drooping of the eyelids (ptosis); poor suck and cry; secondary respiratory infections; and episodic cries precipitated by fever, excitement or vomiting. During crises all symptoms worsen; respiratory muscle weakness results in hypoventilation or apnoea. If untreated the crisis can be fatal, or can produce anoxic cerebral damage. With increasing age the crises become less frequent. After age 10 some patients only complain of easy fatiguability on sustained exertion; others have mild to moderate weakness of cranial, limb and respiratory muscles even at rest, resembling patients with mild to moderate autoimmune myasthenia gravis. The deep tendon reflexes remain normally active, there is no loss of muscle bulk, and a permanent myopathy does not occur. The disease is transmitted by autosomal recessive inheritance (Greer and Schotland, 1960; Conomy *et al.*, 1975; Robertson *et al.*, 1980; Gieron and Korthals, 1985; Engel *et al.*, 1981; Engel, 1986b).

10.3.2. *Electrophysiological aspects*

The electromyogram (EMG) may not show any abnormality in muscles that are not weak when examined. In weak muscles one may detect the non-specific features of neuromuscular transmission defects: (1) an abnormal fluctuation in the shape or size of the motor unit potentials during voluntary effort, due to failure of neuromuscular transmission at a varying proportion of endplates; (2) a progressive decrement in the amplitude of the compound muscle action potential evoked by repetitive, low frequency (2–3 Hz) stimulation, caused by failure of neuromuscular transmission at an increasing number of endplates during depression of n (see above); (3) improvement of the decremental response immediately after a brief period of maximal voluntary exercise, followed within a minute by an increased decremental response; and (4) single fibre EMG abnormalities — consisting of an abnormally prolonged interval between recordings from two muscle fibres served by a single activated motor unit (increased 'jitter'), and failure of a proportion of the impulses to generate an action potential at one of the two fibres ('blocking'). In those patients whose muscles are not weak the weakness and the EMG abnormalities can be induced in some, but not all, muscles either by exercise or by repetitive stimulation at 10 Hz for a few minutes (Engel and Lambert 1987). The EMG decrement, when it is present, can be corrected by the cholinesterase inhibitor, edrophonium (Robertson *et al.*, 1980).

In vitro studies by E. H. Lambert on external intercostal muscles have elucidated the electrophysiological basis of the disorder (Hart *et al.*, 1979; Engel and Lambert, 1987; Mora *et al.*, 1987). Stimulation of small muscle bundles at 10 Hz resulted in an abnormal decrease of the amplitude of the evoked compound muscle action potential (Fig. 10.1), and of the EPP. Unlike in autoimmune myasthenia gravis, the MEPP amplitude was normal in rested muscle but decreased abnormally after 10 Hz stimulation for 5 min. From these findings one can infer that in FIM the safety margin of neuromuscular transmission is compromised by an abnormal decrease of the EPP due to an abnormal decrease in the MEPP amplitude.

The decrease of the MEPP amplitude in the course of prolonged stimulation from an initially normal to an abnormally low level suggests a progressive decrease in the amount of ACh released from synaptic vesicles. An alternative explanation might be an abnormal desensitisation of postsynaptic AChR by physiological amounts of ACh released in the course of stimulation. However, in that case cholinesterase inhibitors, by prolonging the action of ACh, should worsen the defect, but in fact they

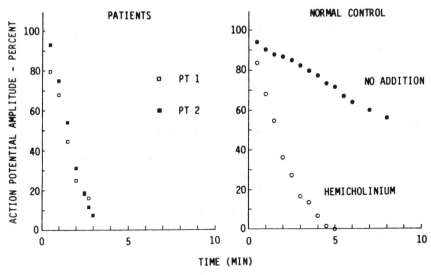

Fig. 10.1. Familial infantile myasthenia (FIM). Effect of 10 Hz stimulation on the amplitude of the evoked compound muscle action potential in external intercostal muscle strips *in vitro* in two FIM patients (left panel) and in a normal subject (right panel). In the presence of 1 mg/dl of hemicholinium-3, the evoked action potential in normal muscle (open circles in right panel), declines as rapidly as the evoked action potential in FIM muscle in the absence of hemicholinium. From Mora *et al.* (1987), by permission.

improve it. The vesicular ACh-depletion hypothesis of FIM is further strengthened by the fact that the response of FIM muscles to electrical stimulation is similar to that of normal muscles treated with hemicholinium (Elmqvist and Quastel, 1965; Jones and Kwanbunbumpen, 1970a, b; Wolters *et al.*, 1974), an inhibitor of choline uptake by the nerve terminal (Fig. 10.1). From these observations one can infer that FIM is caused by a defect in (1) the facilitated uptake of choline by the nerve terminal, (2) ACh resynthesis by choline acetyltransferase, or (3) the transport of ACh molecules into the synaptic vesicles.

10.3.3. *Morphological observations*

Muscle biopsy specimens show no histochemical abnormality. In particular, the usual chequerboard distribution of histochemical fibre types is preserved. AChE-reacted sections demonstrate no abnormality of the NMJ. There are no immune complexes (IgG or complement) at the NMJ. The nerve terminals show normal immunoreactivity for choline acetyltransferase (Engel, 1986b). This, however, does not exclude the possibility of a mutation that alters the kinetic properties of the enzyme.

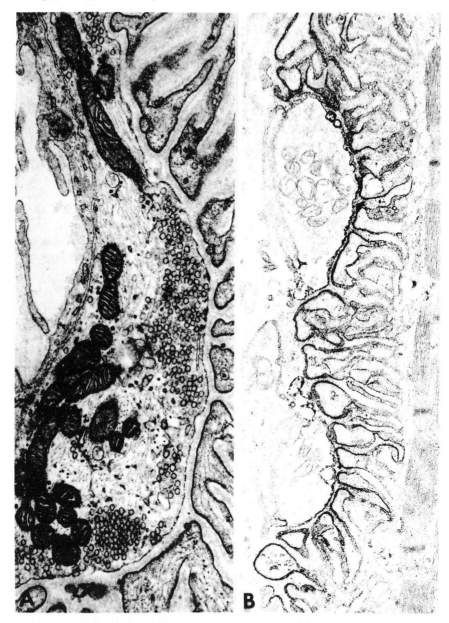

Fig. 10.2. Familial infantile myasthenia (FIM). Electron micrographs of NMJ regions in external intercostal muscle. The specimen shown in panel **A** was prepared for electron microscopy by conventional methods. The nerve terminal and postsynaptic region appear normal. The specimen shown in panel **B** was incubated with peroxidase-labeled α-bungarotoxin before fixation. The black reaction product for peroxidase on the terminal expansions of the junctional folds demonstrates a normal distribution of the acetylcholine receptor on the postsynaptic membrane. **A**, × 28,200; **B** × 16,000.

On electron microscopy the NMJ appears normal on simple inspection (Fig. 10.2A). There is no morphometric abnormality in the size or mitochondrial content of the nerve terminal, the postsynpaptic area of folds and cleft, or the postsynpaptic membrane density. Ultrastructural localisation of AChR with peroxidase-labelled α-bungarotoxin shows normal abundance and distribution of AChR on the terminal expansions of the junctional folds (Fig. 10.2B). Quantitative estimates of the length of the postsynaptic membrane reacting for AChR per nerve terminal (AChR index) and radioimmunochemical estimates of the AChR content per unit wet weight of intercostal muscle are also normal (Hart *et al.*, 1979; Engel *et al.*, 1981).

Recently, Mora *et al.* (1987) searched for a morphological correlate of the failure of neuromuscular transmission in FIM. In previous studies Jones and Kwanbunbumpen (1970a, b) have shown that in the hemicholinium-treated rat diaphragm, nerve stimulation results in an abnormal decrease of the MEPP amplitude and that this is associated with an abnormal decrease in synaptic vesicle size. If in FIM the abnormal decrease of the MEPP amplitude on nerve stimulation was caused by impaired choline uptake by the nerve terminal, or by another defect in ACh synthesis, then the expected morphological concomitant would be a decrease in synaptic vesicle size.

Intercostal muscles from three patients with FIM and three control subjects were studied before and after 10 Hz stimulation for 10 min. In the patients, but not in the controls, neuromuscular transmission failed during stimulation (Fig. 10.1). Synaptic vesicle densities (no/μm^2) and diameters were separately analysed in a superficial 200 nm-wide zone adjacent to the presynaptic membrane, where vesicles are positioned for release, and in the remaining deeper part of the nerve terminal from which vesicles may be mobilised for release. In both patients and controls, stimulation had a similar effect on the density of the superficial and of deep synaptic vesicles, the former decreasing by 20% and the latter by 30–50% of the initial value. For a given site, synaptic vesicle densities did not differ significantly between patients and controls either before or after stimulation. Unexpectedly, the size of the synaptic vesicles was significantly smaller in rested muscle in FIM than in controls. After stimulation, synaptic vesicles increased or did not change size in FIM, and decreased or did not change in size in controls (Fig. 10.3).

There is no simple explanation for the lack of correlation between synaptic vescile size and the MEPP amplitude in FIM. From current knowledge derived from studies of *Torpedo* electric organ synaptic vesicles, ACh is taken up by the synaptic vesicles by a proton-driven ACh translocase that exchanges protons in the vesicles for cytosolic ACh (Anderson *et al.*, 1983; Harlos *et al.*, 1984; Whittaker, 1984). The

EFFECT OF STIMULATION ON SYNAPTIC VESICLE VOLUME

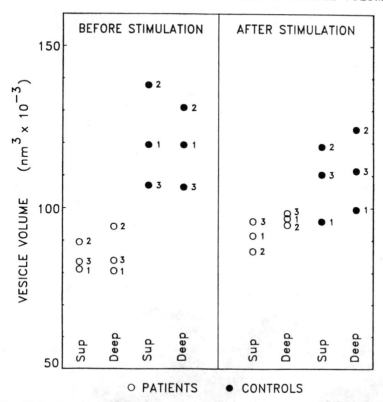

Fig. 10.3. Familial infantile myasthenia. Mean synaptic vesicle volumes in deep and superficial regions of nerve terminals before stimulation and after 10 Hz stimulation for 10 min. Open and closed symbols indicate patients and controls, respectively. From Mora *et al.* (1987), by permission.

accumulation of protons in the vesicles, in turn, depends on a proton translocating ATPase. The synaptic vesicles contain not only ACh and protons, but also a relatively high concentration of ATP, GTP, Ca^{2+}, and Mg^{2+} and a proteoglycan (Whittaker, 1984; Wagner *et al.*, 1978). These observations imply that (1) the number of ACh molecules in the vesicles is not the only determinant of vesicle volume and (2) a defect in any of the mechanisms that regulate the concentrations of any of the osmotically active substances in the synaptic vesicles could affect the vesicle volume. Thus, the fact that in FIM the synaptic vesicles are smaller than normal in rested muscle, and increase paradoxically in size after stimulation, suggests a defect in synaptic vesicle metabolism, but the character of the defect remains undefined.

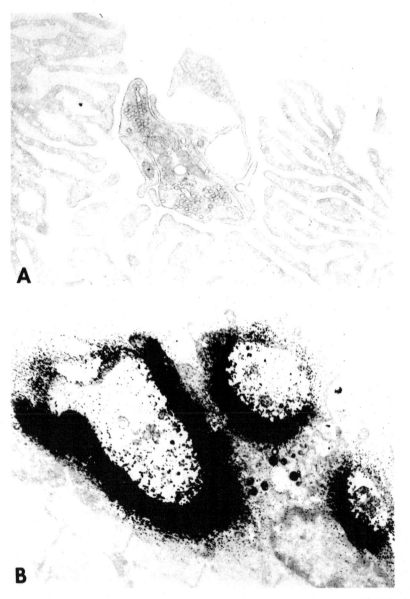

Fig. 10.4.   Electron cytochemical localisation of acetylcholinesterase (AChE) in congenital endplate AChE deficiency. In **A**, patient's endplate shows no reaction after incubation for 1 h at room temperature. In **B**, control endplate is greatly overreacted after incubation for 30 min at room temperature. Here, the black reaction product (lead sulphide) completely covers the synaptic space and junctional folds, and has spread into adjacent regions. **A**, × 20,500; **B** × 8,900. From Engel *et al.* (1977), by permission.

10.3.4. *Treatment*

The muscle weakness, when present, responds well to small or modest doses of anticholinesterase drugs. Some patients are symptomatic or have only minimal weakness except during crises, and require anticholinesterase drugs on an emergency basis only. Parents of affected children must be taught to anticipate sudden worsening of the weakness and possible apnoea with febrile illnesses, excitement or overexertion. The parents also must be familiar with the use of a hand-assisted ventilatory device, and should be able to administer appropriate doses of prostigmine intramuscularly during crises. Patients with febrile illness and a previous history of crisis should be hospitalised for close observation and ventilatory support as needed.

10.4. Congenital endplate acetylcholinesterase deficiency

This disorder was described by Engel *et al.* (1977). Few sporadic male cases and two sisters affected with this disease have been observed to date. Weakness, abnormal fatiguability and a decremental EMG response are present in all voluntary muscles from birth. The symptoms are refractory to anticholinesterase drugs and cause severe disability.

Conventional histological studies of muscle specimens are normal. The basic abnormality is total absence of AChE from the NMJ: no enzyme activity can be demonstrated by light microscopic or electron microscopic cytochemistry (Fig. 10.4) and no immunoreactivity for AChE is detected by polyclonal and several monoclonal AChE antibodies (Engel, 1986b). The total muscle AChE content is also reduced.

Because AChE is absent from the NMJ, ACh–AChR interaction and the duration of the EPP and MEPP are prolonged. This means that the amplitude of the EPP can remain above the threshold required for firing the muscle action potential even after the muscle fibre has recovered from the refractory period of the preceding action potential. As a result one long EPP can evoke two or more muscle fibre action potentials. Consequently, a single supramaximal stimulus applied to a motor nerve can evoke two or more compound muscle action potentials.

The motor nerves are abnormally small (Fig. 10.5A and B) and contain a reduced number of releasable ACh quanta (n). The quantal content of the EPP (m) is reduced because of the smallness of n. The probability of quantal release (p) remains normal. Smallness of the nerve terminals is not as constant as, and is probably secondary to, the AChE deficiency. AChR numbers are normal (Fig. 10.5B) (Engel *et al.*, 1977) or reduced (Engel *et al.*, 1981) at the NMJ. The AChR loss, when present, is caused by degenerative changes in the junctional folds, which can be accounted for by the ACh excess (Engel *et al.*, 1973; Laskowski *et al.*, 1975; Salpeter *et al.*, 1979). However, the ACh excess is mild because ACh release is limited

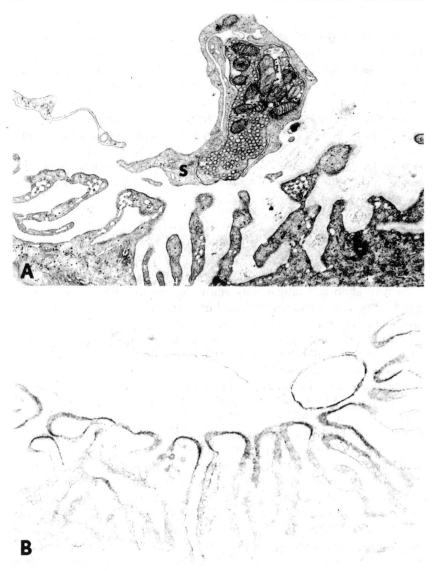

Fig. 10.5. Congenital endplate acetylcholinesterase (AChE) deficiency. In **A**, small nerve terminal, almost completely surrounded by Schwann cell (S), is applied against a small fraction of the postsynaptic region. The junctional folds contain numerous membranous networks. **B** Ultrastructural localisation of the acetylcholine receptor (AChR) with peroxidase-labelled α-bungarotoxin. AChR is normally abundant and is normally distributed on the terminal expansions of the junctional folds. **A**, × 15,400; **B**, × 23,400. From Engel *et al.* (1977), by permission.

by the small size of the nerve terminals. The safety margin of neuromuscular transmission is compromised by lack of releasable ACh quanta and, to a lesser extent, by AChR deficiency.

10.5. **Paucity of synaptic vesicles and reduced quantal release**

In this recently recognised syndrome the safety margin of neuromuscular transmission is compromised by a deficiency in the number of synaptic vesicles in the nerve terminal (Walls *et al.*, 1990; Engel *et al.*, 1990b). The patient, a 23-year-old woman, had fatigable weakness of limb and bulbar muscles since infancy. She improved with anticholinesterase drugs. Tests for anti-AChR antibodies were negative. A decremental EMG response was present at 2 Hz stimulation. In vitro microelectrode studies of an intercostal muscle specimen revealed that the quantal content of the EPP (m) was markedly reduced due to a decrease in the number of immediately releasable quanta (n); the probability of quantal release (p) was normal. Increased $[Ca^{++}]$ in the bath increased m normally. The amplitude and decay time constant of the MEPP were normal and the MEPP frequency increased normally with increased $[K^+]$. NMJ AChR, estimated from the number of alpha-bungarotoxin binding sites, was normal. Quantitative electron microscopy of unstimulated NMJ demonstrated an approximate 80% decrease in synaptic vesicle density (no./μm^2) that was proportionate to the decrease in n. The nerve terminal size, presynaptic membrane length and the postsynaptic region were normal by ultrastructural criteria.

Synaptic vesicles are transported by fast axonal flow from the anterior horn cell perykarion to the motor nerve terminal (see for example Llinas *et al.*, 1989; Booj, 1986) where they undergo exocytosis and recycling (see chapter by Molenaar and Chapter 1). The paucity of synaptic vesicles in this syndrome could be due to an impaired axonal transport of preformed vesicles to the nerve terminal, or to impaired vesicle recycling in the nerve terminal after activity. The fact, however, that the synaptic vesicles were depleted even in the unstimulated NMJ implicates the axonal vesicle transport mechanism.

10.6. **Slow-channel syndrome**

This syndrome was described in 1982 (Engel *et al.*, 1982). Since then one additional report has been published (Oosterhuis *et al.*, 1987). The disease is transmitted by an autosomal dominant gene with high penetrance and variable expressivity. Sporadic cases also occur. The age of onset, the initial and eventual pattern of muscle involvement, the rate of progression, and the degree of weakness and fatiguability vary from case to case. The disease may present in infancy, childhood or adult life. It progresses

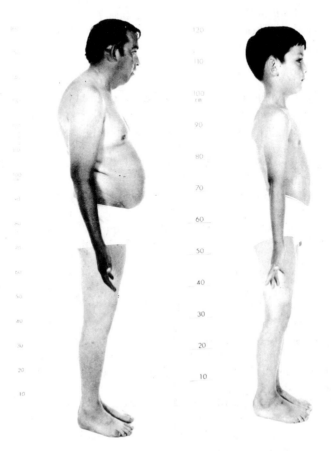

Fig. 10.6. Slow-channel syndrome, father and son. Note atrophy of shoulder and forearm muscles and lordotic stance. From Engel *et al.* (1981), by permission.

gradually or in an intermittent manner, remaining quiescent for years or decades between periods of worsening. Typically there is selective severe involvement of cervical, scapular and finger extensor muscles (Figs. 10.6 and 10.7); mild to moderate weakness of the eyelid elevators and limitation of ocular movements with only occasional double vision; and variable involvement of masticatory, facial and other upper extremity, respiratory and trunk muscles. The lower limbs tend to be spared, or may be less severely affected than the upper ones. The clinically affected muscles are weak, atrophic and fatigue abnormally. The deep tendon reflexes are usually normal but can be reduced in severely affected limbs. Antibodies against the AChR are not present and AChE inhibitors are ineffective. Oosterhuis *et al.* (1987) found flunarazine, a calcium channel blocker, ineffective in one patient.

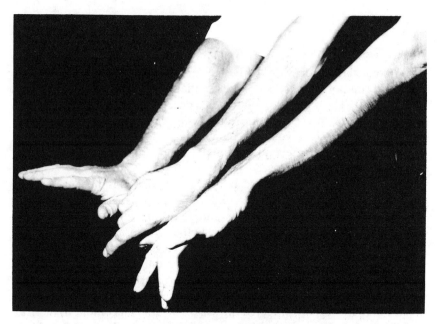

Fig. 10.7. Slow-channel syndrome. Patient attempting to extend wrists and fingers as shown by examiner (with sleeve). Note atrophy of patient's forearm muscles. From Engel *et al.* (1982), by permission.

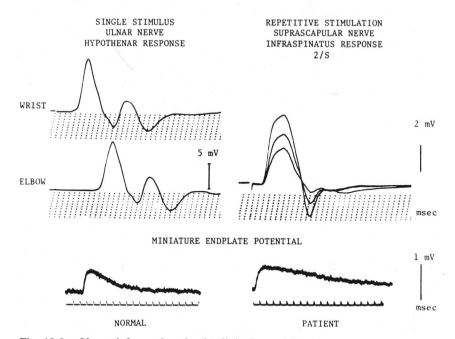

Fig. 10.8. Upper left panels: stimulus-linked repetitive compound muscle action potential in the slow-channel syndrome. Right upper panel: decremental response of infraspinatus muscle action potential during 2 Hz stimulation of suprascapular nerve. Lower panels: the duration and half-decay time of the MEPP are longer in patient than in normal control. From Engel *et al.* (1982), by permission.

10.6.1. *Electrophysiological aspects*

As in congenital endplate AChE deficiency, single nerve stimuli evoke repetitive compound muscle action potentials in all muscles (Fig. 10.8, left upper panel). The consecutive potentials occur at 5–10 ms intervals, each smaller than the preceding one, and disappear after a brief voluntary contraction. Two nerve volleys, 1–3 ms apart, increase rather than inhibit the amplitude of the second action potential, indicating that it is not produced by an axon reflex.

A decremental EMG response at 2–3 Hz stimulation is present, but only in clinically affected muscles (Fig. 10.8, right upper panel). The motor unit potentials fluctuate in shape and amplitude during voluntary activity.

In vitro microelectrode studies indicate that the duration and half-decay time of the intracellularly recorded MEPP (Fig. 10.8, lower panels) and EPP are prolonged in all muscles, and the duration of the potentials is further increased by AChE inhibitors. The amplitude of the MEPP is significantly reduced in some but not all muscles, and the decrease is greater in more severely affected muscles. The quantal content of the EPP is in the normal range. That the prolonged duration of the MEPP and EPP is not due to an alteration in the cable properties of the muscle membrane has been demonstrated by two measures: (1) the duration of the extracellularly recorded MEPP, which is independent of the cable properties of the membrane and reflects the duration of the miniature endplate current (Del Castillo and Katz, 1956), is also markedly prolonged (Engel *et al.*, 1982); (2) miniature endplate currents recorded directly by voltage clamping also display increased decay times (Oosterhuis *et al.*, 1987); (3) in one patient both the depolarisation produced by opening of single channels, and the time constant of the ACh-induced voltage noise at the endplate, were higher than in a control patient (Oosterhuis *et al.*, 1987).

10.6.2. *Morphological studies*

Light microscopic histochemical studies show type 1 fibre predominance, isolated or small groups of atrophic fibres of either histochemical type, tubular aggregates, and vacuoles in fibre regions near motor endplates. Other biopsy specimens show abnormal variation in fibre size, variable fibre splitting and, in some instances, mild to moderate increase of endomysial or perimysial connective tissue.

AChE activity is present at all endplates. The configuration of the endplates is often abnormal, with multiple, small, discrete regions dispersed over an extended length of the muscle fibre. This finding is more pronounced in the more severely affected muscles. Focal calcium deposits were demonstrated at the endplates by Engel *et al.* (1982) in one of four cases in which this test was performed.

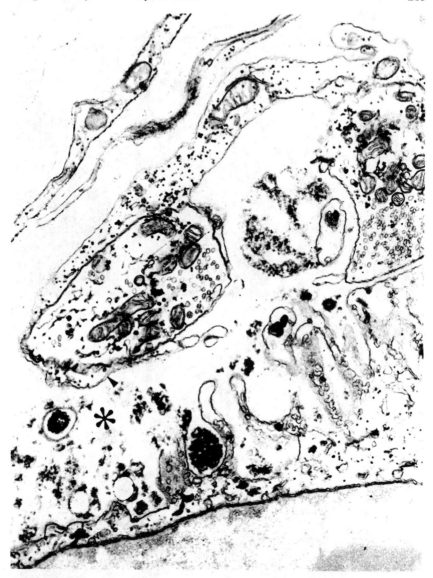

Fig. 10.9. Intercostal muscle endplate in the slow-channel syndrome. Junctional folds have degenerated in the region imaged at left. Highly electron-dense debris marks position of preexisting folds (asterisk). Presynaptic membrane facing degenerated folds is partially covered by Schwann cell (arrowhead). × 20,100. From Engel *et al.* (1982), by permission.

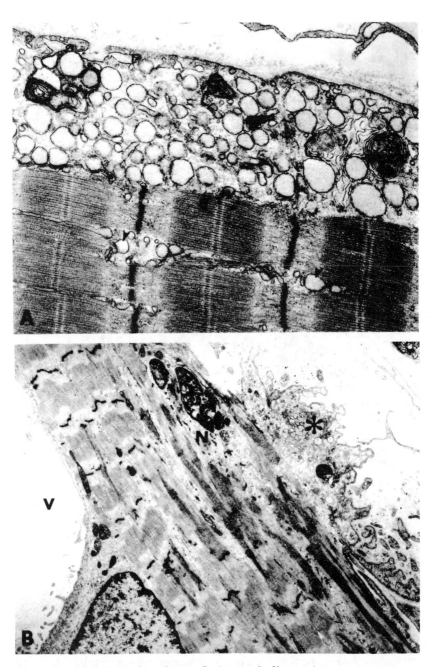

Fig. 10.10.   Slow-channel syndrome. In **A**, muscle fibre region near NMJ displays numerous dilated vesicles of the sarcoplasmic reticulum and occasional myeloid structures. Few dilated components of the sarcoplasmic reticulum also appear between the myofibrils (arrowheads). In **B**, a highly degenerate postsynaptic region denuded of its nerve terminal (asterisk) overlies a fibre region that shows loss of mitochondria, focal myofibrillar degeneration, a disintegrating nucleus (N), and a large membrane-bound vacuole (V). **A** is from infraspinatus muscle; **B** is from finger extensor muscle. From Engel *et al.* (1981), by permission.

On electron microscopic examination, at many NMJs the junctional folds contain myriad pinocytotic vesicles and labyrinthine membranous networks. The junctional folds are frequently degenerating, causing widening of the synaptic space and accumulation of electron-dense debris (Fig. 10.9). Some of the highly abnormal postsynaptic regions are denuded of their nerve terminals (Fig. 10.10B). Unmyelinated nerve sprouts appear near some NMJs. The intramuscular nerves are normal. There are no immune complexes (IgG or complement) at the NMJs, such as are found in myasthenia gravis, but AChR is reduced especially in the more severely affected muscles.

The junctional sarcoplasm often contains membrane-bound vesicles which arise from dilations of the sarcoplasmic reticulum or from the outer membrane of nearby nuclei. In some regions the vesicles are intermingled with small dense bodies, swollen or degenerating mitochondria, myeloid structures and small vacuoles containing degraded membranous organelles. Fibre regions adjacent to endplates often contain tubular aggregates, irregularly arrayed tubules and vesicles (Fig. 10.10A), myeloid structures, degenerating nuclei, and proliferating Golgi elements and transverse tubular system networks. Deeper fibre regions show focal decreases in mitochondria and focal myofibrillar degeneration (Fig. 10.10B). In some muscle fibres there are larger vacuoles near the endplate (Fig. 10.10B). These contain amorphous or granular material or fragmented membranes and are limited by membranes of transverse tubular origin or by proliferating transverse tubular system networks.

Morphometric reconstruction of the endplate shows a 29–43% decrease of nerve terminal size and a 25–37% increase in synaptic vesicle density. The postsynaptic membrane length and density are significantly reduced due to degeneration of the junctional folds.

10.6.3. *Biochemical studies*

Although AChE inhibitors further increased the duration of the MEPP *in vitro*, and although AChE was present at the endplates by cytochemical criteria, a partial deficiency or kinetic abnormality of AChE could still account for the prolonged MEPP. This possibility was excluded by demonstrating that the activity and K_m of AChE were normal in muscle in this syndrome (Engel *et al.*, 1982). Since the catalytic subunit in all forms of muscle AChE is identical (Vigny *et al.*, 1979), the kinetic properties of total muscle AChE are a valid measure of the kinetic properties of endplate AChE.

10.6.4. *Pathogenetic mechanisms*

The prolonged EPP can be attributed to the prolonged MEPP. Since AChE is intact by physiological, histochemical and biochemical criteria, and since the prolonged MEPP cannot be attributed to abnormal cable properties of the muscle fibre plasma membrane, the prolonged MEPP is caused by a prolonged open time of the AChR ion channel.

As in congenital endplate AChE deficiency, the repetitive muscle action potential can be explained by the prolonged EPP. The fact that the repetitive muscle action potential response is present in *all* muscles indicates that the AChR ion channel abnormality is ubiquitous and represents the primary disturbance. Thus, the weakness, wasting and fatiguability which appear in *selected* muscles at variable intervals are secondary phenomena.

The prolonged endplate currents result in an abnormally increased cation flux into the junctional folds and nearby muscle fibre regions. Because a fraction of the current is carried by calcium (Takeuchi, 1963; Evans, 1974; Miledi *et al.*, 1980), transient or permanent calcium excess may occur in the junctional folds and nearby fibre regions. The deleterious effects of the focal calcium excess, which include activation of intracellular proteases and stimulation of membrane-bound phospholipases (Ebashi and Sugita, 1979; Jackson *et al.*, 1984), can readily explain the focal degeneration of the junctional folds and the spectrum of myopathic changes observed in the junctional sarcoplasm and nearby fibre regions. Further, some of the findings are similar to those noted in mouse muscle exposed to carbachol, a cholinergic agonist, and the carbachol-induced changes can be prevented by exclusion of calcium from the extracellular fluid (Leonard and Salpeter, 1979).

The focal degeneration of the junctional folds readily explains the loss of AChR. In addition, it is also possible that AChR synthesis is inhibited, as in cultured muscle exposed to cholinergic agonists (Gardner and Fambrough, 1979). One can infer that the AChR deficiency accounts for the reduced MEPP amplitude and the impaired safety margin of neuromuscular transmission.

The AChR ion channel is also slow in non-innervated muscle fibres and at newly formed endplates (reviewed by Schuetze, 1987). It is therefore possible that the abnormality in the slow-channel syndromes stems from a developmental failure of the slow to fast conversion of the ion channel. It is now known that this conversion is associated with a replacement of the γ subunit of AChR by an ε subunit (Mishina *et al.*, 1986; Witzemann *et al.*, 1987; Gu and Hall, 1988; see Beeson and Barnard, this volume). Therefore, expression of the γ instead of the ε subunit in slow-channel syndrome AChR would be evidence for abnormal developmental regulation. Recent studies, however, indicate that slow-channel AChR is immunoreactive for the ε but not for the γ subunit (Engel, A. G., Gu, Y. and Hall, Z., unpublished data, 1987). The most plausible explanation at this time is that a mutation in a structural gene has so altered endplate AChR that its return from the open to the closed conformation is hindered.

10.7. **High-conductance fast-channel syndrome**

This syndrome has been recently recognized (Engel *et al.*, 1990a and 1990b). The patient, a 9-year-old girl, had poor suck and cry after birth. Since then, she had intermittent weakness of ocular, neck and selected limb muscles on exertion. All symptoms were worsened by exposure to heat. Tests for anti-AChR antibodies were negative. There was no improvement with AChE inhibitors. A decremental EMG response was found in limb muscle after exercise. On electrophysiological studies of an intercostal muscle specimen, the quantal content of the EPP was normal; the MEPP and miniature endplate currents (MEPC) were abnormally large, and their decay time constants were abnormally short. AChR ion channel properties were studied by analysis of the ACh-induced current noise. Mean single channel conductance was increased 1.7-fold and mean channel opentime was 30% shorter than in 5 control muscles (P < 0.001). The number of NMJ AChR, estimated from the number of alpha-bungarotoxin binding sites, was normal. Electron microscopy of most NMJ showed no abnormality, but a few were degenerating or simplified.

The functionally abnormal AChR ion channel is probably due to a mutation in an AChR subunit. Site directed mutagenesis studies indicate that single amino acid substitutions in any subunit that increase negative charges close to the external vestibule of the ion channel enhance the cation flux through the channel (see Dani, 1989; and Beeson and Barnard, this volume). The fact that in this disease the high channel conductance is associated with a shorter than normal channel opentime implies that the mutation has a dual affect on the kinetic properties of the ion channel.

The manner in which the physiologic defect produces clinical symptoms is unclear, but it may be due to the development of an endplate myopathy in severely affected muscles, as occurs in the slow-channel syndrome.

10.8. **Congenital endplate AChR deficiency**

This syndrome is less well characterised and more heterogeneous than those described above.

In three patients studied by Vincent *et al.* (1981) (cases 2, 4, 5) NMJ AChE was preserved and endplate currents were not abnormally long. NMJ AChR, estimated from the number of α-bungarotoxin binding sites, was reduced and the NMJ was elongated on light microscopy. These findings were similar to those in myasthenia gravis (see Vincent) but the weakness was present since birth and the patients did not have anti-AChR antibodies. The AChR deficiency could be due to decreased synthesis, reduced membrane insertion or accelerated degradation of AChR. In case 2 of those investigated by Lecky *et al.* (1986) the NMJ also appeared elongated on light microscopy although NMJ ultrastructure was normal. The number of NMJ α-bungarotoxin binding sites was markedly reduced. No electrophysiological studies were done in this case. In one patient studied by Vincent *et al.* (1981) (case 3), the amount of α-bungarotoxin bound to the NMJ was reduced only after prolonged washing. This may indicate a reduced affinity of AChR for α-bungarotoxin and, by inference, for ACh. Recently, analysis of the ACh-induced current noise in a patient with severe NMJ AChR deficiency revealed normal AChR channel conductance, but the channel open time was 29% shorter than in 5 normal controls ($p < 0.001$) (Nagel *et al.*, 1990; Engel *et al.*, 1990b). The kinetic abnormality of AChR is likely to stem from a mutation in an AChR subunit which, in turn, might result in reduced synthesis of the mutant AChR.

In the patients described above the muscle biopsy did not reveal a myopathy, but in another patient with a congenital myasthenic syndrome observed by us (Lambert, E. H. and Engel, A. G., unpublished data), endplate AChR deficiency and a small MEPP amplitude were associated with a severe myopathy.

In another patient with congenital contractures, studies of the NMJ in the first year of life showed failure of development of the junctional folds, reduced endplate AChR by morphological criteria and a small MEPP (Smit *et al.*, 1984; 1987).

10.9. Abnormal ACh-AChR interaction

In case 1 of those studied by Vincent *et al.*, 1981 the MEPP amplitude was low but the AChR content of the NMJ was normal. This could be due to decreased conductance or open time of the AChR ion channel, decreased number of ACh molecules per quantum, or reduced affinity of AChR for ACh. Specific studies to distinguish between these possibilities were not carried out. In a patient investigated by Lecky *et al.* 1986 (Case 1) a reduced MEPP amplitude was associated with normal alpha-bungarotoxin binding to the postsynaptic membrane, endplate structure, d-tubocurarine affinity, ion channel properties, and passive membrane properties; the effectiveness of ACh to open ion channels, however, was reduced.

Recently, another patient with a decreased MEPP and MEPC amplitude and normal amount of NMJ AChR was investigated by detailed electrophysiological and ultrastructural methods (Uchitel *et al.*, 1990; Engel *et al.*, 1990b). The synaptic vesicles were of normal size which makes a decreased number of ACh molecules per quantum unlikely. AChR ion channel properties were studied by analysis of ACh-induced current noise. Mean single channel conductance was normal. The noise power spectrum was abnormal, containing two components of a different time course. Biexponential AChR ion channel kinetics could result from (1) a dual population of AChR, as in the immature NMJ (Fischbach and Schuetze, 1980); (2) an abnormality of ACh-AChR interaction, such as blocking of the AChR ion channel, or another alteration in ACh-AChR interaction so that the closure of the diliganded channel was no longer rate limiting (see chapter by Colquhoun, and Adams, 1987). A dual population of AChRs with different rate constants of closure is an unlikely explanation because both types of receptors would have to have a low conductance to also explain the small MEPC, but the effective conductance of the population of channels that did open was normal. On the other hand, an abnormal interaction of ACh with AChR can account for both the small MEPC and the biexponetial AChR ion channel kinetics. Single-channel recordings will be required to further characterise the AChR abnormality in this syndrome.

10.10. Less well characterised syndromes

10.10.1. *AChR deficiency with altered affinity for d-tubocurarine*

A patient studied by Morgan-Hughes *et al.* (1981) showed a slight decrease in NMJ AChR and a ten-fold increase in the affinity of AChR for d-tubocurarine. The manner in which the latter abnormality contributed to the defect of neuromuscular transmission was not defined.

10.10.2 *Possible defect in ACh synthesis, mobilisation or storage*

In one infant with a congenital myasthenic syndrome there was marked EMG decrement at all stimulation frequencies and moderate to marked facilitation 15 s after 50 Hz stimulation. Single nerve stimuli did not evoke repetitive compound muscle action potentials and AChE and AChR were normally abundant at the NMJ. Ultrastructural studies of the NMJ suggested a slight decrease in the mean synaptic vesicle diameter. Anticholinesterase and guanidine were ineffective. Although *in vitro* electrophysiological studies of neuromuscular transmission were not carried out, the observations were thought to be consistent with a defect in ACh synthesis, mobilisation or storage (Albers *et al.*, 1984).

10.10.3. *Familial limb-girdle myasthenia*

This is an autosomal recessive syndrome (McQuillen, 1966; Johns *et al.*, 1971; Dobkin and Verity, 1978). Weakness of limb-girdle muscles and easy fatiguability appear during childhood or in the teens. Ocular and other cranial muscles are not affected. The symptoms respond to anticholinesterase drugs but not to prednisone. EMG studies show a decremental response. Joint contractures, cardiac repolarisation defect, type 1 fibre atrophy, and abnormal electrical irritability of the muscle fibres were also noted in one family (Dobkin and Verity, 1978). Histochemical studies have demonstrated tubular aggregates in the muscle fibres. The position of the aggregates relative to the NMJ was not established. Detailed morphological studies of the NMJ, *in vitro* electrophysiological studies of neuromuscular transmission and measurements of NMJ AChR are not available in this syndrome.

Acknowledgements

Work in the author's laboratory was supported in part by Research Grant NS 6277 from the National Institute of Health, and Research Center Grant from the Muscular Dystrophy Association.

References

Adams, P. R. (1987) Transmitter action at endplate membrane. In M. M. Salpeter, ed., *The Vertebrate Neuromuscular Junction*, Alan Liss, New York, pp. 317–359.

Albers, J. W., Faulkner, J. A., Dorovini–Zis, K., Barald, K. F., Must, R. E. and Ball, R. D. (1984) Abnormal neuromuscular transmission in an infantile myasthenic syndrome. *Ann. Neurol.* **16**: 28–34.

Anderson, D. C., King, S. C. and Parsons, S. M. (1983) Pharmacological characterization of the acetylcholine transport system in purefied Torpedo electric organ synaptic vesicles. *Mol. Pharmacol.* **24**: 48–54.

Booj, S. (1986) Axonal transport of synapsin I and cholinergic synaptic vesicle-like material. Further immunohistochemical evidence for transport of axonal cholinergic transmitter vesicles in motor neurons. *Acta Physiol. Scand.* **128**: 155–165.

Conomy, J. P., Levisohn, M. and Fanaroff, A. (1975) Familial infantile myasthenia gravis: a cause of sudden death in young children. *J. Pediatr.* **87**: 428–429.

Dani, J. A. (1989) Site-directed mutagenesis and single-channel currents define the ionic channel of the nicotinic acetylcholine receptor. *TINS* **12**: 125–128.

Del Castillo, J. and Katz, B. (1956) Localization of active spots within the neuromuscular junction of the frog. *J. Physiol.* **132**: 630–649.

Dobkin, B. H. and Verity, M. A. (1978) Familial neuromuscular disease with type 1 fiber hypoplasia, tubular aggregates, cardiomyopathy and myasthenic features. *Neurology* **28**: 1135–1140.

Ebashi, S. and Sugita, H. (1979) The role of calcium in physiological and pathological processes of skeletal muscle. *Ex. Med. ICS* **455**: 73–84.

Elmqvist, D. and Quastel, D. M. J. (1965) Presynaptic action of hemicholinium at the neuromuscular junction. *J. Physiol. (Lond.)* **177**: 463–482.

Engel, A. G. (1986a). The neuromuscular junction. In: *Myology*, A. G. Engel and B. Q. Banker, eds, McGraw–Hill, New York, pp. 209–254.

Engel, A. G. (1986b). Myasthenic syndromes. In: *Myology*, A. G. Engel and B. Q. Banker (eds), McGraw–Hill, New York, pp. 1955–1990.

Engel, A. G. and Lambert, E. H. (1987). Congenital myasthenic syndromes. *Electroenceohalogr. Clin. Neurophysiol.* (Suppl.) **39**, 91–102.

Engel, A. G., Lambert, E. H. and Santa, T. (1973) Study of long-term anticholinesterase therapy. Effects on neuromuscular transmission and on motor endplate fine structure. *Neurology* **23**: 1273–1281.

Engel, A. G., Lambert, E. H. and Gomez M. R. (1977) A new myasthenic syndrome with endplate acetylcholinesterase deficiency, small nerve terminals and reduced acetylcholine release. *Ann. Neurol.* **1**: 315–330.

Engel, A. G., Lambert, E. H., Mulder, D. M., Gomez, M. R., Whitaker, J., Hart, Z. and Sahashi, K. (1981) Recently recognized congenital myasthenic syndromes: (A) Endplate acetylcholine (ACh) esterase deficiency. (B) Putative abnormality of the ACh induced ion channel. (C) Putative defect of ACh resynthesis or mobilization. Clinical features, ultrastructure and cytochemistry. *Ann. N.Y. Acad. Sci.* **377**: 614–639.

Engel, A. G., Lambert, E. H., Mulder, D. M. Torres, C. F., Sahaski, K., Bertorini, T. E. and Whitaker, J. (1982) A newly recognized congenital myasthenic syndrome attributed to a prolonged open time of the acetylcholine-induced ion channel. *Ann. Neurol.* **11**: 553–569.

Engel, A. G., Uchitel, O., Walls, T. J., Nagel, A. and Bodensteiner, J. (1990a) Congenital myasthenic syndrome with high conductance and fast closure of the acetylcholine-induced ion channel. *Neurology* **40** (Suppl. 1): 277.

Engel, A. G., Walls, T. J., Nagel, A. and Uchitel, O. (1990b) Newly recognized congenital myasthenic syndromes: i. Congenital paucity of synaptic vesicles and reduced quantal release. ii. High-conductance fast-channel syndrome. iii. Abnormal interaction of acetylcholine with its receptor. iv. Acetylcholine receptor deficiency and short channel opentime. *Progress in Brain Research* **84**: 125–137.

Evans, R. H. (1974) The entry of labelled calcium into the innervated region of the mouse diaphragm muscle. *J. Physiol. (Lond.)* **240**: 517–533.

Fischbach, G. D. and Schuetze, S. M. (1980) A post-natal decrease in acetylcholine channel open time at rat endplates. *J. Physiol. (Lond.)* **303**: 125–137.

Gardner, J. M. and Fambrough, D. M. (1979) Acetylcholine receptor degradation measured by density labeling: effects of cholinergic ligands and evidence against recycling. *Cell* **16**: 661–674.

Gieron, M. A. and Korthals, J. K. (1985) Familial infantile myasthenia gravis. Report of three cases with follow-up until adult life. *Arch. Neurol.* **42**: 143–144.

Greer, M. and Schotland, M. (1960) Myasthenia gravis in the newborn. *Pediatrics* **26**: 101–108.

Gu, Y. and Hall, Z. W. (1988) Immunological evidence for a change in subunits of the acetycholine receptor in developing and denervated rat muscle. *Neuron.* **1**: 117–125.

Harlos, P., Lee, D. A. and Stadler, H. (1984) Characterization of a Mg^{2+}-ATPase and a proton pump in cholinergic synaptic vesicles from the electric organ of Torpedo marmorata. *Eur. J. Biochem.* **144**: 441–446.

Hart, Z., Sahashi, K., Lambert, E. H., Engel, A. G. and Lindstrom, J. (1979) A congenital, familial, myasthenic syndrome caused by a presynaptic defect of transmitter resynthesis or mobilization (abstract). *Neurology* **29**: 559.

Jackson, M. J., Jones, D. A. and Edwards, R. H. T. (1984) Experimental skeletal muscle damage: The role of calcium activated degenerative processes. *Eur. J. Clin. Invest.* **14**: 369–375.

Johns, T. R., Campa, J. F., Crowley, W. J. and Miller, J. Q. (1971) Familial myasthenia with tubular aggregates (abstract). *Neurology* **21**: 449.

Jones, S. F. and Kwanbunbumpen, S. (1970a) The effects of nerve stimulation and hemicholinium on synaptic vesicles at the mammalian neuromuscular junction. *J. Physiol. (Lond.)* **207**: 31–50.

Jones, S. F. and Kwanbunbumpen, S. (1970b) Some effects of nerve stimulation and hemicholinium on quantal transmitter release at the mammalian neuromuscular junction. *J. Physiol. (Lond).* **207**: 51–61.

Laskowski, M. B., Olson, W. H. and Dettbarn, W. D. (1975) Ultrastructural changes at the motor endplate produced by an irreversible cholinesterase inhibitor. *Exp. Neurol.* **47**: 290–306.

Lecky, B. R. F., Morgan–Hughes, J. A., Murray, N. M. F., Landon, D. N. and Wray, D. (1986) Congenital myasthenia: Further evidence of disease heterogeneity. *Muscle Nerve* **9**: 233–242.

Leonard, J. P. and Salpeter, M. M. (1979) Agonist-induced myopathy at the neuromuscular junction is mediated by calcium. *J. Cell. Biol.* **82**: 811–819.

Linas, R., Sugimori, M., Lin, J. W., Leopold, P. L. and Brady, S. T. (1989) ATP-dependent directional movement of rat synaptic vesicles injected into the presynaptic terminal of squid giant synapse. *Proc. Natl. Acad. Sci. USA*, **86**: 5656–5660.

Magleby, K. L. (1986) Neuromuscular transmission. In: *Myology*. A. G. Engel and B. Q. Banker (eds), McGraw–Hill, New York, pp. 393–418.

McQuillen, M. P. (1966) Familial limb-girdle myasthenia. *Brain* **89**: 121–132.

Miledi, R., Parker, I. and Schalow, G. (1980) Transmitter induced calcium entry across the postsynaptic membrane at frog endplates measured using arsenazo III. *J. Physiol. (Lond.)* **300**: 197–212.

Mishina, M., Takai, T., Imoto, K., Noda, M., Takahashi, T., Numa, S., Methfessel, C. and Sakmann, B. (1986) Molecular distinction between fetal and adult forms of muscle acetylcholine receptor. *Nature* **321**: 406–411.

Mora, M., Lambert, E. H. and Engel, A. G. (1987) Synaptic vesicle abnormality in familial infantile myasthenia. *Neurology* **37**: 206–214.

Morgan–Hughes, J. A., Lecky, B. R. F., Landon, D. N. and Murray, N. M. F. (1981) Alterations in the number and affinity of junctional acetylcholine receptors in a myopathy with tubular aggregates. A newly recognized receptor defect. *Brain* **104**: 279–295.

Nagel, A., Engel, A. G., Walls, T. J., Harper, M. C. and Waisburg, H. (1990) Congenital myasthenic syndrome with endplate acetylcholine receptor deficiency and short channel opentime. *Neurology* **40** (Suppl. 1): 277–278.

Oosterhuis, H. J. G. H., Newsom–Davis, J., Wokke, J. H. J., Molenaar, P. C., Weerden, T. V., Oen, B. S., Jennekens, F. G. I., Veldman, H., Vincent, A., Wray, D. W., Prior C. and Murray, N. M. F. (1987). The slow channel syndrome. Two new cases. *Brain* **110**: 1061–1079.

Robertson, W. C., Chun, R. W. M. and Kornguth, S. E. (1980). Familial infantile myasthenia. *Arch. Neurol.* **37**: 117–119.

Salpeter, M. M. (1987) Vertebrate neuromuscular junctions: General morphology, molecular organization and functional consequences. In: *The Vertebrate Neuromuscular Junction*, Salpeter, M. M., ed., Alan Liss, New York, pp. 1–54.

Salpeter, M. M., Kasprzak, H., Feng, H. and Fertuck, H. (1979) Endplates after esterase inactivation *in vivo*: correlation between esterase concentration, functional response and fine structure. *J. Neurocytol.* **8**: 95–115.

Schuetze, S. M. (1987). Developmental regulation of acetylcholine receptors. *Ann. Rev. Neurosci.* **10**: 403–457.

Smit, S. M. E., Jennekens, F. G. I., Veldman, H. and Barth, P. G. (1984) Paucity of secondary synaptic clefts in a case of congenital myasthenia with multiple contractures: ultrastructural morphology of a developmental disorder. *J. Neurol. Neurosurg. Psyçhiatry* **47**: 1091–1097.

Smit, L. M. E., Veldman, H., Jennekens, F. G. I., Molenaar, P. C. and Oen, B. S. (1987) A congenital myasthenic disorder with paucity of secondary synaptic clefts: Deficiency and altered distribution of acetylcholine receptors. *Ann. N.Y. Acad. Sci.* **505**: 346–356.

Takeuchi, N. (1963) Effects of calcium on the conductance change of the endplate membrane during the action of the transmitter. *J. Physiol. (Lond.)* **167**: 141–155.

Uchitel, O., Engel, A. G., Walls, T. J., Nagel, A., Bril, V. and Trastek, V. F. (1990) Congenital myasthenic syndrome attributed to abnormal acetylcholine-acetylcholine receptor interaction. *Neurology* **40** (suppl. 1): 278.

Vigny, M., Bon, S., Massoulie, J. and Gisiger, V. (1979) The subunit structure of mammalian acetylcholinesterase: catalytic subunits, dissociating effects of proteolysis and disulphide reduction on the polymeric forms. *J. Neurochem.* **33**: 559–565.

Vincent, A., Cull–Candy, S. G., Newsom–Davis, J., Trautmann, A., Molenaar, P. C. and Polak, R. L. (1981) Congenital myasthenia: endplate acetylcholine receptors and electrophysiology in five cases. *Muscle Nerve* **4**: 306–318.

Wagner, J. A., Carlson, S. C. and Kelly, R. B. (1978). Chemical and physical characterization cholinergic synaptic vesicles. *Biochemistry* **17**: 1199–1206.

Walls, T. J., Engel, A. G., Nagel, A., Harper, M. C. and Trastek, V. F. (1990) Congenital myasthenic syndrome with paucity of synaptic vesicles and reduced quantal release. *Neurology* **40** (Suppl. 1): 278.

Whittaker, V. P. (1984) The structure and function of cholinergic synaptic vesicles. *Biochem. Soc. Trans.* **12**: 561–578.

Witzemann, V., Barg, B., Nishikawa, Y., Sakmann, B. and Numa, S. (1987) Differential regulation of muscle acetylcholine receptor gamma and epsilon-subunit mRNAs. *FEBS Lett.* **223**: 104–112.

Wolters, Ch. M. J., Leeuwin, R. S. and Van Wijngaarden, K. V. (1974) The effect of prednisolone on the rat phrenic nerve–diaphragm preparation treated with hemicholinium *Eur. J. Pharmacol.* **29**: 165–167.

Myasthenia gravis — an autoimmune disorder of neuromuscular transmission

11.1. Introduction

One of the dramatic advances which has resulted from investigation of neuromuscular transmission is the recognition of different forms of neuromuscular disorder, and their classification into both autoimmune and inherited aetiologies. This chapter and the following describe the autoimmune disorders which affect neuromuscular transmission, and show how their pathogeneses have been established by using the wide range of techniques available today. More detailed reviews can be found in Lindstrom *et al.* (1988) and Willcox and Vincent (1988).

Myasthenia gravis is a condition in which the patient complains of weakness and a tendency to become easily fatigued during activities which require repetitive or sustained actions such as dressing, eating, drinking or reading. Diplopia (double vision) stemming from fatigue of the extrinsic eye muscles, and ptosis (drooping of the eyelids) are frequent presenting symptoms. Generalised weakness including respiratory problems is also common in the more seriously affected cases.

Weakness in myasthenia gravis is usually improved by rest and often dramatically by anti-acetylcholinesterase drug treatment. The diagnosis is now made by a combination of clinical history, short-lived improvement following the i.v. injection of anticholinesterase (Tensilon test), the presence of serum anti-AChR antibodies and investigation of the compound muscle action potential following nerve stimulation *in vivo* (electromyography); this typically shows a normal initial action potential which decreases during repetitive stimulation at low rates (e.g. 3 Hz, see Fig. 2.3). This 'decrement' indicates failure of neuromuscular transmission at an increasing number of endplates during the run-down in the number of packets released from the nerve terminal. The reason that this normal run-down is evident in MG, but not in control individuals, is because the safety factor for transmission is reduced (see also Engel, this volume) due to the loss of acetylcholine receptors (AChR); during a train of impulses the EPP at many endplates becomes subthreshold.

Several observations led Simpson in 1960 to suggest an autoimmune basis for MG. MG is frequent in young females, and often associated with other autoimmune conditions or the presence of autoantibodies to various tissue antigens including muscle proteins; the thymic gland is frequently abnormal and thymectomy leads to clinical improvement; mothers with MG sometimes give birth to infants who develop a self-limiting form of the disease. This latter observation strongly implicates a humoral immune factor. One can now add to these observations the fact that antibodies to muscle AChR are present, and both plasma exchange, which reduces circulating Immunoglobulins (Ig), and drugs that suppress the immune system also produce clinical improvement. Moreover, immunisation with AChR produces an experimental model of the human disease (EAMG, see De Baets, this volume).

MG has been divided into three groups based on the thymic pathology, age of onset and associations with different polymorphisms of the human leucocyte antigen (HLA) genes (Compston *et al.*, 1980; see Table 11.1). Since anti-AChR is present in all three groups, it seems likely that the immunogenetic associations underlie susceptibility to particular precipitating factors in aetiology, rather than differences in pathogenetic mechanisms. Unfortunately, defining the factors involved in the aetiology of MG has been difficult.

11.2. Pathology of myasthenia gravis

MG is caused principally by autoantibodies that bind to the AChRs at the neuromuscular junction and cause loss of functional AChRs mainly from a combination of complement-dependent lysis and an increased rate of

Table 11.1. Subgroups of patients with myasthenia gravis

	Hyperplasia	*Thymoma*	*Atrophy*
Thymic pathology			
Age at onset (years)	< 40 Young onset	30–60	> 40 Old onset
Sex (M:F)	1:3	1:1	2:1
HLA association	B8;DR3	none	B7;DR2
Percentage of antibodies binding to each region[a]			
Regions			
1	55	50	51
2	24	21	21
3	55**	20	20
4	59*	57*	39
5	23	39	31

[a] Defined by competition with anti-human AChR monoclonal antibodies (see Fig. 11.10).
** Significantly different from thymoma or old-onset group, $p < 0.005$; *.significantly different from old-onset group, $p < 0.05$.

degradation. The thymus gland is clearly involved in the autoimmune
response but its role is still unclear.

11.2.1. *Experimental observations on biopsied muscle*

It was shown in 1964 that MEPPs in MG muscle biopsies were abnormally
small, less than one-third of the normal amplitude (Elmqvist *et al.*, 1964;

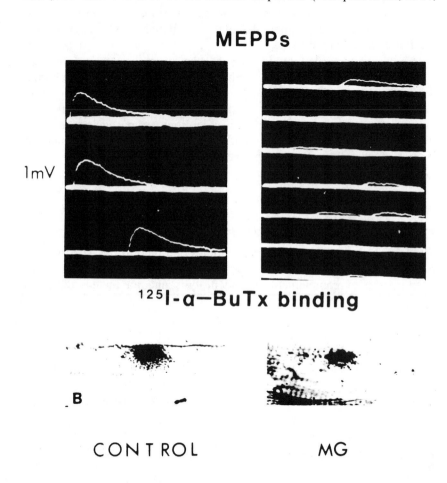

Fig. 11.1.   MEPPs and ^{125}I-α-BuTX autoradiograms of muscles from control and
MG patients. The MEPPs were measured in the presence of an anticholinesterase
drug to increase the amplitude. Both MEPP amplitudes and the number of
^{125}I-α-BuTX binding sites are decreased in MG. Adapted from Ito *et al.*, 1978 with
permission.

see Fig. 11.1). This was sufficient to account for the defect in neuromuscular transmission since at many endplates the EPP was too small to fire the action potential, while at others the EPP fell below the firing threshold during a train of stimuli at low frequency. The reduced MEPP amplitude was found to correlate well with a reduced number of AChRs, as measured by the binding of ^{125}I-α-BuTX (Fambrough *et al.*, 1973; Ito *et al.*, 1978; Fig. 11.1) and of peroxidase-conjugated α-BuTX (Engel *et al.*, 1976). Moreover IgG and complement components C3 and C9 were shown to be localised at the postsynaptic regions of MG endplates, which frequently show signs of focal destruction, clearly indicating their involvement in the loss of AChR (Engel *et al.*, 1977; Sahashi *et al.*, 1980; see Fig. 11.2). Further studies on biopsied muscle have shown that the induced release of ACh is actually increased in MG (Ito *et al.*, 1976), possibly as a compensatory mechanism,

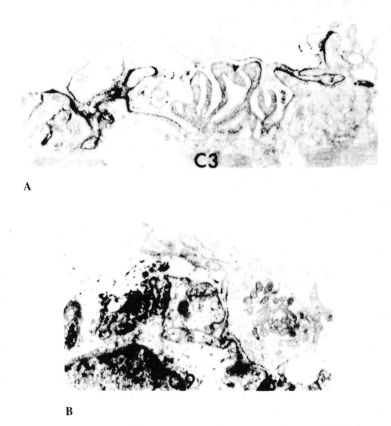

A

B

Fig. 11.2. Immunohistochemistry of the neuromuscular junction. Using peroxidase-labelled antibodies to C3 (**A**) or C9 (**B**) Engel and his associates clearly showed the presence of complement at MG endplates. **A** was taken with permission from Engel *et al.*, 1977; **B** is courtesy of Dr A. Engel. Copyright Mayo Foundation.

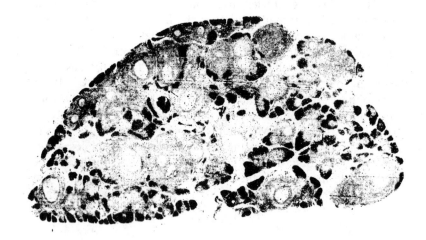

Fig. 11.3.   A section through an MG thymus showing germinal centres. Courtesy of Prof. K. Henry.

while the AChRs, though reduced in number, function normally (Cull-Candy *et al.*, 1979).

11.2.2. *Thymic pathology*

There are several findings that suggest an important aetiological role for the thymus. Patients presenting under 40 years of age frequently have thymic hyperplasia (see Fig. 11.3). In these patients thymectomy often leads to improvement, and thymic lymphocytes taken from the hyperplastic glands can be shown to synthesise anti-AChR antibodies *in vitro* (Scadding *et al.*, 1981). The amount of specific antibody correlates with the serum titre and with the presence of T cell areas and germinal centres in the thymic medulla (Schluep *et al.*, 1988). However, after thymectomy, anti-AChR antibody titres fall to a varying extent, and it is clear that the thymus is not the only site of anti-AChR production (Vincent *et al.*, 1983).

The hyperplasia reflects large areas of T cell and germinal centre invasion of the thymic medulla. These areas are separated from the medulla by a fenestrated laminin layer (for review see Willcox and Vincent, 1988). In the medulla of both MG and normal thymi there are muscle-like cells, first recognised by histologists and shown to contain striated muscle antigens, that express AChR (Schluep *et al.*, 1987; Fig. 11.4). Thus the medulla is the site of the appropriate antigen. Moreover the myoid cell AChR binds monoclonal antibodies raised against purified human muscle AChR, suggesting that it is a true muscle-type AChR, probably identical to that present on embryonic muscle (Fig. 11.4a).

F8

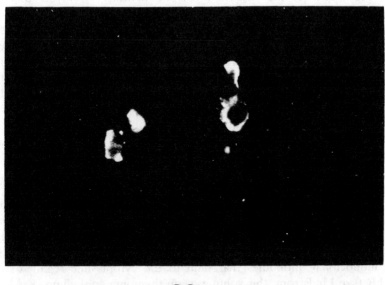

C3

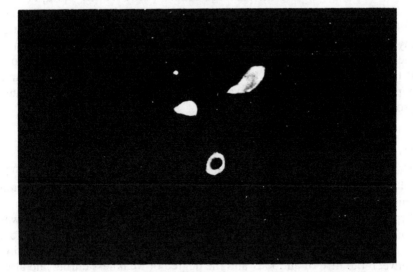

Fig. 11.4. AChRs demonstrated in MG thymus by immunofluorescence using monoclonal anti-AChR antibodies F8 and C3. In muscle F8 binds only to extrajunctional or embryonic AChRs; C3 does not descriminate between junctional and extrajunctional AChRs. In the thymus both antibodies bound to all myoid cells. Courtesy of Dr M. Schluep.

These findings would appear to provide strong circumstantial evidence that the origin of the disease is in the thymus. However, there is controversy as to whether there are immunohistological features consistent with involvement of the myoid cells. The latter do not express HLA class II antigens (Schluep *et al.*, 1987), as found in for instance thyroid cells undergoing autoimmune attack, and are separated from the germinal centres where the antibody synthesis is presumed to take place; on the other hand, Kirchner *et al.* (1988a,b) reported that they were embedded in an HLA class II environment and in contact with interdigitating cells that could be responsible for initiating an immune process.

About 10% of MG patients have a thymoma. Thymic tumours are usually associated with a later age of onset of the disease (Table 11.1). They are lymphoepithelial in nature but the lymphocytes appear to be secondary to the presence of proliferating epithelium in the medulla. The latter, unusually, frequently demonstrates simultaneous expression of cell surface markers for medullary, subcortical and cortical epithelium, suggesting that the tumour may arise from an epithelial precursor (Willcox *et al.*, 1987). AChR is not present in thymoma tissue (Schluep *et al.*, 1987) but monoclonal antibodies that bind to the cytoplasmic region of the AChR (see Lindstrom, this volume) stain thymoma epithelium (Kirchner *et al.*, 1988b) suggesting the presence of an 'AChR-related' epitope.

The lymphocytes in thymoma tissue are generally immature T cells, rather than B cells, and anti-AChR synthesis does not occur in the thymoma tissue itself. However, there is often some thymic hyperplasia in the surrounding tissue which may, therefore, be a secondary phenomenon. If this is the case then one has to consider the possibility that the thymic hyperplasia in non-thymoma cases is also secondary to the autoimmune process, rather than causative.

11.3. Use of passive transfer to investigate MG

The presence of anti-AChR antibodies in MG was first shown in 1973 following the observations by Patrick and Lindstrom on experimental animals immunised against purified AChR (see De Baets, this volume). Typical results from MG patients are shown in Fig. 11.5. Although it was quickly recognised that the antibodies were diagnostic for MG (Lindstrom *et al.*, 1976), and within an individual there was a strong correlation between the titre of antibody and the degree of weakness during and after plasma exchange which removes circulating antibodies (Newsom-Davis *et al.*, 1978), there was a rather poor relationship between titre and clinical state (see Fig. 11.5).

One way to assess the clinical relevance of the antibodies was to use 'passive transfer' in which immunoglobulins (Ig) are injected into animals in order to confirm their pathogenicity. Toyka *et al.* (1977) injected IgG

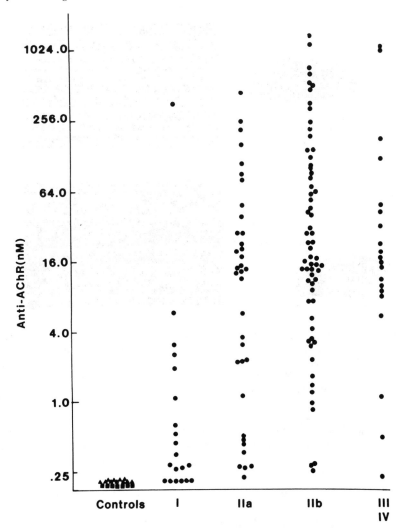

Fig. 11.5. Anti-AChR antibody results in MG patients with different grades of disease compared with normal healthy controls (■) or patients with other neurological disorders (▲). The assay is performed by immunoprecipitation of ^{125}-I-α-BuTX-labelled human muscle AChR (see Chapter 3).

from MG patients into mice, and were able to reproduce the main physiological findings: muscle from the injected animals showed small MEPPs and reduced ^{125}I-α-BuTX binding (Fig. 11.6). The loss of AChRs appeared to be partly dependent on complement, since C5-deficient animals were resistant to the effects of MG IgG.

Another cause of the loss of AChR was clearly established when it was

a

b

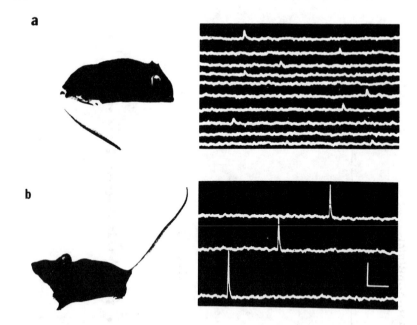

Fig. 11.6. Demonstration of the pathogenic role of antibodies in MG. IgG preparations from MG (**a**) or control (**b**) were injected into mice for several days. The MEPP amplitudes were very small in the MG IgG-injected animals, some of which were weak. AChR numbers measured by ^{125}I-α-BuTX binding to the muscle endplates were also reduced. Taken with permission from Toyka *et al.*, 1977.

shown that during passive transfer the degradation rate of AChRs increased (Stanley and Drachman, 1978). This was done by labelling MG IgG-treated mouse diaphragm muscle AChRs *in vivo* by intrathoracic injection of ^{125}I-α-BuTX and counting the radioactive label remaining at different time intervals over a period of days. Results from a similar experiment are shown in Fig. 11.7. However, in some cases the increased degradation rate appeared to be compensated for by an increase in synthesis rate, so that the overall loss of AChRs, at least after several days, was not substantial (Wilson *et al.*, 1983).

A proportion of patients with typical symptoms of MG do not have detectable anti-AChR antibody. However, plasma exchange and immuno-suppressive drug treatment, both of which reduce circulating antibodies, are often effective in reducing symptoms. Passive transfer of Ig from these patients to mice showed that a humorally mediated defect in neuromuscular transmission resulted (Mossman *et al.*, 1986). This was demonstrated by looking at decremental responses to nerve stimulation in the presence of d-tubocurarine to reduce the safety factor for transmission (Figs. 11.8, 11.9). The nature of this defect, however, is not clear. The AChRs extracted from the muscle are not reduced in number and do not appear to have any

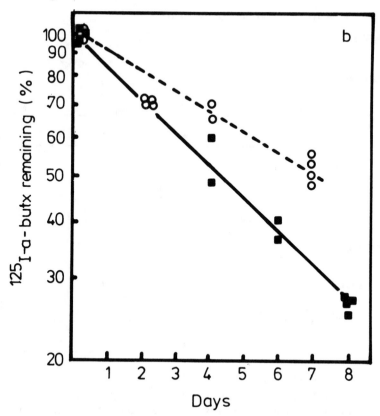

Fig. 11.7. Increased degradation rate of endplate AChRs in mice injected with MG IgG (squares) compared to control IgG (circles). The AChRs were first labelled by intrathoracic injection of ^{125}I-α-BuTX and the amount of radioactivity remaining determined at each time interval. Taken from Wilson *et al.*, 1983 with permission.

attached Ig (Fig. 11.8b); therefore, any binding that does occur must rapidly reverse as soon as the AChRs are extracted from the membrane. Alternatively, the antibodies may be binding to some other determinants at the neuromuscular junction. Interestingly, similar studies using anti-AChR 'positive' Ig preparations (e.g. Fig. 11.9) showed in some cases a lack of correlation between decrement and antibody binding to AChRs; thus similar antibodies may contribute to the defect in neuromuscular transmission even in anti-AChR positive MG (Mossman *et al.*, 1988).

11.4. Acute effects of MG IgG *in vitro*

To confirm the pathogenic effect of anti-AChR and to investigate further their characteristics and the mechanisms by which they reduce the number of functional AChRs, various *in vitro* approaches have been used.

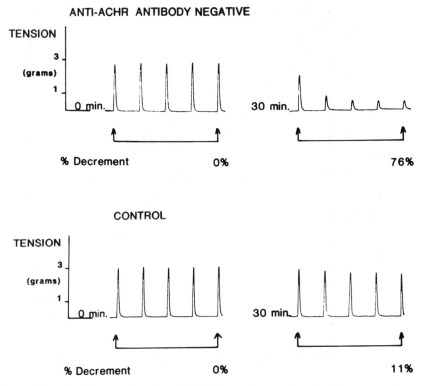

Fig. 11.8. Passive transfer of anti-AChR negative and control Ig preparations. After 3 days of injecting 60 mg/day Ig intraperitoneally into mice the diaphragms were examined *in vitro* for decrement in the twitch tension during five successive stimuli at 3 Hz before (left) and after (right) applying 0.8 µg/ml of d-tubocurarine. Anti-AChR negative Ig produced a highly significant decrement (top) compared with control Ig (bottom). Courtesy Dr S. Mossman.

11.4.1. *On intact muscle*

It would be convenient to be able to assess the pathogenic effect of anti-AChR antibodies *in vitro* on a nerve–muscle preparation, in the way in which pharmacological drugs are tested. The results of such studies, however, have been quite varied; indeed there are few reports (e.g. Burges *et al.*, 1990) that clearly show the presence of direct 'immunopharmacological' block that can be attributed to antibody. This is not so surprising when one considers that most of the antibodies in MG bind to sites on the AChR that do not seem to be related to function (see below), and probably achieve their effect by a combination of complement-dependent lysis and increased degradation. In addition, it may be difficult for a sufficient number of anti-AChR antibodies to reach the AChRs that are present at very high concentration at the neuromuscular junction.

11.4.2. *On cultured muscle*

Rather more successful has been the use of cultured cell lines or primary muscle cultures that express human or mouse AChR to investigate antibody-mediated changes in AChR numbers or ion flux through the AChR. Initial studies, performed by prelabelling surface AChRs with ^{125}I-α-BuTX and monitoring both the loss of label and the appearance of degraded products in the culture fluid, clearly showed that the presence of MG serum or IgG in the culture medium at 37°C increased the rate of AChR degradation from a $t_{\frac{1}{2}}$ of about 16 h to about 8 h (e.g. Bevan *et al.*, 1977). This process was shown to be temperature- and energy-dependent, i.e. it depended on metabolic processes.

The importance of crosslinking of AChRs by divalent antibodies was illustrated on cultured cells by experiments in which divalent (Fab′)$_2$ fragments increased degradation, whereas Fab′ monomers did not, unless an anti-human IgG which crosslinked the monomeric Fab′ preparation was also injected (Drachman *et al.*, 1978).

The possibility of an immunopharmacological block of AChR function has been tested on various cell lines. Pretreatment of cultures with MG preparations reduced the carbachol-induced Na$^+$ flux into cells. The fact that this occurred at room temperature, where an increase in the temperature-dependent degradation rate should not be a major factor, and was associated with block of ^{125}I-α-BuTX binding, suggested that some antibodies could inhibit ion channel function by blocking the ACh/α-BuTX site, or even the ion channel itself (Lang *et al.*, 1988). However, one must remember that cultured cell lines express extrajunctional-type AChR, and that this is partially different from junctional AChR (see Chapter 1); this difference may account for some of the discrepancy between the effect of MG Ig preparations on cultured cells compared with intact muscle preparations.

11.5. Antibody binding to solubilised AChR

The availability of a snake toxin that binds specifically and irreversibly to nicotinic AChRs from most species, and monoclonal antibodies (mAbs) that are specific for different regions of the AChR, has made it possible to analyse the binding of MG antibodies in considerable detail.

In the routine diagnostic assay human muscle is extracted in detergent and the solubilised AChRs labelled with ^{125}I-α-BuTX. The binding of MG antibodies can be detected by immunoprecipitation with an anti-human IgG serum (Lindstrom *et al.*, 1976; Vincent and Newsom–Davis, 1985; Fig. 11.5). This assay can be adapted in many ways: different species of AChR can be used in order to see to what extent MG antibodies are specific for human receptor; different anti-IgG preparations can be used, e.g. anti-light chain or anti-subclass-specific, in order to investigate the

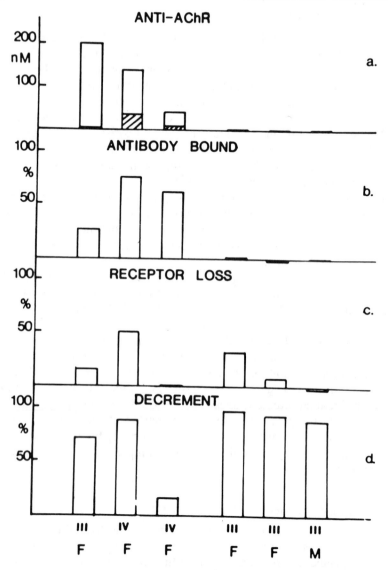

Fig. 11.9. Results of passive transfer of MG Ig to mice in six patients. (a) Three (left columns) of the six patients illustrated had clearly elevated anti-AChR titres. The other three (right columns) were negative. After passive transfer the mice were assessed for (b) antibody bound to extracted leg muscle AChR, (c) endplate AChR loss, and (d) decrement in the presence of d-tubocurarine as described in Fig. 11.8. Although there was no evidence of antibody bound to AChRs in the mice given anti-AChR negative Ig, and AChR loss was not substantial, the degree of decrement was as great or greater than that produced by anti-AChR positive Ig preparations. Hatched bars, antibody cross-reacting with mouse AChR. Data from Mossman *et al.* 1986, 1988.

immunochemical characteristics of the anti-AChR antibodies; and the assay can be performed under conditions that test the affinity of the antibodies or the proportion of antibodies that inhibit the binding of ^{125}I-α-BuTX.

The results showed that each patient has a different spectrum of antibodies (Vincent and Newsom–Davis, 1982). Most patients had anti-AChR in all subclasses of IgG, and of both lamda and kappa light chain. Moreover, they showed heterogeneity as regards their specificity for different mammalian AChRs and for binding to the α-BuTX binding site on the AChR.

Another way in which to look at the characteristics of the antibodies is to use inhibition by monoclonal anti-AChR as first performed by Tzartos *et al.*, 1982. We used mAbs raised against purified human AChR which bound to five partially overlapping regions on the extracellular surface of the receptor. These are representated graphically in Fig. 11.10 (Heidenreich *et al.*, 1988a). Region 1 is specific for extrajunctional AChR, and region 4 is identical to the main immunogenic region (MIR) to which a large, but variable, proportion of antibodies in both MG and EAMG sera bind (see Lindstrom, this volume).

The effect of saturating ^{125}I-α-BuTX-labelled AChR with each mAb, before adding MG serum in limiting amounts, enabled us to assess, by inhibition, the proportion of a patient's antibodies that bound to the same site as the mAb. The results showed considerable variation between each serum (Fig. 11.10) but, overall, patients with young-onset disease had more antibody directed at region 3 than did those with thymoma or with old-onset MG (Heidenreich *et al.*, 1988b; see Table 11.1). The meaning of this result is not yet clear; one possibility is that the young-onset patients have been 'sensitised' to a different form of the AChR, or the differences may merely reflect the nature of the immune response to the same antigen in different groups of patients with diverse immunogenetic backgrounds.

The difference in anti-AChR specificity in young-onset cases might be due to involvement of the thymus, in which some of the anti-AChR is made (see above). However, thymic culture supernatants contained anti-AChR antibody which was of identical specificity to that in the individual's serum (Fig. 11.10), and therefore the thymus did not appear to be contributing a particular specificity. Moreover, after thymectomy when the anti-AChR fell in many individuals, the specificity of the serum anti-AChR did not change appreciably (Heidenreich *et al.*, 1988c). Thus these studies, rather than indicating a special role for the thymus in MG, would be perfectly consistent with a secondary role.

11.5.1. *Idiotypes and anti-idiotypes in MG*

Further evidence for the heterogeneity of anti-AChR antibodies came from studies on anti-AChR idiotypes. The idiotype is the variable part of

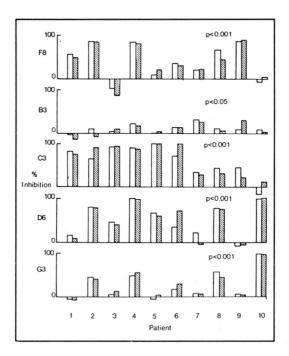

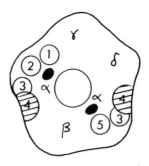

a

b

Fig. 11.10. (a) Inhibition of anti-AChR antibody binding to human AChR by monoclonal antibodies directed against five different regions of the AChR. Results are shown for serum (open columns) and thymic culture supernatants (hatched columns) for 10 different patients. Although the degree of inhibition with each monoclonal antibody varies between patients, the results of individual serum and culture supernatants are strongly correlated (*p* values). Taken with permission from Heidenreich *et al.*, 1988c. (b) Scheme of topology of human AChR (viewed from above, see Lindstrom, this volume) showing the five mAb binding regions determined by competition experiments. The degree of competition between the antibodies is denoted by overlapping of the regions. None of the antibodies interferred with α-BuTX binding (filled ovals). Region 1 antibodies only bound to extrajunctional or embryonic AChR. A moncolonal antibody directed against region 4 (hatched) competed directly with anti-MIR antibody 35 (see Lindstrom, this volume) and bound to peptide α 64–78 of the human AChR. A region 5 mAb bound to another peptide representing sequence α 125–143 (Wood *et al.*, 1989). Taken from Heidenreich *et al.*, 1988a.

the immunoglobulin molecule that is responsible for the binding to the antigen, and may consist of several different 'idiotopes'. Antibodies raised against the idiotypes of purified anti-AChR antibodies from one individual did not bind appreciably to anti-AChR from others. Thus the idiotypes appeared to differ between individuals (Lang *et al.*, 1985).

According to the network theory proposed by Jerne (1974) each idiotype (or idiotope) has a complementary anti-idiotype (see De Baets, Fig. 13.5, this volume), and some of these anti-idiotypes may be the idiotypes for another antigen. Dwyer *et al.* (1986) reported the presence of anti-AChR idiotype antibodies, that also bound to the bacterial polysaccharide α-1,3 dextran, in a high proportion of MG patients, and suggested that MG might arise as a result of perturbation of the idiotype network stemming from a bacterial infection. However, the presence of abnormal levels of anti-AChR idiotypes in MG, although found by some (e.g. Lefvert, 1981), has been disputed by others (Vincent, 1988), and their specificity for other antigens has yet to be confirmed.

11.6. Use of recombinant and synthetic peptides

One of the exciting developments in the clinical application of basic science has been the use of molecular biological techniques to investigate the nature of the immune response. T cells are thought to recognise antigen only after its processing by antigen-processing cells (APC), and only when the resulting peptides are expressed on the surface of the APC bound to self-MHC antigens (Fig. 11.11). B cells, on the other hand, tend to recognise native antigen molecules, and the antibodies that they produce are mainly directed against conformationally dependent determinants that are not necessarily intact after processing, or after denaturation. Thus in the initial stages of the immune response some antigen is processed and presented by APC, and both B cells responding to the native molecule and T cells recognising the processed peptides proliferate at the site of antigen. Subsequently, proliferating B cells may process and present the antigen themselves. The T cells secrete lymphokines which stimulate the B cells to make the specific antibody (see Fig. 11.11).

B cell epitopes recognised by anti-AChR antibodies in MG are not very easy to identify at the level of the amino acid sequence, largely because, as mentioned above, they depend on the native conformation of the molecule which will not necessarily be represented by short synthetic peptide sequences. The only successful studies so far have been with monoclonal anti-AChR antibodies. Some antibodies directed at the MIR were shown to bind to a polypeptide, synthesised as a fusion protein in *E. coli* representing the sequence 6–85 of the α subunit of the mouse receptor (Barkas *et al.*, 1987), and the binding site located more precisely to the sequence 67–76 by using short synthetic peptides of the human AChR (Tzartos *et al.*, 1988; see also Lindstrom, this volume and Fig. 11.10).

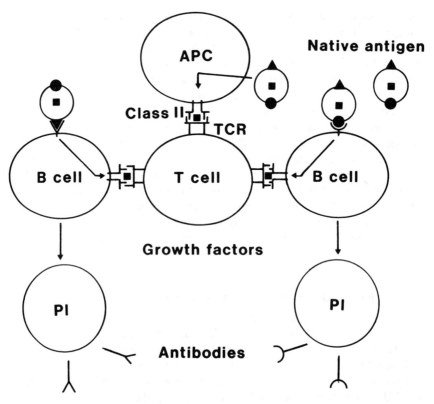

Fig. 11.11.   Scheme to illustrate cooperation between T and B lymphocytes in the immune response. Native antigen is taken up and processed by antigen processing cells (APC). The processed peptides associate with HLA class II molecules (HLA DR, DP and DQ) and are presented on the surface of the APC. They will be recognised only by T cells which have the appropriate receptors (TCR) for binding of the class II/peptide complexes. The T cells secrete growth factors (e.g. interleukins) which stimulate neighbouring B cells to divide. B cells, which express class II molecules, can also take up the native antigen via the specific immunoglobulins on the B cell surface, and present the peptide to the relevant T cell. The B cell then matures into an antibody secreting plasma cell (Pl). There are several important results of this complex process: (a) the class II molecules are polymorphic and some may not be able to bind peptides derived from a particular antigen. (b) Some individuals might not possess the particular T cells that can recognise the class II/peptide complex. Both (a) and (b) would tend to limit the response. (c) The peptides recognised by T cells can be short linear sequences and are not necessarily related to the sites recognised by the antibodies, which are likely to be much more conformationally dependent and exposed on the surface of the native antigen. In addition, recognition by a single T cell probably turns on antibody production by several different B lymphocytes, thus diversifying the response.

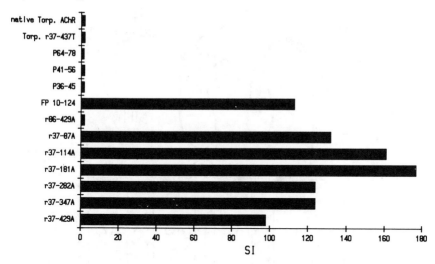

Fig. 11.12. Responses of a T cell clone raised from an MG patient against recombinant human AChR α subunit. The cloned T cells were stimulated by the full-length α subunit and by smaller fragments. Response to synthetic peptides had not yet been demonstrated with this clone. Taken with permission from Newsom–Davis *et al.*, 1989.

Identification of T cell epitopes is of considerable interest because this could lead to specific therapy aimed at killing or deleting the particular lymphocytes (see also De Baets, this volume). Purified AChR from *Torpedo* electric organ can be shown to stimulate T cells *in vitro*, indicating the presence of specifically sensitised cells (Hohlfeld *et al.*, 1984; Melms *et al.*, 1988). Several short synthetic sequences of the human α subunit have been identified that stimulate T cells from MG patients in culture (Harcourt *et al.*, 1988; Brocke *et al.*, 1988; Hohlfeld *et al.*, 1988).

Recently we and others (Melms *et al.*, 1989) have begun to use recombinant AChR polypeptides expressed in *E. coli* (see Beeson and Barnard, this volume) to stimulate and clone the relevant T cells from MG patients (Fig. 11.12). These cells can then be tested for their reactivity to shorter recombinant fragments and synthetic peptides. In this way we are beginning to identify the epitopes at the amino acid level (Newsom–Davis *et al.*, 1989). The epitopes may not be the same in all patients, since only some sequences will be recognised and bound by the individual's MHC antigens (see above). Indeed, as summarised in Fig. 11.13, there seems to be some heterogeneity of T cell epitopes both within and between individuals. Nevertheless, if a few major epitopes can be identified it may be possible to kill the responding T cells by cell-directed toxicity using toxin–peptide conjugates. Alternatively antibodies might be raised against the T cell receptors (the specific cell surface proteins that recognise the

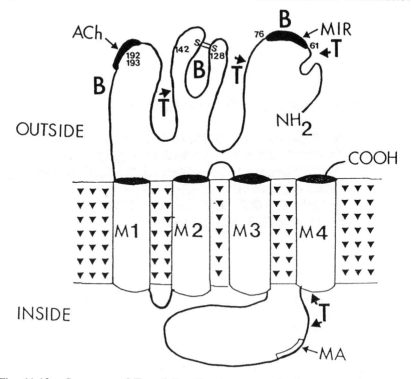

Fig. 11.13. Summary of T and B cell epitopes on the human α subunit. The transmembrane topology of the α subunit sequence is represented, including the 25 amino acid insert identified in the human sequence (see chapter by Beeson and Barnard). A few antibody-binding sites (B) have been identified by ELISA assays (Tzartos *et al.*, 1988; Wood *et al.*, 1989). Several T cell sites (T) have now been mapped, using recombinant AChR and synthetic peptides, for AChR specific T cell clones from MG patients; one site includes part of the 25 amino acid loop (Harcourt, G., Ong, B., Nagvekar, N., Willcox, N., Vincent, A. and Newsom–Davis, J. 1990, unpublished observations).

peptide/MHC complex, see Fig. 11.11) leading to anti-clonotypic antibodies; in the presence of complement these would destroy the antigen-specific T cells and prevent further B cell activation.

If any of these approaches can be achieved in humans they will represent a major advance in treating an autoimmune disease. These approaches should be applicable to other autoimmune conditions when the target antigens are better defined.

Acknowledgements

I am grateful to the Medical Research Council of Great Britain for support.

References

Barkas, T., Mauron, A., Roth, B., Alliod, C., Tzartos, S. and Ballivet, M. (1987) Mapping the main immunogenic region and toxin binding site of the nicotinic acetylcholine receptor. *Science* **235**: 77–80.

Bevan, S., Kullberg, R. and Heinemann, S. (1977) Human myasthenic sera reduce acetylcholine sensitivity of human muscle cells in tissue culture. *Nature* **267**: 263–265.

Brocke, S., Brautbar, C., Steinman, L., Abramsky, O., Rothbard, J., Neumann, D., Fuchs, S. and Mozes, E. (1988) *In vitro* proliferative responses and antibody titers specific to human acetylcholine receptor synthetic peptides in patients with myasthenia gravis and relation to HLA class II genes. *J. Clin. Invest.* **82**: 1894–1900.

Burges, J., W.-Wray, D., Pizzighella, S., Hall, Z. and Vincent, A. (1990) A myasthenia gravis immunoglobulin reduces miniature endplate potentials at human endplates *in vitro*. *Muscle Nerve* **13**: 407–413.

Compston, D. A. S., Vincent, A., Newsom–Davis, J. and Batchelor, J. R. (1980) Clinical, pathological HLA antigen and immunological evidence for disease heterogeneity in myasthenia gravis. *Brain*, **103**: 579–601.

Cull–Candy, S., Miledi, R. and Trautmann, A. (1979) Endplate currents and acetylcholine noise at normal and myasthenic endplates. *J. Physiol. (Lond).* **287**: 247–265.

Drachman, D. B., Angus, D. W., Adams, R. N., Michelson, J. D. and Hoffman, G. J. (1978) Myasthenia antibodies cross-link acetylcholine receptors to accelerate degradation. *N. Engl. J. Med.* **198**: 1116–1122.

Dwyer, D. S., Vakil, M. and Kearney, J. F. (1986) Idiotypic network connectivity and a possible cause of myasthenia gravis. *J. Exp. Med.* **164**: 1310–1318.

Elmqvist, D., Hofman, W. W., Kugelberg, J. and Quastel, D. M. (1964) An electrophysiological investigation of neuromuscular transmission in myasthenia gravis. *J. Physiol.* **174**: 417–434.

Engel, A. G., Lindstrom, J. M., Lambert, E. H. and Lennon, V. A. (1976) Ultrastructural localization of the acetylcholine receptor in myasthenia gravis and in its experimental autoimmune model. *Neurology* **27**: 307–315.

Engel, A. G., Lambert, E. H. and Howard, F. M. (1977) Immune complexes (IgG and C3) at the motor endplate in myasthenia gravis. Ultrastructural and light microscopic localization and electrophysiologic correlations. *Mayo Clin. Proc.* **52**: 267–280.

Fambrough, D. M., Drachman, D. B. and Satyamurti, S. (1973) Neuromuscular junction in myasthenia gravis. Decreased acetylcholine receptors. *Science* **182**: 293–295.

Harcourt, G., Sommer, N., Rothbard, J., Willcox, N. and Newsom–Davis, J. (1988) A juxta-membrane epitope on the human acetylcholine receptor recognized by T cells in myasthenia gravis. *J. Clin. Invest.* **82**: 1295–1300.

Heidenreich, F., Vincent, A., Roberts, A. and Newsom–Davis, J. (1988a) Epitopes on human acetylcholine receptor defined by monoclonal antibodies and myasthenia gravis sera. *Autoimmunity* **1**: 285–297.

Heidenreich, F., Vincent, A. and Newsom–Davis, J. (1988b) Differences in fine specificity of anti-acetylcholine receptor antibodies between subgroups of spontaneous myasthenia gravis of recent onset, and of pencillamine-induced myasthenia. *Autoimmunity* **2**: 31–37.

Heidenreich, F., Vincent, A., Willcox, N. and Newsom–Davis, J. (1988c) Anti-acetylcholine receptor antibody specificities in serum and in thymic culture supernatants from myasthenia gravis patients. *Neurology* **38**: 1784–1788.

Hohlfeld, R. K., Toyka, K. V., Heininger, K., Gross–Wilde, H. and Kalies, I. (1984) Autoimmune human T lymphocytes specific for acetylcholine receptor. *Nature* **310**: 244–246.

Hohlfeld, R. K., Toyka, K., Miner, L., Walgrave, S. and Conti–Tronconi, B. (1988) Amphipathic segment of the nicotinic acetylcholine receptor alpha subunit contains epitopes recognized by T lymphocytes in myasthenia gravis. *J. Clin. Invest.* **81**: 657–660.

Ito, Y., Miledi, R., Molenaar, P., Newsom–Davis, J. and Vincent, A. (1976) Acetylcholine in human muscle. *Proc. Roy. Soc. Lond. B* **192**: 475–480.

Ito, Y., Miledi, R., Vincent, A. and Newsom–Davis, J. (1978) Acetylcholine receptors and endplate electrophysiology in myasthenia gravis. *Brain* **101**: 345–368.

Jerne, N. K. (1974) Towards a network theory of the immune system. *Ann. Immunol. (Paris)* **125C**: 373–389.

Kirchner, T., Hoppe, F., Schalke, B. and Muller–Hermelink, H. K. (1988a) Microenvironment of thymic myoid cells in myasthenia gravis. *Virch. Archiv. B Cell Pathol.* **54**: 395–402.

Kirchner, T., Tzartos, S., Hoppe, F., Schalke, B., Wekerle, H., Muller–Hermelink, H. K. (1988b) Pathogenesis of myasthenia gravis. Acetylcholine receptor-related antigenic determinants in tumour-free thymuses and thymic epithelial tumours. *Am. J. Pathol.* **130**: 268–280.

Lang, B., Roberts, A. J., Vincent, A. and Newsom–Davis, J. (1985) Anti-acetylcholine receptor idiotypes in myasthenia gravis analysed by rabbit anti-sera. *Clin. Exp. Immunol.* **60**: 637–644.

Lang, B., Richardson, G., Rees, J., Vincent, A. and Newsom–Davis, J. (1988) Plasma from myasthenia gravis patients reduces acetylcholine receptor agonist-induced Na^+ flux into TE671 cell line. *J. Neuroimmun.* **19**: 141–148.

Lefvert, A. K. (1981) Anti-idiotype antibodies against the receptor antibodies in myasthenia gravis. *Scand. J. Immunol.* **49**: 257–265.

Lindstrom, J., Seybold, M. E., Lennon, V. A., Whittingham, S. and Duane, D. D. (1976) Antibody to acetylcholine receptor in myasthenia gravis. *Neurology* **26**: 1054–1059.

Lindstrom, J., Shelton, D. and Fujii, Y. (1988) Myasthenia gravis. *Adv. Immunol.* **42**: 233–284.

Melms, A., Schalke, B. C. G., Kirchner, T., Muller–Hermelink, H. K., Albert, E. and Wekerle, H. (1988) Thymus in myasthenia gravis: isolation of T-lymphocyte lines specific for the nicotinic acetylcholine receptor from thymuses of myasthenia patients. *J. Clin. Invest.* **81**: 902–908.

Melms, A., Chrestel, S., Schalke, B. C. G., Wekerle, H., Mauron, A., Ballivet, M. and Barkas, T. (1989) Autoimmune T lymphocytes in myasthenia gravis. Determination of target epitopes using T lines and recombinant products of the mouse nicotinic acetylcholine receptor gene. *J. Clin. Invest.* **83**: 785–790.

Mossman, S., Vincent, A. and Newsom–Davis, J. (1986) Myasthenia gravis without acetylcholine-receptor antibody: a distinct disease entity. *Lancet* **i**: 116–118.

Mossman, S., Vincent, A. and Newsom–Davis, J. (1988) Passive transfer of myasthenia gravis by immunoglobulins: lack of correlation between AChR with antibody bound, acetylcholine receptor loss and transmission defect. *J. Neurol. Sci.* **84**: 15–28.

Newsom–Davis, J., Pinching, J. A., Vincent, A. and Wilson, S. G. (1978) Function of circulating antibody to acetylcholine receptor in myasthenia gravis investigated by plasma exchange. *Neurology* **28**: 266–272.

Newsom–Davis, J., Harcourt, G., Sommer, N. O., Beeson, D., Willcox, N. and

Rothbard, J. B. (1989) T cell reactivity in myasthenia gravis. *J. Autoimmun.* **2** (Suppl.): 101–108.

Patrick, J. and Lindstrom, J. (1973) Autoimmune response to acetylcholine receptors. *Science* 180: 871–872.

Sahashi, K., Engel, A. G., Lambert, E. H. and Howard, F. M. Jr (1980) Ultrastructural localization of the terminal and lytic complement component (C9) at the motor end-plate in myasthenia gravis. *J. Neuropathol. Exp. Neurol.* **39**: 160–172.

Scadding, G. K., Vincent, A., Newsom–Davis, J. and Henry, K. (1981) Acetylcholine receptor antibody synthesis by thymic lymphocytes: correlation with thymic histology. *Neurol. (Minneap.)* **28**: 502–507.

Schluep, M., Willcox, N. H., Vincent, A., Dhoot, G. K. and Newsom–Davis, J. (1987) Acetylcholine receptors in human myoid cells *in situ*: an immunohistological study. *Ann. Neurol.* **22**: 212–222.

Schluep, M., Willcox, H. N. A., Ritter, M. A., Newsom–Davis, J., Larche, M. and Brown, A. N. (1988) Myasthenia gravis thymus; clinical, histological and culture correlations. *J. Autoimmun.* **1**: 445–467.

Simpson, J. A. (1960) Myasthenia gravis. A new hypothesis. *Scot. Med. J.* **5**: 419–436.

Stanley, E. F. and Drachman, D. B. (1978) Effect of myasthenic immunoglobulin on acetylcholine receptors of intact neuromuscular junctions. *Science* **200**: 1285–1286.

Toyka, K. V., Drachman, D. B., Griffen, D. E., Pestronk, A., Winkelstein, J. A., Fischbeck, K. H. and Kao, I. (1977) Myasthenia gravis. Study of humoral immune mechanisms by passive transfer to mice. *N. Engl. J. Med.* **296**: 125–131.

Tzartos, S., Seybold, M. E. and Lindstrom, J. M. (1982) Specificities of antibodies to acetylcholine receptors in sera from myasthenia gravis patients measured by monoclonal antibodies. *Proc. Natl. Acad. Sci. USA* **79**: 188–192.

Tzartos, S. J., Kokla, A., Walgrave, S. and Conti–Tronconi, B. M. (1988) Localization of the main immunogenic region of human muscle acetylcholine receptor to residues 67–76 of the α subunit. *Proc. Natl. Acad. Sci. USA* **85**: 2899–2903.

Vincent, A. (1988) Are spontaneous anti-idiotypic antibodies against anti-acetylcholine receptor antibodies present in myasthenia gravis? *J. Autoimmun* **1**: 131–142.

Vincent, A. and Newsom–Davis, J. (1982) Acetylcholine receptor antibody characteristics in myasthenia gravis. 1. Patients with generalised myasthenia or disease restricted to ocular muscles. *Clin. Exp. Immunol*, **49**: 257–265.

Vincent, A. and Newsom–Davis, J. (1985) Acetylcholine receptor antibody as a diagnostic test for myasthenia gravis: result in 153 validated cases and 2967 diagnostic assays. *J. Neurol. Neurosurg. Psychiatry*, **48**: 1246–1252.

Vincent, A., Newsom–Davis, J., Newton, P. and Beck, N. (1983) Acetylcholine receptor antibody and clinical response to thymectomy in myasthenia gravis. *Neurology* **33**: 1276–1282.

Willcox, H. N. A. and Vincent, A. (1988) Myasthenia gravis as an example of organ-specific autoimmune disease. In: *The B Lymphocyte in Human Disease*, A. G. Bird and J. E. Calvert, eds, Oxford University Press, London, pp. 469–506.

Willcox, H. N. A., Schluep, M., Ritter, M. A., Schurman, H. J., Newsom–Davis, J. and Christensson, B. (1987) Myasthenic and nonmyasthenic thymoma: an expansion of a minor cortical epithelial cell subset? *Am. J. Pathol.* **127**: 447–460.

Wilson, S., Vincent, A. and Newsom–Davis, J. (1983) Acetylcholine receptor in mice with passively transferred myasthenia gravis. II. Receptor synthesis. *J.*

Neurol. Neurosurg. Psychiatry, **46**: 383–387.

Wood, H., Beeson, D., Vincent, A. and Newsom–Davis, J. (1989). Epitopes on human acetylcholine receptor α-subunit: binding of monoclonal antibodies to recombinant and synthetic peptides. *Biochem. Soc. Trans.* **17**: 220–221.

The Lambert–Eaton myasthenic syndrome

12.1. Introduction

Investigation of the aetiology and pathology of myasthenia gravis (see Vincent, this volume) has demonstrated the power of immunological approaches to the study of possible autoimmune disorders. Another disease which affects neuromuscular transmission is the Lambert–Eaton myasthenic syndrome (LEMS). This chapter describes the main features of LEMS and illustrates how a combination of *in vivo* and *in vitro* investigations has led to our present understanding of the underlying pathology.

12.2. Main features of the disorder

LEMS is a disorder of neuromuscular transmission characterised by a reduction in nerve-stimulated release of acetylcholine (ACh). The reduction in ACh release leads to skeletal muscle weakness, typically most evident in the muscles of the trunk and girdle, and muscle strength often improves with prolonged effort. In about 30% of patients, autonomic dysfunction also occurs, such as dry mouth, impotence and constipation, while in 65% of patients there is associated small-cell carcinoma of the lung, which often postdates muscle weakness. The muscle weakness often improves if the small cell tumour is treated.

The features of this disorder clearly contrast with those of myasthenia gravis, which is an autoimmune postsynaptic disorder with a different pattern of muscle weakness and no autonomic dysfunction (Vincent, this volume). In this chapter, evidence is discussed from a wide variety of experimental techniques that has led to the conclusion that LEMS is also an autoimmune disorder, due to autoantibodies against nerve terminal calcium channels.

In LEMS patients, electromyography shows a reduction in the amplitude of the compound muscle action potential following nerve stimulation. This comes about because the reduced ACh release leads to smaller end-plate potentials (EPPs) than normal; hence many muscle fibres do not fire action potentials, and thus muscle weakness is produced.

Another characteristic feature of the disorder observed in electromy-

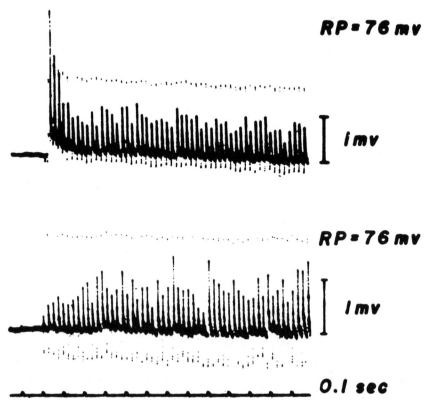

Fig. 12.1. Microelectrode recordings of EPPs in biopsied human muscle. The nerve was stimulated at 40 Hz. Top: normal muscle, bottom: LEMS muscle. From Lambert and Elmqvist, 1971.

ography of LEMS patients is a progressive increase in the amplitude of compound muscle action potentials during high-frequency repetitive nerve stimulation, either electrical or voluntary. This effect is due to an increase in amplitude of EPPs during the train ('facilitation') (see Fig. 12.1), leading to progressively more muscle fibres firing action potentials, which in turn increases muscle tension and is the mechanism responsible for the improved muscle strength during prolonged effort referred to above. Facilitation of EPP amplitudes in LEMS muscles occurs because of progressive increase in the number of ACh packets released by each nerve stimulus during the train, due to progressive accumulation of intracellular Ca^{2+} at the nerve terminals (see also Chapter 2 and the chapter by Engel, this volume). On the other hand, for normal muscle, depression of EPP amplitudes occurs in high-frequency trains (Fig. 12.1) due to depletion of available packets of ACh for release from the nerve terminal. Depression does not usually occur for LEMS patients' muscles because the low release rate of packets of ACh does not deplete the nerve terminals; indeed facilitatory effects predominate.

Besides the passive transfer experiments discussed below, there are several clinical indications that this is an autoimmune disorder. For instance, patients show short-term electromyographical and clinical improvement in response to plasma exchange (Newsom–Davis and Murray, 1984), which temporarily reduces circulating antibody levels. Furthermore, immunosuppressive drugs (azathioprine and prednisolone) lead to clinical improvement in LEMS patients. A feature of autoimmune disorders in general is their association with other autoimmune disorders; in LEMS patients autoantibodies are found against thyroid, stomach and skeletal muscle components (Lennon *et al.*, 1982). Furthermore, autoimmune disorders in general tend to associate with certain histocompatibility antigens, and this is also the case for LEMS, where the HLA antigen B8 is present in 60% of LEMS patients as compared to a control frequency of 20% (Willcox *et al.*, 1985).

12.2.1. In vitro *studies of LEMS muscles*

ACh release can be measured electrophysiologically in biopsied muscle from LEMS patients using microelectrodes to record EPPs. From such measurements the quantal content (i.e. the number of packets of ACh released per nerve stimulus) can be obtained, and is found to be reduced in

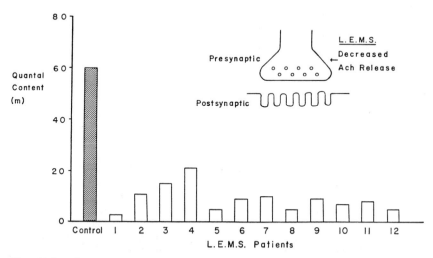

Fig. 12.2. Quantal content values for biopsied human muscles. Nerves were stimulated once per second, EPPs recorded by microelectrode and quantal content (i.e. the number of packets of ACh released per nerve impulse) calculated. Data for control muscle and for 12 LEMS patients' muscles, from Lambert and Elmquist, 1971.

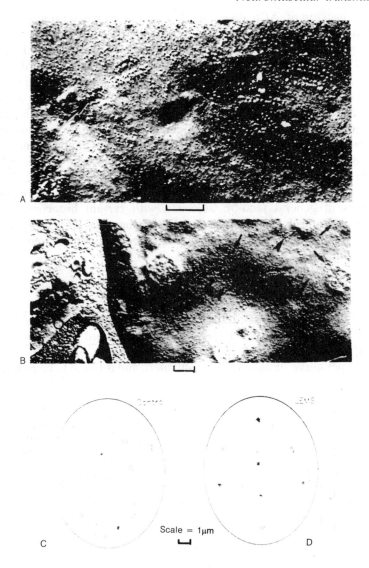

Fig. 12.3. Active zones in presynaptic membrane faces observed by freeze-fracture electron microscopy of human neuromuscular junctions. **A**: In control muscle there are active zones consisting of double parallel rows of particles and a few which display less than four rows, or clusters (arrows). **B**: In LEMS muscles there are far fewer particles in either active zones or clusters (arrowheads). **C** and **D** are schematic reconstructions based on the mean results of nine patients and 14 controls. Taken with permission from Fukunaga *et al.*, (1982). Courtesy of Dr A. Engel.

LEMS patients (Fig. 12.2; Lambert and Elmqvist, 1971). Chemical measurements of ACh release also show a reduction for LEMS patients' muscle (although levels of ACh and choline acetyltransferase in the nerve terminal are normal) (Molenaar *et al.*, 1982). The other main feature of *in vitro* electrophysiological microelectrode recordings in LEMS muscle (i.e. facilitation of EPP amplitudes at high-frequency nerve stimulation, Fig. 12.1) has been discussed above.

In LEMS patients' muscles, miniature endplate potential (MEPP) amplitude is normal, indicating lack of postsynaptic abnormality. Unstimulated quantal release is also normal, as measured by the frequency of occurrence of MEPPs. However, when release is stimulated by high K^+ concentration solutions, LEMS patients' muscles show a significant reduction in MEPP frequency compared to controls.

Under the light microscope, neuromuscular junctions appear normal for biopsied muscle from LEMS patients. However, freeze-fracture electron-microscopy of the nerve terminal membrane reveals abnormalities of the active zones (Fukunaga *et al.*, 1982). In normal terminals, arrays of double parallel lines of particles 10–12 nm in diameter form the active zones (Fig. 12.3). However, in LEMS patients these arrays are disorganised and the total number of particles is reduced.

12.3 Use of passive transfer experiments to investigate the autoimmune basis of LEMS

As for myasthenis gravis (see Vincent, this volume), the autoimmune nature of the Lambert–Eaton myasthenic syndrome (LEMS) was clearly demonstrated by 'passive transfer' experiments (Lang *et al.*, 1983). For this, mice were injected intraperitoneally (i.p.) with the IgG fraction from LEMS patients or with control IgG. Microelectrode recordings were made from diaphragm muscles taken from the mice. The phrenic nerve was stimulated and end-plate potentials recorded. It was found that there was a reduction in the quantal content by the LEMS IgG (Fig. 12.4). Furthermore, for mice injected with LEMS IgG, high-frequency nerve stimulation led to facilitation (or less marked depression) of EPP amplitudes (Fig. 12.5). Both these features are characteristic of the disorder in patients themselves (cf. Figs 12.1 and 12.2). Thus LEMS IgG transferred the electrophysiological features of the disorder to the mice. These experiments therefore provide strong evidence for the involvement of auto-antibodies in this disorder.

In the above experiments mice were injected with either 10 mg/day IgG for 30–99 days or with 50–60 mg/day for 2 days. The time-course of the effect was studied in further experiments (Prior *et al.*, 1985); different mice were injected daily with 10 mg LEMS IgG over a range of times and

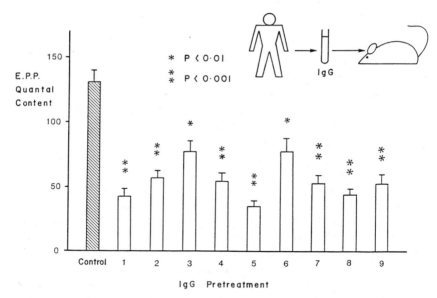

Fig. 12.4. Quantal content values for mouse muscles injected with IgG. Nerves were stimulated once every 2 s, EPPs recorded by microelectrode and quantal content calculated. Data for control IgG (left column) and for IgG from each of nine LEMS patients (other columns), different patients from those in Fig. 12.2. Significance levels are also shown.

CONTROL IgG

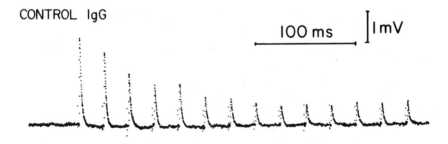

IgG FROM MYASTHENIC SYNDROME

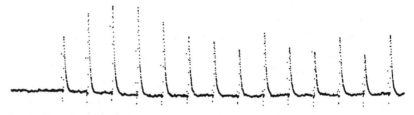

Fig. 12.5. Microelectrode recordings of EPPs in mouse muscle. The nerve was stimulated at 40 Hz. Top: muscle treated with control IgG, bottom: muscle treated with LEMS IgG (Newsom–Davis et al., 1982).

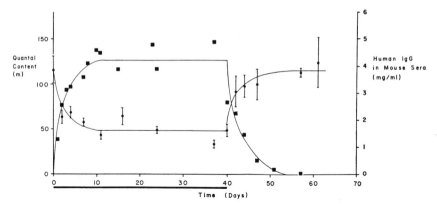

Fig. 12.6. Time-course of the effect of daily injections of LEMS IgG on quantal content in mice (circles). Also shown is the serum level of human IgG in the mice (squares). LEMS IgG was given for 40 days (as shown by the horizontal bar — Prior *et al.*, 1985).

quantal content again measured (Fig. 12.6). At 10 days the LEMS IgG had its maximal effect, with half-maximal effect at 1–2 days. When the injections were stopped, quantal content recovered to its normal levels over a period of several days. Serum levels of total human IgG in the mice were also measured and found to correlate with the reduction in quantal content (Fig. 12.6), further supporting the idea that LEMS IgG autoantibody acts to reduce ACh release. Moreover, reduction in stimulated ACh release in LEMS IgG-treated mice has been confirmed by chemical measurements of ACh release (Lang *et al.*, 1984).

The above effects of LEMS IgG to reduce quantal content and to cause facilitation of EPP amplitudes are presynaptic in origin. There are no postsynaptic actions of this antibody; so for instance MEPP amplitudes are not affected in patients or in mice treated with LEMS IgG (Lang *et al.*, 1983).

Antibodies in general can act by activating the complement cascade. The possible role of mouse complement was investigated by injecting LEMS IgG into mice genetically deficient in the fifth component of complement (C5). LEMS IgG was as effective in reducing quantal content in these animals as in normal animals (Prior *et al.*, 1985). This suggests that complement components (C5, and components activated by C5) are not involved in this disorder. In further experiments, mice were injected with LEMS IgG or with whole plasma containing the same amount of IgG. Both caused similar reductions in quantal content. Thus, whole plasma was no more effective than IgG in transferring the disorder to the mice, further supporting the idea that non-IgG components are not involved in the disease.

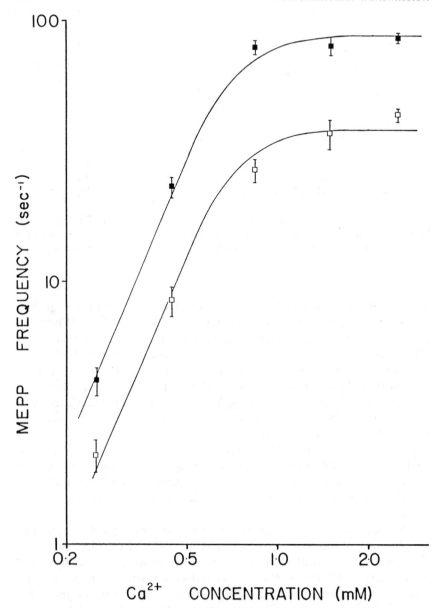

Fig. 12.7. Effect of LEMS IgG on MEPP frequency at high K^+ concentration. MEPP frequency is plotted for mice treated with control IgG (closed squares) and with IgG from two LEMS patients. MEPP frequency was significantly reduced ($p < 0.002$) by LEMS IgG at each calcium concentration used (Lang *et al.*, 1987a).

Passive transfer experiments have also been used to study the nature of the site of action of LEMS IgG at the nerve terminal (Lang *et al.*, 1987a). Acetylcholine release was stimulated by using high K^+ solutions to depolarise mouse nerve terminals, so that the effect of LEMS IgG could be investigated in the absence of nerve action potentials. Release was measured by recording the frequency of occurrence of MEPPs. As found for biopsied patients' muscles (see above), release was reduced in the mice by LEMS IgG under these conditions. This suggests that the action of LEMS IgG does not involve the propagation of the action potential in the nerve.

Further experiments were carried out to investigate the site of action of LEMS IgG at the mouse nerve terminal. Using a fixed high K^+ concentration to evoke release, the Ca^{2+} concentration was varied. In control muscles the MEPP frequency increased to a plateau as the Ca^{2+} concentration was increased (Fig. 12.7), because more Ca^{2+} can enter the nerve terminal via voltage-dependent Ca^{2+} channels at higher Ca^{2+} concentrations. In LEMS treated muscles, the MEPP frequency also increased with increasing Ca^{2+} concentration, but at each Ca^{2+} concentration release was significantly lower so that the curve was shifted downwards (Fig. 12.7). An action of LEMS IgG as an antagonist of Ca^{2+} entry into the terminal or of its intraterminal binding would cause such a shift in the curve. Evidence for such an action of LEMS IgG at mouse nerve terminals was also found by studying nerve-evoked release. EPPs were recorded over a range of Ca^{2+} concentrations and quantal content determined. In LEMS IgG-treated animals the curve of quantal content versus Ca^{2+} concentration was shifted to the right (Fig. 12.8). A similar shift in this curve is known to be produced by magnesium ions which act to antagonise calcium ions (Jenkinson, 1957), again consistent with the idea that LEMS IgG acts as a Ca^{2+} antagonist. To distinguish between antagonism of Ca^{2+} entry and antagonism of intraterminal binding of Ca^{2+}, studies were made of MEPPs from mouse muscles in Ca^{2+}-free solutions. Release under these conditions is determined by processes not involving Ca^{2+} entry. LEMS IgG did not affect MEPP frequency (Lang *et al.*, 1987a), suggesting that it does not have an intraterminal action. Furthermore, other agents such as ouabain and lithium, which cause an increase in MEPP frequency without a concomitant increase in Ca^{2+} entry, were investigated (Lande *et al.*, 1985). The increases in MEPP frequencies produced by these drugs in mouse muscle were unaffected by treatment with LEMS IgG, again indicating that LEMS IgG does not act via intraterminal mechanisms involved in ACh release. Thus the overall conclusion is that LEMS IgG acts to antagonise Ca^{2+} entry into the nerve terminal rather than to interfere with intraterminal binding of Ca^{2+}. Antagonism of Ca^{2+} entry probably comes about by loss of function of nerve terminal voltage-dependent Ca^{2+} channels by the antibody.

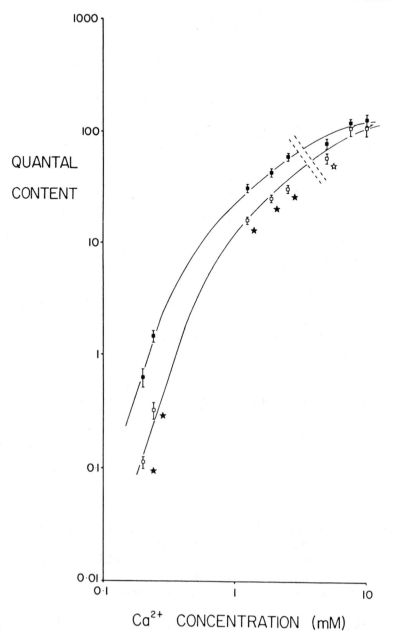

Fig. 12.8. Effect of LEMS IgG on quantal content. Mice were treated with control IgG (closed squares) and with LEMS IgG (open squares). Significant reductions by LEMS IgG: $p < 0.05$, $p < 0.001$ (Lang *et al.*, 1987a)

In LEMS patients' muscles active zone particles found at nerve terminals are disorganised and reduced in number (see above). This feature of the disorder can also be transferred to mice by injecting LEMS IgG; particles move closer together, become disorganised and reduced in number (Fukunaga *et al.*, 1983). This again supports the autoimmune basis of the disorder. The particles are thought to be Ca^{2+} channels and their loss probably underlies the loss of function of Ca^{2+} channels implied by the electrophysiological experiments described above.

Passive transfer of LEMS IgG to the mouse has also been used to study the binding of LEMS IgG at mouse nerve terminals (Engel *et al.*, 1987). For this, after injecting mice with LEMS IgG for 2–15 days, muscles were removed and treated with goat antihuman antibody to bind the LEMS IgG. The goat antibody was in turn localised with ferritin or peroxidase. In this way it was shown (Fig. 12.9) that LEMS IgG binds to presynaptic membrane active zone regions, although it has not yet been possible to resolve whether the antibody binds directly to the active zone particles themselves or to an associated membrane component.

Ca^{2+} channels are also found in the heart, and we investigated whether LEMS IgG interfered with Ca^{2+} entry via these channels (Lang *et al.*,

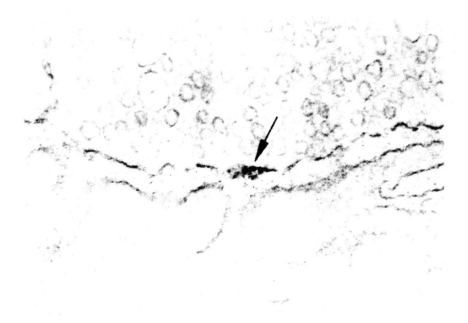

Fig. 12.9. Immunoperoxidase localisation of human IgG in mice treated with LEMS IgG. Arrows indicate immunostained active zones. ×50,000 (Engel *et al.*, 1989).

1988). Recordings were made from ventricular muscle taken from the mice in which LEMS IgG was shown to produce a reduced quantal content at the neuromuscular junction. In the presence of high K^+ concentration solutions, fast Na^+ channels are inactivated and Ca^{2+} channel currents underlie 'slow' action potentials which can be recorded with microelectrodes. LEMS IgG did not affect such action potentials, indicating a lack of action on heart Ca^{2+} channels. This finding implies that antigenic differences exist between the Ca^{2+} channels in the heart and at the motor nerve terminal.

12.4. Acute effects of LEMS antibodies in vitro

12.4.1. *Effect on neuromuscular transmission*

This section discusses effects of exposing mouse muscles *in vitro* to LEMS IgG. After incubating muscles for 2 h with LEMS IgG in the bath, at a similar concentration to that effective in injected mice, EPPs were recorded (Prior *et al.*, 1985). Under these conditions LEMS IgG was without effect, suggesting that direct pharmacological block of Ca^{2+} channels by LEMS IgG is not the mechanism. As indicated by the morphological experiments described above, antibody-induced loss of channels seems a more likely mechanism, and indeed marked effects were produced in 1–2 days in injected mice (see above). Furthermore *in vitro* application

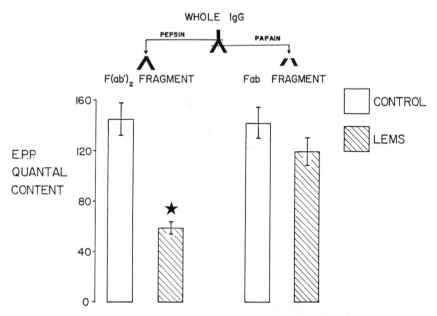

Fig. 12.10. Quantal content of mouse muscles treated *in vitro* with antibody fragments. Values are shown for divalent F(ab')₂ and monovalent Fab fragments from control and LEMS IgG. Significant difference from control: $p < 0.001$.

of LEMS IgG for 24 h at room temperature to mouse muscle was as effective as i.p. injections in causing reductions in quantal content (Lang *et al.*, 1987b). A possible way in which channel loss can occur is by the antibody crosslinking adjacent Ca^{2+} channels and thereby increasing their rate of degradation. This was studied by *in vitro* incubation of mouse muscles with antibody fragments. Digestion of LEMS IgG with pepsin produces divalent fragments ($F(ab')_2$), while digestion with papain leads to monovalent fragments (Fab). The divalent fragments caused significant reductions in quantal content while the monovalent fragments had no effect (Lang *et al.*, 1987b; Fig. 12.10). Therefore, the divalent structure of LEMS IgG is essential for its effect; crosslinking of adjacent Ca^{2+} channels causing their loss. This conclusion is supported by morphological studies of nerve terminals in mouse muscles incubated *in vitro* as above for 24 h; LEMS IgG caused active zone particles to move closer together (as for injected mice, see above), consistent with crosslinking prior to their loss (Engel *et al.*, 1989). Furthermore, divalent antibody fragments, but not monovalent fragments, have a similar *in vitro* effect on active zone particles moving them closer together, again consistent with the idea of cross-linking.

12.4.2. *Effect on cultured cell lines*

(a) $^{45}Ca^{2+}$ flux measurements in cultured cells

Since many LEMS patients have small cell carcinoma, it may be that these are the primary antigenic determinant for those patients. Indeed Ca^{2+} channels appear to be present on these cells since they exhibit Ca^{2+}-dependent action potentials. *In vitro* effects of LEMS IgG on cultured human small cell carcinoma cells were therefore studied, using measurements of $^{45}Ca^{2+}$ uptake (Roberts *et al.*, 1985). Depolarising cells with high K^+ concentrations (96 mM) stimulated the influx of Ca^{2+}, presumably via voltage-dependent Ca^{2+} channels since this effect was blocked by micromolar concentrations of the Ca^{2+} channel antagonists nifedipine or methoxyverapamil. Cells cultured for 7 days in LEMS IgG showed a significantly reduced K^+-stimulated Ca^{2+} flux as compared with controls (Fig. 12.11). This reduction was found not only for LEMS IgG from patients with associated carcinoma but also for those completely free of carcinoma. These results suggest that in patients with associated carcinoma the primary antigenic determinant could be the Ca^{2+} channels in the small cells. For patients without carcinoma the primary antigenic determinant may be the nerve terminal Ca^{2+} channels themselves or some other cell expressing Ca^{2+} channels.

(b) Effect of LEMS IgG on NG 108 15 cells

Direct electrical recordings of Ca^{2+} channel currents at the skeletal muscle nerve terminal are not possible, but such recordings can be made from

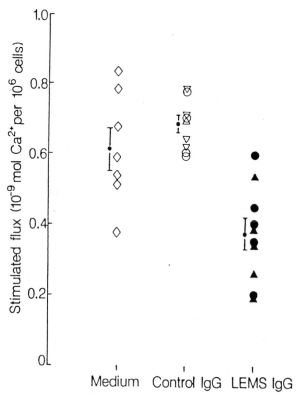

Fig. 12.11.   The effect of LEMS IgG on K$^+$-stimulated calcium flux in small-cell carcinoma cells. Cells were cultured in medium alone ($\Diamond$), in control IgG (from normals, $\bigcirc$, and non-LEMS patients, $\triangledown$, $\triangle$), and in LEMS IgG (with, $\blacktriangle$, or without, $\bullet$, associated small-cell carcinoma). Means $\pm$ standard errors are also shown (Roberts *et al.*, 1985).

cultured cells where the action of LEMS IgG on Ca^{2+} channels can be investigated.

In the whole cell patch clamp technique a micropipette is sealed to the membrane and suction applied to rupture the membrane at its tip (Fig. 12.12, see also Chapter 3). The micropipette is then in electrical contact with the interior of the cell which can be voltage-clamped by standard techniques at a variety of potentials. When voltage steps are applied, inward currents are observed corresponding to currents through Ca^{2+} channels. For instance, in NG 108 15 neuroblastoma cells, voltage steps from -80 mV to around -30 mV evoke transient currents, attributed to openings of 'T-type' Ca^{2+} channels, while voltage steps from -40 mV to around 0 mV evoke sustained currents due to openings of 'L-type' channels (Fig. 12.12).

NG 108 15 cells were incubated for 24–48 h with control or LEMS IgG

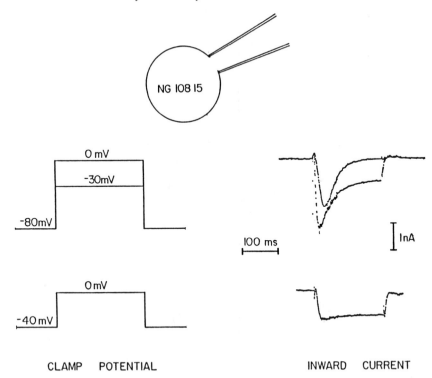

CLAMP   POTENTIAL   INWARD   CURRENT

Fig. 12.12.   Whole-cell patch clamp recordings of calcium currents in NG 108 15 cells. Top: schematic drawing of recording technique. The patch electrode is first sealed on to the membrane of the cell, the membrane is then broken by suction so that the inside of the cell is in contact with the electrode. Inward currents flowing across the cell membrane leave via the electrode where they are recorded. Sodium and potassium channels were blocked with tetrodotoxin and tetraethylammonium + caesium respectively, while barium was the charge carrier via calcium channels. Bottom: sample recordings of calcium channel currents; left: potential steps used, right: corresponding inward currents observed (Lang *et al.*, 1989).

(Lang *et al.*, 1987c, 1989). Using voltage steps which elicit sustained (L-type) currents, LEMS IgG caused marked reductions in these currents (Fig. 12.13). On the other hand, under conditions where only T-type channels are activated, LEMS IgG was without effect (Fig. 12.14). Thus, in NG 108 15 cells, LEMS IgG selectively blocks current flow through L-type channels while leaving T-type channels unaffected.

The cross-reactivity of LEMS antibody with Ca^{2+} channels at motor nerve terminals and with L-type Ca^{2+} channels in NG 108 15 cells suggests that there are regions of antigenic similarities between these channel proteins. However, the channels are not completely identical since organic Ca^{2+} channel agonists and antagonists have little or no effect on nerve

A

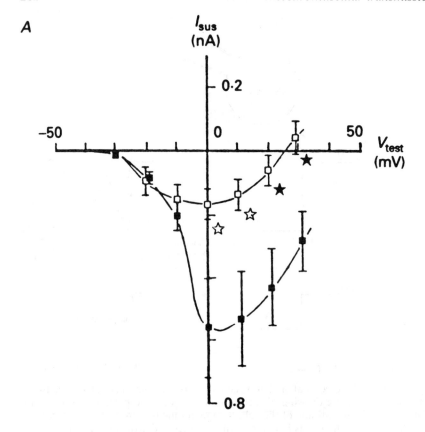

Fig. 12.13.   Effect of LEMS IgG on L-type calcium currents in NG 108 15 cells. The figure shows a plot of sustained current (I_{sus}) evoked by voltage steps from a potential of -40 mV to more depolarised potentials (V_{test}). The recording techniques were as in Fig. 12.12. Control IgG: ■, LEMS IgG: □ Significant reductions by LEMS IgG: ☆ $p < 0.02$, ★ $p < 0.005$ (Peers *et al.*, 1990).

terminal Ca^{2+} channels; therefore the latter do not appear to be L-type (Burges and W.-Wray, 1989).

LEMS IgG appears to cross-react preferentially with cells of neuronal origin. So for instance, besides cross-reacting with Ca^{2+} channels at motor nerve terminals and NG 108 15 cells, it cross-reacts with Ca^{2+} channels in chromaffin (Kim and Neher, 1988), pituitary cells (Login *et al.*, 1987) and small-cell carcinoma cells (derived from the neuroectoderm). Moreover, the autonomic dysfunction which occurs with many LEMS patients may be due to an action of LEMS IgG on Ca^{2+} channels at postganglionic parasympathetic nerve endings. On the other hand, mouse cardiac muscle and insect skeletal muscle (Pearson *et al.*, 1989) Ca^{2+} channels appear to be unaffected by LEMS IgG. The preferential action of LEMS IgG on

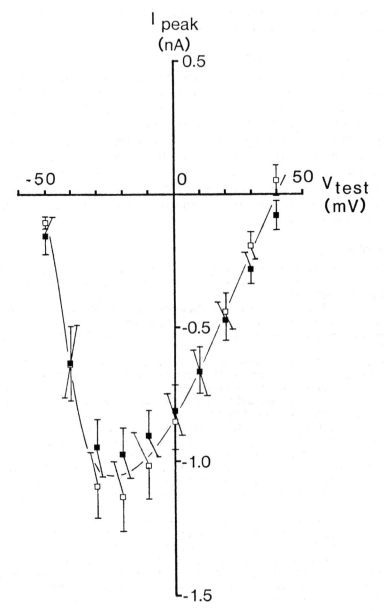

Fig. 12.14. Lack of effect of LEMS IgG on T-type calcium channels in NG 108 15 cells. The figure shows a plot of transient current (I_{peak}) evoked by voltage steps from a potential of -80 mV to more depolarised potentials (V_{test}). Nitrendipine was present to block L-type channels. The recording techniques were as in Fig. 12.12. Control IgG: ■, LEMS IgG: □ (Peers *et al.*, 1990).

neuronal tissues indicates that Ca^{2+} channels from a variety of neuronal tissues share a common determinant.

12.4.3. *An assay for LEMS antibody*

The 27 amino acid polypeptide, ω-conotoxin (ω-CgTX), from the marine snail *Conus geographus* binds to and blocks neuronal Ca^{2+} channels (see Norman, this volume). By prelabelling Ca^{2+} channels from a human neuronal cell line with ^{125}I-ω-CgTX, subsequent binding of LEMS antibody to these channel complexes has now been demonstrated by immunoprecipitation (Sher *et al.*, 1989). This forms the basis for a specific diagnostic assay for LEMS, the value of which may prove to be similar to that of the analogous immunoprecipitation assay using ^{125}I-α-bungarotoxin for the detection of anti-AChR antibodies in myasthenia gravis (see Vincent, this volume).

References

Burges, J. and W.-Wray, D. (1989) Effect of the calcium channel agonist CGP 28392 on transmitter release at mouse neuromuscular junctions. *Ann. N.Y. Acad. Sci.* **560**: 297–300.

Engel, A. G., Fukuoka, T., Lang, B., Newsom–Davis, J., Vincent A. and Wray, D. (1987). Lambert–Eaton myasthenic syndrome IgG: early morphologic effects and immunolocalization at the motor end-plate. *Ann. N.Y. Acad. Sci.* **505**: 333–344.

Engel, A. G., Nagel, A., Fukuoka, T., Fukunaga, H., Osame, M., Lang, B., Newsom–Davis, J., Vincent, A., W.-Wray, D. and Peers, C. (1989) Motor nerve terminal calcium channels in Lambert–Eaton myasthenic syndrome: morphologic evidence for depletion and that the depletion is mediated by autoantibodies. *Ann. N.Y. Acad. Sci.* **560**: 278–290.

Fukunaga, H., Engel, A. G., Osame, M. and Lambert, E. H. (1982) Paucity and disorganization of presynaptic membrane active zones in the Lambert–Eaton myasthenic syndrome. *Muscle and Nerve* **5**: 686–697.

Fukunaga, H., Engel, A. G., Lang, B., Newsom–Davis, J. and Vincent, A. (1983) Passive transfer of Lambert–Eaton myasthenic syndrome with IgG from man to mouse depletes the presynaptic membrane active zones. *Proc. Natl. Acad. Sci.* **80**: 7636–7640.

Jenkinson, D. H. (1957) The nature of the antagonism between calcium and magnesium ions at the neuromuscular junction. *J. Physiol.* **138**: 434–444.

Kim, Y. I. and Neher, E. (1988) IgG from patients with Lambert–Eaton syndrome blocks voltage-dependent calcium channels. *Science* **439**: 405–408.

Lambert, E. H. and Elmqvist, D. (1971). Quantal components of endplate potentials in the myasthenic syndrome. *Ann. N.Y. Acad. Sci.* **183**: 183–199.

Lande, S., Lang,.B., Newsom–Davis, J. and Wray, D. (1985) Site of action of Lambert–Eaton myasthenic syndrome antibodies at mouse motor nerve terminals. *J. Physiol.* **371**: 61P.

Lang, B., Newsom–Davis, J., Prior, C. and Wray, D. (1983) Antibodies to nerve terminals: an electrophysiological study of a human myasthenic syndrome transferred to mouse. *J. Physiol.* **344**: 335–345.

Lang, B., Molenaar, P. C., Newsom–Davis, J. and Vincent, A. (1984) Passive transfer of Lambert–Eaton myasthenic syndrome in mice: decreased rates of resting and evoked release of acetylcholine from skeletal muscle. *J. Neurochem.*

42: 658–662.

Lang, B., Newsom–Davis, J., Peers, C., Prior, C. and W.-Wray, D. (1987a) The effect of myasthenic syndrome antibody on presynaptic calcium channels in the mouse. *J. Physiol.* **390**: 257–270.

Lang, B., Newsom–Davis, J., Peers, C. and W.-Wray, D. (1987b) The action of myasthenic syndrome antibody fragments on transmitter release in the mouse. *J. Physiol.* **390**: 173P.

Lang, B., Newsom–Davis, J., Peers, C. and W.-Wray, D. (1987c) Selective action of Lambert–Eaton myasthenic syndrome antibodies on Ca^{2+} channels in the neuroblastoma × glioma hybrid cell line NG 108 15. *J. Physiol.* **394**: 43P.

Lang, B., Newsom–Davis, J. and W.-Wray, D. (1988) The effect of Lambert–Eaton myasthenic syndrome antibody on slow action potentials in mouse cardiac ventricle. *Proc. R. Soc. B* **235**: 103–110.

Lennon, V. A., Lambert, E. H., Wittingham, S. and Fairbanks, V. (1982) Autoimmunity in the Lambert–Eaton myasthenic syndrome. *Muscle and Nerve* **5**: S21–S25.

Login, I. S., Kim, Y. I., Judd, A. M., Spangelo, B. L. and Macleod, R. M. (1987) Immunoglobulins of Lambert–Eaton myasthenic syndrome inhibit rat pituitary hormone release. *Ann. Neurol.* **22**: 610–614.

Molenaar, P. C., Newsom–Davis, J., Polak, R. L. and Vincent, A. (1982) Eaton–Lambert syndrome: acetylcholine and choline acetyltransferase in skeletal muscle. *Neurology* **32**: 1062–1065.

Newsom–Davis, J. and Murray, N. M. F. (1984) Plasma exchange and immunosuppressive drug treatment in the Lambert–Eaton myasthenic syndrome. *Neurology* **34**: 480–485.

Newsom–Davis, J., Murray, N., Wray, D., Lang, B., Prior, C., Gwilt, M. and Vincent, A. (1982) Lambert–Eaton myasthenic syndrome: electrophysiological evidence for a humoral factor. *Muscle Nerve* **5**: S17–S20.

Pearson, H. A., Newsom–Davis, J., Lees, G. and W.-Wray, D. (1989) Lack of action of Lambert–Eaton myasthenic syndrome antibody on calcium channels in insect muscle. *Ann. N.Y. Acad. Sci.*, **560**: 291–293.

Peers, C., Lang, B., Newsom–Davis, J. and Wray, D. (1990) Selective action of myasthenic syndrome antibodies on calcium channels in rodent neuroblastoma × glioma cell line. *J. Physiol.* **421**: 293–308.

Prior, C., Lang, B., Wray, D. and Newsom–Davis, J. (1985) Action of Lambert–Eaton myasthenic syndrome IgG at mouse motor nerve terminals. *Ann. Neurol.* **17**: 587–592.

Roberts, A., Perera, S., Lang, B., Vincent, A. and Newsom–Davis, J. (1985). Paraneoplastic myasthenic syndrome IgG inhibits $^{45}Ca^{2+}$ flux in a human small cell carcinoma line. *Nature* **317**: 737–739.

Sher, E., Gotti, C., Canal, N., Scopetta, C., Piccolo, G., Evoli, A. and Clementi, F. (1989) Specificity of calcium channel autoantibodies in Lambert–Eaton myasthenic syndrome. *Lancet*, ii: 640–643.

Willcox, N., Demaine, A. G., Newsom–Davis, J., Welsh, K. I., Robb, S. A. and Spiro, A. G. (1985) Increased frequency of IgG heavy chain marker Glm(2) and of HLA–B8 in Lambert–Eaton myasthenic syndrome with and without associated lung carcinoma. *Hum. Immunol.* **14**: 29–36.

Experimental autoimmune myasthenia gravis

13.1. Introduction

The development of an animal model of a disease is an important step towards investigating pathological mechanisms, the influence of genetic factors, and possible approaches to treatment. The idea that antibodies to a membrane receptor could be a cause of disease was first put forward by Carnegie (1971), and subsequently referred to as immunopharmacological disease (Lennon and Carnegie, 1981). In the early 1970s Patrick and Lindstrom (1973) showed that rabbits immunised against the nicotinic acetylcholine receptor (AChR) purified from electric organs of the electric eel developed a defect of neuromuscular transmission, which was due to anti-AChR antibodies. The rabbits' condition responded dramatically to anti-acetylcholinesterase treatment, just as patients with myasthenia gravis do. Experimental autoimmune myasthenia gravis (EAMG), as it was termed, can be induced in experimental animals by injection of AChR from many species, and because of the availability of the antigen this model serves as a prototype for autoimmune receptor disease in many fields of medicine (Table 13.1). This chapter will describe the main features of EAMG and summarise the ways in which it has provided a useful model for studying the human disease.

The autoimmune nature of EAMG was first investigated by Lennon *et al.* (1975) and the demonstration of antibodies against AChR in myasthenia gravis (see Vincent, this volume) confirmed the relevance of the experimental disease to the human disorder. Since then several other autoimmune receptor diseases have been identified clinically, mainly through the development of assays to measure antibodies to various cell surface proteins.

13.2. The autoantigen

Advances in the study of organ-specific autoimmune disease eventually require detailed knowledge of the molecular structure of the target autoantigen. The acetylcholine receptor is a transmembrane protein consisting of four different subunits assembled in the stoichiometry, α_2, β, γ (or ε), δ. The primary amino acid sequence of the four subunits of AChR

Table 13.1. Anti-receptor autoimmune disease

Discipline	Receptor for	Disease
Neurology	AChR	Myasthenia gravis
Endocrinology	TSH	Graves' disease (TSI)
		Myxoedema (TGI block)
		Goitre (TGI)
	Insulin	Hyperglycaemia
		Hypoglycaemia
	FSH	Amenorrhoea
Nephrology	PTH	Secondary hyperparathyroidism in patients with renal failure
Haematology	Transferrin	Anaemia
Gastroenterology	Gastrin	Pernicious anaemia, achylia
Immunology	IgA	IgA deficiency
	β_2-adrenergic agonists	Asthma/allergic rhinitis

TSI = thyroid stimulating immunoglobulins; TGI = thyroid growth promoting immunoglobulins; TGI block = thryoid growth blocking; FSH = follicle stimulating hormone; PTH = parathyroid hormone. For a review of other anti-receptor mediated disorders see De Baets, 1988.

of several species, including humans, has been elucidated, and although the three-dimensional structure has not yet been elaborated in detail, various models of the transmembrane orientation of the four subunits have been proposed. These are discussed fully elsewhere (see chapters by Beeson and Barnard, and by Lindstrom).

13.3. Induction of experimental autoimmune myasthenia gravis

EAMG can be induced in mammals, birds and reptiles by injection of purified AChRs from electric organ or muscle incorporated in complete Freund's adjuvant (CFA) with or without additional adjuvants such as *Bordetella pertussis* vaccine. The species used to date include rabbit, rat, guinea pig, goat, monkey, frogs and hens (Lindstrom *et al.*, 1988).

Interestingly, the clinical symptoms and severity of the disease vary widely among these species; this partly reflects their different safety factors for neuromuscular transmission (see Chapter 2, and Engel, this volume). With few exceptions rabbits develop flaccid paralysis 1 week after a second injection of *Torpedo* AChR (100 μg). The affected animals are unable to support their weight, have difficulty in breathing and swallowing, and usually die within 1–2 days from respiratory insufficiency. Anticholinesterase treatment produces a marked but temporary improvement, reminiscent of the response found in MG patients (see Vincent, 1980). Monkeys develop signs that are particularly similar to the human disease with lid ptosis, dysphagia, facial weakness and ophthalmoplegia (Tarrab–Hazdai *et al.*, 1975). However, most studies of the autoimmune mechanisms have been concentrated on EAMG in rodents, particularly rats and mice.

13.3.1. *EAMG in rats*

Rats, in contrast to mice (see below), are susceptible to the clinical signs of EAMG because they have a lower safety factor for neuromuscular transmission. Signs of myasthenia have been induced in several strains (Biesecker and Koffler, 1988).

Lewis rats immunised with additional adjuvants such as *B. pertussis* develop a biphasic illness: an acute transient condition characterised by severe paralysis begins 7–10 days after immunisation; about 1 month later a chronic disease develops. EAMG can also be passively transferred to non-immunised litter mates by injection of small amounts of serum (e.g. 200 µl) from the immunised animals (Lindstrom *et al.*, 1976b) indicating that a serum antibody is involved.

The clinical signs in rats are typically the consequence of weakness in the upper limbs, head and neck. The animal lays his head and chest on the floor, the back is exaggeratedly humped and the thighs partially abducted. The digits or forelimbs are flexed and fail to extend when the rat is placed on a flat surface (Fig. 13.1). Anticholinesterase drugs reverse these

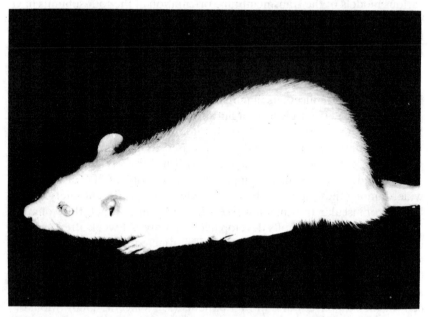

Fig. 13.1. Posture of a myasthenic rat. The animal lays his head and chest on the floor, the back is exaggeratedly humped with the thighs partially abducted.

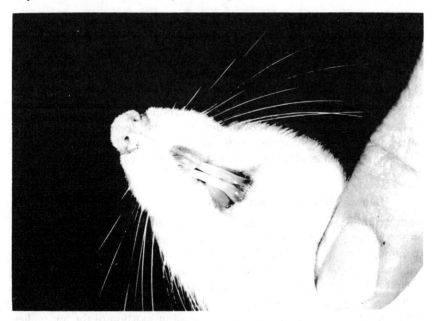

Fig. 13.2. Close-up of the head of a myasthenic rat. Note the excessive growth of the teeth due to impairment of the masticatory muscles.

symptoms. During the chronic stage respiratory disease becomes manifest as loud expiratory wheezes and brown porphyrin staining of nasal secretion and tears. Excessive growth of the teeth suggests impairment of masticatory muscles (Fig. 13.2) and the rats finally die from malnutrition. Death can be delayed by trimming the teeth and placing soft food within reach.

13.3.2. *EAMG in mice*

Mice, like rats, develop EAMG after injection of AChR in FCA, and some features of the disease have also been obtained in mice immunised without adjuvants (Scadding *et al.*, 1986; Jermy *et al.*, 1989a). Mice may develop muscular weakness after the second injection of AChR but this is highly variable. In order to distinguish between myasthenic and non-myasthenic animals various tests of muscle strength can be applied, and injection of low doses of d-tubocurarine, which lowers the safety factor for transmission by blocking a proportion of the AChRs, may precipitate weakness in affected animals (Berman and Patrick 1980a, b).

The susceptibility to EAMG in inbred and genetically defined strains of mice is linked to genes on the major histocompatibility complex and the genes of the IgCh locus (Berman and Patrick 1980a,b; Christadoss *et al.*, 1982). In some strains, including C57B1/6, SJL and AKR, 50–70% of the mice develop clinical EAMG, while in Balb/cke, SWR/J and C3H/HC only 3–15% of the mice become paralysed. It appears, therefore, that immunogenetic influences determine susceptibility to the disease and these studies indicate the involvement of the immune system both at the level of immune responsiveness (H-2) and of the immunoglobulin molecule itself (IgCh locus). However, attempts to analyse the underlying basis for these differences in terms of the antibody response have not been very conclusive (see below). Moreover, differences between the strains in the safety factor for transmission were minimal, and did not appear to be involved in susceptibility (Berman and Patrick 1980a).

13.4. Humoral immune response to AChR

Immunisation of animals with AChR results in the production of antibodies against the AChR which can be measured by double antibody immunoprecipitation using ^{125}I-α-BuTX-labelled AChR. Alternatively antibodies can be measured by enzyme-linked immunoassay (ELISA) (see Chapter 3). The presence of ^{125}I-α-BuTX bound to the AChR in the immunoprecipitation assay does not markedly interfere with the binding of antibodies to the receptor, since only a small proportion of the antibodies bind to the α-BuTX binding site.

Rats immunised against *Torpedo* AChR produce antibody against the immunogen which cross-react with their own AChR (Lennon *et al.*, 1975). The primary immune response measured against *Torpedo* AChR reaches a peak about 20 days after immunisation (Fig. 13.3), but the serum titre against rat AChR appears later and does not exceed about 1% of that to *Torpedo* AChR. On the face of it this difference in the time-course suggests that the cross-reactive antibodies are produced later on during the response. However, it is more likely that the delay is due to selective absorption of anti-rat AChR by rat muscle AChR at the neuromuscular junction during the early stages of the disease, when total anti-rat AChR antibody is low. Indeed antibodies can be demonstrated at the neuro-muscular junction complexed to the AChR at times when they cannot be easily detected in the animal's serum (Lindstrom *et al.*, 1976b).

Many of the antibodies against *Torpedo* AChR that cross-react with the animal's own AChRs are directed against a highly conserved region, present on each of the α subunits of the receptor, termed the 'main immunogenic region' (MIR) (Tzartos and Lindstrom, 1980). Antibodies against this region (anti-MIR) are found in all EAMG animals and appear to be responsible for much of the loss of AChR that characterises this condition. However, since these anti-MIR antibodies are circulating in excess over the amount of AChR in the muscle, parameters other than titre or antibody specificity must be important in determining disease severity.

Other antigenic epitopes can play a role in EAMG since persistent

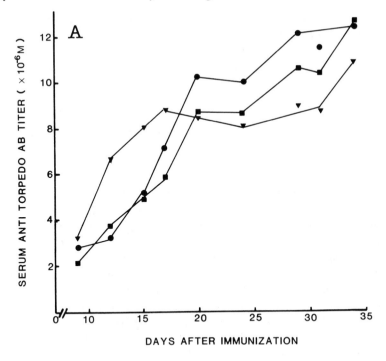

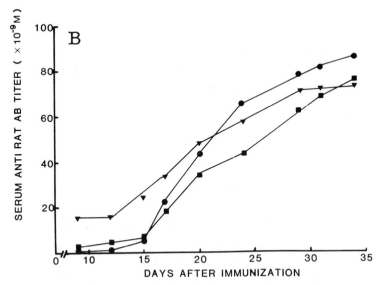

Fig. 13.3. Kinetics of the immune response against *Torpedo* and rat AChR. These rats were immunised once with 15 µg *Torpedo* AChR. Anti-*Torpedo* AChR (**A**) and anti-rat AChR titres (**B**) were measured at given time intervals after immunisation. Note the difference in scales between **A** and **B**.

immunisation with any of the four isolated subunits of the AChR, which do not adopt a 'native' conformation, can cause weakness (Lindstrom *et al.*, 1978), and monoclonal antibodies (mAbs) directed at specific epitopes, e.g. the ACh/α-BuTX binding site, can be shown to induce EAMG when injected into normal animals (Gomez and Richman, 1983). Indeed antibodies against the ACh/α-BuTX binding site cause an immediate paralysis, presumably by competition with released ACh, whereas anti-MIR mAbs do not directly affect AChR function but produce an effect about 48 h later.

13.5. Pathology of neuromuscular transmission

Electrophysiological studies in rats with chronic EAMG revealed that the amplitude of the first evoked compound muscle action potential was usually normal, but in rats with clinical weakness a decremental electromyographic response was seen at low frequences of stimulation (Seybold *et al.*, 1976; for explanation see Chapter 2). The amplitude of the miniature endplate potential (MEPP), produced by the spontaneous release of single quanta of acetylcholine, was decreased (Lambert *et al.*, 1976). These electrophysiological abnormalities are also seen in other species, e.g. rabbit (see Vincent, 1980), and are provoked by several immunopathological mechanisms, discussed below, all of which lead to a loss of functional AChR.

13.5.1. *Cellular invasion of the endplate*

In acute EAMG in rats light microscopy showed a marked inflammatory exudate of mononuclear cells confined to the endplates. Under electron microscopy the postsynaptic membrane was split away from the underlying muscle fibres and the junctional folds destroyed by macrophages. However, this cellular invasion was found only in acute EAMG and not in chronic EAMG (Engel *et al.*, 1976).

13.5.2. *Complement-mediated lysis of the postsynaptic membrane*

In chronic EAMG there were no changes on light microscopy but intense degeneration of the postsynaptic folds which were simplified in morphology. The increased membrane density, that signifies the presence of AChRs, was clearly reduced overall (Engel *et al.*, 1976), consistent with the reduction in total AChR as determined by ^{125}I-α-BuTX binding (Lindstrom *et al.*, 1976a).

Immunoglobulin G and complement (C3) have been demonstrated by immunoelectron microscopy on the terminal expansions of the junctional folds of the postsynaptic membrane in rats with chronic EAMG. The distribution is similar to that of AChRs localised by peroxidase-labelled α-BuTX. These findings strongly support an immune-mediated destruction of the muscle membrane (Engel *et al.*, 1977; Sahashi *et al.*, 1978).

Complement induces membrane destruction and cell death through the formation of the lytic membrane attack complex, a polymer of C9 molecules which spans the cell membrane and forms an ion channel. The activation of the complement cascade also generates anaphylatoxins (C3a and C5a) which attract polymorphonuclear leucocytes and macrophages (Hugli and Muller–Eberhard, 1978). These cells are not present in chronic EAMG (or in MG) but are found at the endplate in acute EAMG and passively transferred acute EAMG. Depletion of C3 with cobra venom factor prevents the AChR deficiency and inflammatory infiltration (Lennon *et al.*, 1978).

The failure to induce acute EAMG by passive transfer of anti-AChR to complement-depleted rats or C4-deficient guinea pigs indicates that complement plays a central role. The importance of the role of complement is also indicated in chronic EAMG; C4-deficient guinea pigs which had been immunised with AChR in CFA did not show clinical signs of EAMG, in spite of the presence of antibody–AChR complexes at the neuromuscular junction (De Baets, unpublished observations).

13.5.3. *Antigenic modulation of AChR*

The rate of degradation of AChRs can be measured in cultured muscle cells by labelling the surface AChRs with ^{125}I-α-BuTX and monitoring the appearance of degraded products of ^{125}I-α-BuTX in the culture medium. This is because the ^{125}I-α-BuTX–AChR complexes are internalised and degraded by lysosomal enzymes. This is an energy-dependent process which is inhibited by low temperature, DNP, NaF and inhibitors of cytoskeletal interactions (Heinemann *et al.*, 1977).

Anti-AChR antibody applied in the culture medium increases the rate of degradation of AChR on cultured muscle cells *in vitro* from a $t_{\frac{1}{2}}$ of about 16 h to about 8 h. This reduces the number of available AChRs on the muscle surface membrane as measured by subsequent ^{125}I-α-BuTX binding. The effect does not require complement but depends critically on the divalent nature of antibodies, and can be shown to result from crosslinking of AChRs on the muscle surface (Heinemann *et al.*, 1977). Similar findings apply in cultures treated with serum from myasthenia gravis patients (see Vincent, this volume).

In diaphragms taken from EAMG animals, or treated with EAMG serum *in vitro*, a similar increased rate of AChR degradation occurs. However, at the intact endplate the normal degradation rate occurs with a $t_{\frac{1}{2}}$ of over 10 days (see Chapter 1), and the effect of anti-AChR antibodies is to reduce this value to about 4–6 days (Heinemann *et al.*, 1978).

13.5.4. *Direct block of AChR function by antibody*

Conceptually, antibodies to the ACh binding site should be strong
inhibitors of ACh function and might play a large role in the pathology of
EAMG and MG. Agonist-induced depolarisation of eel electric organ or of
frog neuromuscular junctions was shown to be reduced by preincubation in
excess anti-AChR antibody, although some of the antibodies may have
bound to sites that had an allosteric (indirect) effect on AChR function
(Lindstrom, 1976).

Monoclonal antibodies can be shown to inhibit α-BuTX binding and to
compete with cholinergic ligands for binding to the ACh binding site, and
some of these block neuromuscular transmission or ACh-induced ion flux.
In one study two of 25 mAbs were able to block carbamylcholine-induced
$^{22}Na^+$ flux into liposomes containing reconstituted purified AChR (see
Lindstrom, this volume). However, there is little evidence that such
antibodies make an important contribution to the overall pathogenicity of
EAMG sera, as they probably represent only a minor fraction of the total,
and the concentration of anti-ACh site antibodies does not correlate
closely with severity of the disease in most instances (De Baets and Van
Breda Vriesman, 1985).

13.6. **Role of antibody diversity in EAMG**

Isoelectric focusing (IEF) is a method frequently used to analyse the
diversity of antibodies involved in an immune response. In all EAMG sera
tested, the immune response to *Torpedo* and rat AChR was polyclonal, i.e.
antibodies against the antigenic determinants on AChR are produced by
quite distinct B cell clones and therefore form separate bands on IEF. The
full spectrotype of antibodies was expressed early after immunisation and
remained during the period of study (Bionda *et al.*, 1984). Moreover the
population of antibodies bound to receptors in muscle is similar to the
population circulating in the animal's serum (Fig. 13.4), indicating that
most or all of the serum antibody specificities are capable of binding to the
AChR *in situ*.

There have been several attempts to account for differences in disease
susceptibility between strains of mice or rats by analysing the specificities
and/or pathogenicities of the serum antibodies (e.g. Berman and Heinemann, 1984; Christadoss *et al.*, 1985; Brown and Krolick, 1988). So far no
particular antibody specificity or mechanism of antibody-mediated loss of
AChR function has been clearly demonstrated to underlie strain susceptibility.

Since immunological factors such as antibody titres, antibody specificity
and diversity do not appear to determine the severity of the disease, other
factors such as the capacity of the neuromuscular junction to regenerate
AChRs or postsynaptic membrane may be more important. Animals in

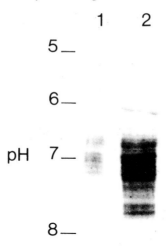

Fig. 13.4. Comparison of IEF profiles of serum antibodies versus antibodies eluted from a diseased animal (EAMG). After focusing, both serum (lane 2) and tissue eluate (lane 1) were reacted with ^{125}I-α-BuTX–*Torpedo* AChR and the gels autoradiographed.

which the AChR synthesis in muscle is increased artificially by denervation, are protected against AChR loss in the denervated muscle after immunisation with AChR in CFA (De Baets *et al.*, 1988). Since muscle is capable of large increases in receptor synthesis during embryonic development or after denervation, a compensatory increase in AChR gene expression should be looked for by measuring mRNA for the AChR subunits.

13.7. Idiotype networks in EAMG and MG

The variable region of an antibody (antibody 1) which contains the antigen combining site, may itself act as an antigenic determinant. Antibodies (antibody 2) that are directed to this may have a regulatory role *in vivo*. Antigenic determinants on antibody 1 are called idiotypes and their complementary antibodies (antibody 2) are termed anti-idiotypes. The idiotype is most frequently localised on the combined heavy and light chains of the immunoglobulin molecule. Jerne (1974) postulated that idiotypes and anti-idiotypes, connected in a functional regulatory network, maintain an immunological homeostasis.

Antoimmune diseases are the result of loss of tolerance against self. Perturbations in the natural balance between autoantibodies and their

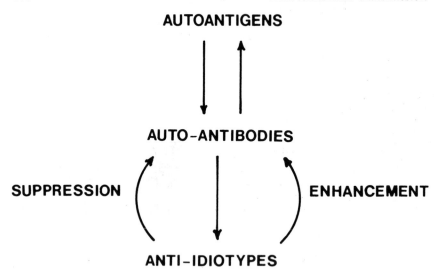

Fig. 13.5.   The autoimmune network. Modified from Zanetti 1986.

complementary anti-idiotypes (an autoimmune network, see Fig. 13.5) could be an important aetiological mechanism in autoimmune disorders (Zanetti, 1986). One finding in favour of this concept is that autoantibodies in several human diseases express idiotypes (not necessarily directly part of the antigen-combining site) that are found on other autoantibodies, even those that are specific for other autoantigens. This is because the autoantibodies appear to use a limited number of Ig variable heavy chain (VH) genes (Monestier *et al.*, 1986).

Perturbation of an autoimmune network might be achieved by idiotypic interactions or by molecular mimicry of autoantigens, idiotypes or exogenous antigens including viruses. For instance certain human anti-dextran antibodies (which would be part of the response against bacterial polysaccharides) are apparently connected to anti-acetylcholine receptor antibodies via idiotypic interactions (Dwyer *et al.*, 1983; Dwyer, 1988 see Fig. 13.6).

Rabies virus has been shown to bind to AChR (Lentz *et al.*, 1985), which serves to localise the virus at the neuromuscular junction where it is taken up into the nerve endings. Anti-id(65) (an anti-idiotype antibody raised against a monoclonal anti-AChR antibody, see below) was found to bind to rabies viral proteins. Thus in this system antibodies to virus could perturb an anti-AChR regulatory network (Fig. 13.6). Although rabies is not likely to be involved in the initiation of MG, perhaps, on the contrary, patients with MG might be resistant to rabies virus because of the presence of anti-idiotypic antibodies.

The potential relevance of network perturbations in EAMG was clearly

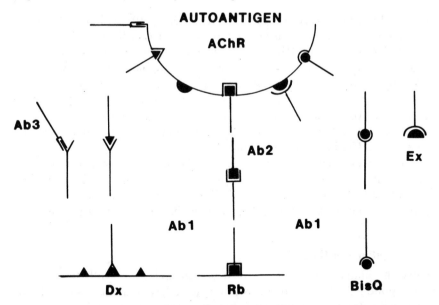

Fig. 13.6. Autoimmunity via idiotype networks and cross-reactivity. Antibodies (Abl) to epitopes on exogenous antigens (for instance bacterial polysaccharides (Dx), rabies virus (Rb) or a cholinergic ligand (BisQ) stimulate the formation of anti-idiotypes (Ab2) which happen to cross-react with the antoantigen. In other cases the Abl antibodies may bind directly to the autoantigen (direct cross-reactivity with the exogenous antigen, Ex) or further idiotypic interactions may lead to Ab3 which recognises an unrelated epitope.

illustrated by the demonstration that rabbits immunised against BisQ, an AChR agonist, developed antibodies to BisQ which in turn could stimulate the production of antibodies to the AChR itself (Wasserman *et al.*, 1982). In this case, presumably, the antigen (BisQ), being complementary to the ACh binding site on the AChR, stimulates the production of antibodies that mimic the shape of the AChR and lead to an anti-idiotype response which is also anti-AChR (Fig. 13.6). However, it should be pointed out that in the two situations described briefly above, anti-AChR antibodies derived as a result of idiotypic interactions would be directed against a distinct region on the AChR, e.g. the rabies binding site or the ACh binding site. There is no evidence that either of these sites is of particular importance as epitopes for human autoantibodies in MG.

The possibility of manipulating the immune system via the network has been analysed in a number of reports. For instance anti-idiotype antibodies can prevent the induction of EAMG in chicks in which EAMG was induced by passive transfer of a highly pathogenic monoclonal antibody (Souroujon *et al.*, 1986). In other cases anti-idiotype treatment has enhanced production of the idiotype. For instance, rats were injected neonatally with increasing amounts (5, 50, 5×10^3 and 5×10^4 ng) of anti-Id(65) previously raised against an anti-AChR mAb (mAb 65, directed towards the MIR). At 11 weeks of age they were immunised against 15 µg AChR to see whether their response to the AChR was affected. Neonatal administration of 'physiological' doses of anti-id(65) induced a long-lasting *enhancement* of idiotype expression. The group given 50 ng of anti-id(65) had four-fold higher serum anti-AChR antibody titres against both *Torpedo* and rat AChR and the most severe myasthenic symptoms. The other doses had no effect.

These experiments indicate that the autoimmune network can be manipulated in various ways via the idiotype network. However, the possibility that autoantibodies in MG or in other autoimmune disorders result from perturbation of idiotype circuits has not yet been proven.

13.8. Epitopes of the AChR

Once the amino acid sequence of a protein is known synthetic peptides corresponding to short sequences can be tested as immunogens in order to try and localise the immunologically relevant sites, and to raise antibodies that can be used to study the structure and transmembrane orientation of the molecule (see Lindstrom, this volume). The use of short synthetic or larger recombinant peptides makes it possible to map not only the regions to which some antibodies bind, but also the short sequences involved in immune recognition of the antigen by T helper cells.

Mulac–Jericevic *et al.* (1987) have analysed the antibody response to purified *Torpedo* AChR by testing mouse sera for binding to short, overlapping synthetic peptides. In this way they have shown the presence of several antigenic regions on the primary sequence. Lindstrom and his colleagues have similarly mapped monoclonal antibodies and shown that many bind to regions that are situated intracytoplasmically in the native molecule (see Lindstrom, this volume). In contrast few of the mAbs raised against intact AChR bound to isolated peptide sequences. Thus it is clear, as pointed out by Lindstrom, that the results obtained by this sort of approach will not necessarily be representative of the total immune response.

Immunisation of animals with a synthetic peptide corresponding to residues 125–147 of *Torpedo* electric organ AChR α subunit induced a delayed-type hypersensitivity response (indicative of activated T cells), antibodies to native AChR and experimental evidence of EAMG (reduced MEPP amplitude) (Lennon *et al.*, 1985). Peptides containing the α-BuTX binding site were also able to induce EAMG (Takamori, 1988). Curiously a recombinant fusion peptide (see Chapter 3) containing the main immunogenic region (see Lindstrom, this volume) did not induce EAMG in rabbits in spite of the production of high titres of antibody to the protein

(Barkas *et al.*, 1987). This failure to induce clinical disease can be largely explained by the absence of a native three-dimensional folding of the fusion protein, and the lack, therefore, of antibodies that cross-react with the animals' own AChRs. Indeed when mice were immunised against recombinant human α subunit most of the antibodies formed were directed against intracytoplasmic determinants and did not bind to the AChR *in situ* or in solution (Jermy *et al.*, 1989b). This illustrates one of the major problems in working with recombinant subunits of oligomeric proteins.

In summary, peptides are valuable tools to dissect the specificities of the immune response, but the lack of a native structure makes it difficult to map all the antibody specificities. On the other hand this is not a major restriction when applied to T cell work since T lymphocytes recognise short, denatured sequences rather than highly conformational epitopes (see below).

13.9. Cellular immune responses in EAMG

T lymphocytes can be divided into T helper cells that enhance the immune response, T suppressor cells that suppress the immune response, and cytotoxic T cells. T cells only recognise antigens in the context of the animals' own MHC; the antigens are first degraded proteolytically and then presented on the surface of antigen-presenting cells where they are bound to either class I (for presentation to cytotoxic T cells) and/or class II (for presentation to helper T cells) MHC gene products.

Although EAMG is an antibody-mediated disease several T cell-mediated immune reactions can be observed such as positive skin tests (Lennon *et al.*, 1976) and T cell proliferation in the presence of the antigen (Christadoss *et al.*, 1982; De Baets, *et al.*, 1982). The possible contribution of defined lymphocyte populations to the pathogenesis of the disease, however, was tested by passive transfer experiments which served to emphasise the fact that T cell involvement was largely due to the need for T cell help in the production of antibody by B cells (Wekerle *et al.*, 1981). There was little evidence of a direct attack on the neuromuscular junction by cytolytic T cells.

These studies were of interest, however, in relation to the genetic control of disease susceptibility. Christadoss *et al.*, (1979) tested the proliferative response of lymph node cells to *Torpedo* AChR using different strains of mice. These indicated that an immune response gene located in the I-A subregion of the MHC (class II) was important during the induction phase of EAMG. Lymphocyte responses could be eliminated by blocking I-A antigens on lymphocytes with anti-I-A sera (Christadoss *et al.*, 1983a), and a spontaneous mutation at the I-A subregion converted high responders to low responders (Christadoss *et al.*, 1982). Removal of adherent antigen-presenting cells had the same effect, suggesting that the associated Ia molecule was limiting the response (De Baets *et al.*, 1982;Christadoss *et al.*, 1983b).

Establishment of systems for looking at T cell-directed antibody production *in vitro* by specific B cells is an essential step towards the investigation of possible therapeutic strategies (see below). Lymphocytes from EAMG rats or mice proliferate *in vitro* when AChR is added to the culture medium, and AChR-reactive T lymphocytes can be isolated from rats with chronic EAMG (Hohlfeld *et al.*, 1981; Wekerle *et al.*, 1981; De Baets *et al.*, 1982). Culture of these in the presence of the antigen resulted in the selection of autoreactive T cell clones. These clones, which predominantly recognised the α subunit of the AChR, could transfer EAMG to unprimed rats, but only if injected with AChR and AChR-primed B cells (Wekerle *et al.*, 1981). Thus, as indicated above, the role of helper T cells is to direct the production of antibody by specific B cells, and the T cells are unable to do this in the absence of the antigen.

Using these EAMG-primed T cells and lymph node B cells we showed antibody production *in vitro*. This required smaller amounts of antigen than were required for the initial T cell proliferation experiments, and indeed larger amounts inhibited antibody synthesis (De Baets, 1982; see also Fujii and Lindstrom, 1988). This may be due to the generation of specific suppressor T cells at high antigen concentrations (Bogen *et al.*, 1984).

These studies show that it is relatively easy to demonstrate immuno-competent T and B cells that can recognise the antigen. Moreover, immunisation in adjuvant is not necessary to induce an antibody response (Scadding *et al.*, 1986; Jermy *et al.*, 1989a). The lack of autoantibodies to AChR in normal animals, and humans (see Vincent, this volume), may therefore relate to the absence of circulating antigen. In contrast, in

Table 13.2. Relationship between levels of self-proteins in the serum, immune status of T and B cells to autoantigens and autoimmune disease

Experimental[a] *autoimmune*	*Autoantigen*[b] *(concentration)*	*Immune status of*[c]		*Effector cells*
		T cell	*B cell*	
Thyroiditis (EAT)	Thyroglobulin (low)	TOL	IC	T/B
Encephalomyelitis (EAE)	Myelin basic protein (undetectable)	IC	IC	T
Myasthenia (EAMG)	AChR (undetectable)	IC	IC	B

[a] EAT = experimental autoimmune thyroiditis; EAE = experimental encephalomyelitis; EAMG = experimental autoimmune myasthenia gravis.

[b] The degree of tolerance in both T and B cell compartments is dependent on the concentration of the self-antigen in the microenvironment. For the examples given, the autoantigen concentration is low, or the autoantigen is not detectable.

[c] TOL = tolerant; IC = immunocompetent.

Table 13.3.   Comparison between chronic EAMG and MG

			EAMG	MG
A.	Clinical			
	(1)	weakness	+	+
	(2)	fatiguability	+	+
	(3)	eyelid ptosis	+/−	+
B.	Electrophysiological			
	(1)	decremental electromyogram	+	+
	(2)	effect of acetylcholinesterase inhibitors	+	+
	(3)	reduced MEPP amplitude	+	+
	(4)	increased curare sensitivity	+	+
	(5)	decreased acetylcholine sensitivity	+	+
C.	Immunological			
	(1)	anti-AChR antibodies in serum	+	+
	(2)	anti-AChR antibodies at the endplate	+	+
	(3)	complement components at the postsynaptic membrane	+	+
	(4)	antigenic modulation by antibody	+	+
	(5)	antibodies directed to ACh binding site	+	+
	(6)	anti-MIR antibodies	+	+
	(7)	neonatal transfer of disease	+	+
	(8)	cellular immunity of AChR	+	+
	(9)	thymic abnormalities	−	+

experimental autoimmune thyroiditis the T cells are actually tolerised by the low circulating thyroglobulin levels in the serum, and this tolerance has to be over-ridden by adjuvant in order to stimulate antibody production (see Table 13.2; Weigle and Romball, 1980; De Baets, 1988).

13.10. Relevance of EAMG as a model for myasthenia gravis and specific immunotherapy

Only monkeys develop myasthenic signs and symptoms that are highly reminiscent of those in MG patients (Tarrab–Hazdai *et al.*, 1975), but in all species weakness can be shown to be enhanced by effort, and relieved by rest and anticholinesterase treatment, and in all other respects EAMG shows great similarity to the human disease (see Table 13.3).

The great potential of a model such as EAMG for a human disease lies in its use in the testing of new therapeutic approaches. As in the human disease, myasthenia gravis, non-specific immunosuppression via drugs such as azathioprine, steroids, cyclophosphamide and cyclosporin A are usually effective in reducing antibody levels and clinical expression of the disease (see Pachner, 1987). More interesting was the *in vivo* treatment with anti-I-A mAbs which suppressed the immune response to AChR in

EAMG (Waldor *et al.*, 1983). However, treatment with anti-I-A antibodies is rather non-specific and could lead to general immunosuppression.

A more specific approach to treatment would be aimed at suppressing only those antibodies or cells that were specific for the antigen, AChR. Specific therapy could be achieved by several approaches: (1) by anti-idiotypic suppression (see above); (2) by specific killing of anti-AChR-producing B cells; (3) by specific killing of AChR-specific T cells; (4) by induction of antigen-specific suppressor T cells. Various examples of these can be found in the literature (see Pachner, 1987). For instance AChR-ricin conjugates can reduce antibody production by B cells *in vitro* (Killen and Lindstrom, 1984), but T cells are less sensitive than antibody-producing cells. Induction of antigen-specific suppression has been demonstrated by a number of groups (Sinigaglia *et al.*, 1984; Bogen *et al.*, 1984; McIntosh and Drachman, 1986) but the mechanisms by which these cells work, and the possible application to *in vivo* studies, is not yet clear.

Most of these procedures have not been found effective if given after the induction of the disease. The hope for the future lies in deletion of T cells specific for the antigen, which are clearly involved in initiating and maintaining the disease state in both EAMG and in MG.

References

Barkas, T., Mauron, A., Roth, B., Alloid, C., Tzartos, S. J. and Ballivet, M. (1987) Mapping of the main immunogenic region and toxin-binding site of the nicotinic acetylcholkine receptor. *Science* **235**: 77–80.

Berman, P. W. and Patrick, J. (1980a) Experimental myasthenia gravis. A murine system. *J. Exp. Med.* **151**: 204–223.

Berman, P. W. and Patrick, J. (1980b) Linkage between the frequency of muscular weakness and loci that regulate immune responsiveness in murine experimental myasthenia gravis. *J. Exp. Med.* **152**: 507–520.

Berman, P. W. and Heinemann, S. F. (1984) Antigenic modulation of junctional acetylcholine receptor is not sufficient to account for the development of myasthenia gravis in receptor immunized mice. *J. Immunol.* **132**: 711–717.

Biesecker, F. and Koffler, D. (1988) Resistance to experimental autoimmune myasthenia gravis in genetically inbred rats. *J. Immunol.* **140**: 3406–3410.

Bionda, A., De Baets, M. H., Tzartos, S. J. (1984) Lindstrom, J. M., Weigle, W. O. and Theophilopoulos, A. N. Spectrotypic analysis of antibodies to acetylcholine receptors in experimental autoimmune myasthenia gravis. *Clin. Exp. Immunol.* **57**: 41–50, 1984.

Bogen, S., Mozes, E. and Fuchs, S. (1984) Induction of acetycholine receptor-specific suppression. *J. Exp. Med.* **159**: 292–304.

Brown, R. and Krolick, K. A. (1988) Selective idiotype suppression of an adoptive secondary anti-acetylcholine receptor antibody response by immunotoxin treatment before transfer. *J. Immunol.* **140**: 893–898.

Carnegie, P. F. (1971) Properties, structure and possible neuroreceptor role of the encephalitogenic protein of human brain. *Nature* **229**: 25–28.

Christadoss, P., Lennon, V. A., Kroo, C. J. and David, C. S. (1982) Genetic control of experimental autoimmune myasthenia gravis in mice. III. Ia molecules mediate cellular immune responsiveness to acetylcholine receptors. *J. Immunol.*

128: 1141–1444.

Christadoss, P., Dauphine, M. and Lindstrom, J. (1983a) Deficient T cell mitogen response in murine experimental autoimmune myasthenia gravis: a defect in the adherent cell population. *Cell. Immunol.* **79**: 358–366.

Christadoss, P., Lindstrom, J. and Talal, N. (1983b) Cellular immune response to acetylcholine receptors in murine experimental myasthenia gravis inhibition with monoclonal anti-I-A antibodies. *Cell. Immunol.* **81**: 1–8.

Christadoss, P., Lennon, V. A. and David, C. (1979) Genetic control of experimental autoimmune myasthenia gravis in mice. I. Lymphocyte proliferative response to acetylcholine receptors is under H-2 linked IR gene control. *J. Immunol.* **123**: 2540–2543.

Christadoss, P., Lindstrom, J., Munro, S. and Talal, N. (1985) Muscle acetylcholine receptor loss in murine experimental autoimmune myasthenia gravis: correlated with cellular, homoral and clinical responses. *J. Neuroimmunol.* **8**: 29–41.

De Baets, M. H. (1984) Autoimmunity to cell surface receptors. Ph.D. thesis, Maastricht, The Netherlands.

De Baets, M. H. (1988) Specificities of autoantibodies in autoimmune receptor diseases. *Immunol Rev.* **7**: 218–231.

De Baets, M. H., Einarson, B., Lindstrom, J. M. and Weigle, W. O. (1982) Lymphocyte activation in experimental autoimmune myasthenia gravis. *J. Immunol.* **128**: 2228–2235.

De Baets, M. H., Verschuuren, J., Daha, M. R. and van Breda Vriesman, P. J. C. (1988) Effects of the rate of acetylcholine receptor synthesis on the severity of experimental autoimmune myasthenia gravis. *Immunol. Res.* **7**: 200–211.

De Baets, M. H. and van Breda Vriesman, P. J. C. (1985) Autoimmunity to cell membrane receptors. *Surv. Synth. Pathol. Res.* **4**: 185–215.

Dwyer, S. D., Bradley, R. J., Urquhart, C. K. and Kearney, J. F. (1983) Naturally occuring anti-idiotypic antibodies in myasthenia gravis patients. *Nature* **301**: 611–614.

Dwyer, D. S. (1988) Idiotype network interactions. In: *B Lymphocytes in Human Disease*, G. Bird and J. E. Calvert, eds, Oxford University Press, Oxford, pp. 393–408.

Engel, A. G., Tsujihata, M., Lindstrom, J. M. and Lennon, V. A. (1976) The motor endplate in myasthenia gravis and in experimental autoimmune myasthenia gravis. A quantitative ultrastructural study. *Ann. N.Y. Acad. Sci.* **274**: 60–79.

Engel, A. G., Lindstrom, J. M., Lambert, E. H. and Lennon, V. A. (1977) Ultrastructural localization of the acetylcholine receptor in myasthenia gravis and in its experimental autoimmune model. *Neurology* **27**: 307–315.

Fujii, Y. and Lindstrom, J. (1988) Specificity of the T cell immune response to acetylcholine receptor in experimental autoimmune myasthenia gravis. *J. Immunol.* **140**: 1830–1837.

Gomez, C. and Richman, D. (1983) Anti-acetylcholine receptor antibodies directed against the alpha-bungarotoxin binding site induce a unique form of experimental myasthenia. *Proc. Natl. Acad. Sci. USA* **80**: 4089–4093.

Heinemann, S., Bevan, S., Kullberg, R., Lindstrom, J. and Rice, J. (1977) Modulation of acetylcholine receptor by antibody against the receptor. *Proc. Natl. Acad. Sci. USA* **74**: 3090–3094.

Heinemann, S., Merlie, J. and Lindstrom, J. (1978) Modulation of acetylcholine receptor in rat diaphragm by antireceptor sera. *Nature (Lond.)* **274**: 65–67.

Hohlfeld, R., Kalies, I., Heinz, F., Kalden, J. R. and Wekerle, H. (1981) Autoimmune rat T-lymphocytes monospecific for acetylcholine receptors. *J.*

Immunol. **126**: 1355–1359.

Hugli, T. E. and Muller-Eberhard, J. J. (1978) Anaphylatoxins: C3a and C5a. *Adv. Immunol.* **26**: 1–53.

Jermy, A., Fisher, C., Vincent, A., Willcox, N. and Newsom–Davis, J. (1989a) Experimental autoimmune myasthenia gravis induced in mice without adjuvants: genetic susceptibility and adoptive transfer of weakness. *J. Autoimmun.* **2**: 675–688.

Jermy, A., Beeson, D., Vincent, A., Willcox, N. and Newsom–Davis, J. (1989b) Mice immunised with recombinant a subunit of the human acetylcholine receptor develop anti-AChR antibodies but not experimental autoimmune myasthenia gravis. *Abst. J. Autoimmun.* **2**: 903–904.

Jerne, N. K. (1974) Towards a network theory of the immune system. *Ann. Immunol.* **125c**: 373–385.

Killen, J. A. and Lindstrom, H. M. (1984) Specific killing of lymphocytes that cause experimental autoimmune myasthenia gravis by RICIN toxin–acetylcholine receptor conjugates. *J. Immunol.* **133**: 2549–2553.

Lambert, E. H., Lindstrom, J. M. and Lennon, V. A. (1976) End-plate potentials in experimental autoimmune myasthenia gravis in rats. *Ann. N.Y. Acad. Sci.* **274**: 300–318.

Lennon, V. A. and Carnegie, P. R. (1971) Immunopharmacological disease: a break of tolerance to receptor sites. *Lancet* i: 630–633.

Lennon, V. A., Lindstrom, J. and Seybold, M. E. (1975) Experimental autoimmune myasthenia gravis: a model of myasthenia gravis in rats and guinea pigs. *J. Exp. Med.* **141**: 1365–1375.

Lennon, V. A., Lindstrom, J. M. and Seybold, M. E. (1976) Experimental autoimmune myasthenia gravis: cellular and humoral immune responses. *Ann. N.Y. Acad. Sci.* **274**: 283–299.

Lennon, V. A., Seybold, M. E., Lindstrom, J. M., Cochrane, C. and Ulevitch, R. (1978) Role of complement in the pathogenesis of experimental autoimmune myasthenia gravis. *J. Exp. Med.* **147**: 973–983.

Lennon, V. A., McCormick, D. J., Lambert, E. H., Griesman, G. E. and Atassi, M. Z. (1985) Region of peptide 125–147 of acetylcholine receptor alpha subunit is exposed at neuromuscular junction and induces experimental autoimmune myasthenia gravis, T-cell immunity, and modulating autoantibodies. *Proc. Natl. Acad. Sci. USA* **82**: 8805–8809.

Lentz, T. L., Chester, J., Benson, R. J. J., Hawrod, E., Tignor, G. H. and Smith, A. L. (1985) Rabies virus binding to cellular membranes measured by enzyme immunoassay. Muscle and Nerve **8**: 336–345.

Lindstrom, J. M. (1976) Immunological studies of acetylcholine receptors. *J. Supramol. Struct.* **4**: 389–403.

Lindstrom, J. M., Einarson, B. L., Lennon, V. A. and Seybold, M. E. (1976a) Pathological mechanisms in experimental autoimmune myasthenia gravis. I. Immunogenicity of syngeneic muscle acetylcholine receptor and quantitative extraction of receptor and antibody–receptor complexes from muscles of rat with experimental autoimmune myasthenia gravis. *J. Exp. Med.* **144**: 726–738.

Lindstrom, J. M., Engel, A. G., Seybold, M. E., Lennon, V. A. and Lambert, E. H. (1976b) Pathological mechanisms in experimental autoimmune myasthenia gravis. II. Passive transfer of experimental autoimmune myasthenia gravis in rats with anti-acetylcholine receptor antibodies. *J. Exp. Med.* **144**: 739–753.

Lindstrom, J., Shelton, D. and Fujii, Y. (1988) Myasthenia gravis. *Adv. Immunol.* **42**: 233–284.

Lindstrom, J. M., Einarson, B. and Merlie, J. (1978) Immunization of rats with polypeptide chains from *Torpedo* acetylcholine receptor causes an autoimmune response to receptors in rat muscle. *Proc. Natl. Acad. Sci.* **75**: 769–773.

McIntosh, K. R. and Drachman, D. B. (1986) Induction of suppressor cells specific for AChR in experimental autoimmune myasthenia gravis. *Science* **232**: 401–403.

Monestier, M., Manheimer–Lory, A., Bellon, B., Painter, C., Dang, H., Talal, N., Zanetti, M., Schwartz, R., Pisetsky, D., Kuppers, R., Rose, N., Borchier, J., Klareskog, L., Holmdahl, R., Erlanger, B., Alt, F. and Bona, C. (1986) Shared idiotypes and restricted V_H genes characterize murine autoantibodies of various specificities. *J. Clin. Invest.* **78**: 753–759.

Mulac–Jericeric, B., Kurisaki, J., and Atassi, M. Z. (1987) Profile of the continuous antigenic regions on the extracellular part of the alpha chain of an acetylcholine receptor. *Proc. Natl. Acad. Sci. USA* **84**: 3633–3637.

Pachner, A. R. (1987) Experimental models of myasthenia gravis: lessons in autoimmunity and progress toward better forms of treatment. *Yale J. Biol. Med.* **60**: 169–177.

Patrick, J. and Lindstrom, J. M. (1973) Autoimmune response to acetylcholine receptor. *Science* **180**: 871–872.

Sahashi, K., Engel, A. G., Lindstrom, J. M., Lambert, E. H. and Lennon, V. A. (1978) Ultrastructural localization of immune complexes (IgG and C3) and the endplate in experimental autoimmune myasthenia gravis. *J. Neuropathol. Exp. Neurol.* **37**: 212–223.

Scadding, G. K., Calder, L., Vincent, A., Prior, C., Wray, D. and Newsom–Davis, J. (1986) Anti-acetylcholine receptor antibodies induced in mice by syngeneic receptor without adjuvants. *Immunology* **58**: 151–155.

Seybold, M. E., Lambert, E. H., Lennon, V. A. and Lindstrom, J. M. (1976) Experimental autoimmune myasthenia gravis: clinical, neurophysiologic and pharmacologic aspects. *Ann. N.Y. Acad. Sci.* **274**: 275–282.

Sinigaglia, F., Gotti, C., Castagnoli, R. and Clementi, F. (1984) Acetylcholine receptor-specific suppressive T cell factor from a retrovirally transformed T-cell line. *Proc. Natl. Acad. Sci. USA* **81**: 7569–7573.

Souroujon, M. C., Pachner, A. R. and Fuchs, S. (1986) The treatment of passively transferred experimental myasthenia with anti-idiotypic antibodies. *Neurology* **36**: 622–625.

Takamori, M. (1988) Myasthenogenic significance of synthetic α-subunit peptide 183–200 of *Torpedo californica* and human AChR. *J. Neurol. Sci.* **85**: 121–129.

Tarrab–Hazdai, R., Aharonov, A., Silman, I., Fuchs, S. and Abramsky, O. (1975) Experimental autoimmune myasthenia gravis induced in monkeys by purified acetylcholine receptor. *Nature* **256**: 128–130.

Tzartos, S. J. and Lindstrom, J. M. (1980) Monoclonal antibodies used to probe acetylcholine receptor structure: localization of the main immunogenic region and detection of similarities between subunits. *Proc. Natl. Acad. Sci. USA* **77**: 755–759.

Vincent, A. (1980) Immunology of acetylcholine receptors in relation to myasthenia gravis. *Physiol. Rev.* **60**: 756–824.

Waldor, M. K., Sriram, S. B., McDevitt, H. O. and Steinman, L. (1983) *In vivo* therapy with monoclonal anti-I-A antibody suppresses immune responses to acetylcholine receptor. *Proc. Natl. Acad. Sci USA* **80**: 2713–2717.

Wassermann, N. H., Penn, A. S., Freimuth, P. I., Treptow, N., Wentzel, S., Cleveland, W. L. and Erlanger, B. F. (1982) Anti-idiotypic route to anti-acetylcholine receptor antibodies and experimental myasthenia gravis. *Proc. Natl. Acad. Sci. USA* **79**: 4810–4814.

Weigle, W. O. and Romball, C. G. (1980) Relationship among the levels of self proteins, immune status of T and B cells and autoimmunity. In: *Autoimmune*

Aspects of Endocrine Disorders, A. Pinchera, D. Doniach, G. F. Fenzi and L. Baschieri, eds, Academic Press, New York, pp. 39–55.

Wekerle, H., Hohlfeld, R., Ketelsen, U. P., Kalden, J. R. and Kalies, I. (1981) Thymic myogenesis, T-lymphocytes and the pathogenesis of myasthenia gravis. *Ann N.Y. Acad. Sci.* **377**: 455–476.

Zanetti, M. (1986) Idiotype network and its relevance to autoimmune diseases: functional considerations. In: *Concepts in Immunopathology*, vol. 3, J. M. Cruse, and R. E. Lewis, eds, Karger AG, Basel, 1986, pp. 253–284.

Index